PAEDIATRIC NURSING

NURSES' AIDS SERIES

Altschul's Psychology for Nurses
Anatomy and Physiology for Nurses
Cardiac Nursing
Caring for Women
Gastroenterological Nursing
Geriatric Nursing
Mathematics in Nursing
Medical Nursing
Microbiology for Nurses
Multiple Choice Questions, Book 1
Multiple Choice Questions, Book 2
Multiple Choice Questions, Book 3
Multiple Choice Questions, Book 4
Ophthalmic Nursing
Orthopaedic Nursing
Paediatric Nursing
Personal and Community Health
Pharmacology for Nurses
Practical Nursing
Psychiatric Nursing
Sociology for Nurses
Surgical Nursing
Theatre Technique

PAEDIATRIC NURSING

Seventh Edition

Barbara F. Weller
RSCN, SRN, RNT
Lecturer (Paediatric Nursing),
the Norfolk College of Nursing and Midwifery, Norwich,
formerly Nursing Officer, Department of Health,
Elephant and Castle, London

Sheila Barlow
RSCN, SRN, RNT
Director of Nurse Education, The Hospitals for Sick Children,
Charles West School of Nursing, 24 Great Ormond Street, London

BAILLIERE TINDALL
London Philadelphia Toronto Sydney Tokyo

Baillière Tindall
W.B. Saunders

24–28 Oval Road,
London NW1 7DX

The Curtis Center,
Independence Square West,
Philadelphia, PA 19106–3399, USA

55 Horner Avenue,
Toronto, Ontario M8Z 4X6, Canada

Harcourt Brace Jovanovich (Australia) Pty Ltd,
32–52 Smidmore Street,
Marrickville, NSW 2204, Australia

Harcourt Brace Jovanovich (Japan) Inc.
Ichibancho Central Building, 22-1 Ichibancho
Chiyoda-ku, Tokyo 102, Japan

First published 1961
Sixth edition 1983
Seventh edition 1991

Photoset by Best-set Typesetter Ltd
Printed in Great Britain by Clays Ltd, St Ives plc

British Library Cataloguing in Publication Data
Weller, Barbara F.
  Paediatric Nursing.—7th ed.—(Nurses' aids series)
  1. Paediatric nursing
  I. Title. II. Barlow, Sheila III. Series
  610.73′62   RJ245
ISBN 0-7020-1415-X

Contents

Preface   vii

PART I: Principles of Child Health
1   The healthy child   3
2   The newborn   26
3   The infant at risk   50
4   The sick child: home and hospital   79

PART II: Principles of Care
5   The child with respiratory problems   129
6   The child with cardiovascular problems   174
7   The child with rheumatic and collagen problems   197
8   The child with haematological problems   208
9   The child with gastrointestinal problems   226
10 The child with metabolic problems   273
11 The child with endocrine problems   291
12 The child with neurological problems and
    learning difficulties   308
13 The child with dermatological problems   339
14 The child with orthopaedic problems   356
15 The child with genitourinary problems   373
16 The child with infection problems   408

Appendix 1: Safety   432
Appendix 2: 'Play Matters'   437

Appendix 3: Useful addresses   439
Appendix 4: Normal values and conversion tables   442

Index   444

Preface

When the first edition, written by Margaret Duncombe, of *Aids to Paediatric Nursing* was published in 1961, it was the first textbook on paediatric nursing written by a paediatric nurse. At that time in nurse education it was considered sufficient to give the medical facts as they related to the care provided, but the first edition went further than this and included the wider, holistic dimension of the nursing of sick children, emphasizing an awareness and sensitivity to their special needs as developing individuals and as members of their families. The first edition therefore has continued to set a standard for each succeeding edition.

The growth in knowledge and increasing sophistication of paediatric nursing has been dramatic since 1961. Whilst fewer sick children are now cared for in the hospital setting and the length of stay has been considerably reduced, other changes have been noted. Many more children with congenital abnormalities and chronic health problems live longer, often requiring repeated hospital admission and long-term support from the community nursing services. Smaller and more vulnerable infants now survive and many conditions untreatable in 1961 are managed with a minimum of intervention. The impact of the Human Immunodeficiency Virus on the health of families too has been considerable during this period. We have also seen sociological changes, both in the family and in our communities, living as we do now in a multicultural society.

The authors for this seventh edition have sought to in-
corporate the recognition of these changes and of those
occurring currently within nursing and nurse education
into the text to provide a challenging and exciting framework to child health. The student reader new to this
speciality will, we hope, recognize that caring for a child is
not an easy option but one which demands highly skilled
and knowledgeable professionals.

Producing a text of this kind, like paediatric nursing,
requires partnership and teamwork with others and we
should like to record our gratitude to all those who have
offered helpful comments and suggestions, and especially
to Francis Hardy, Ward Sister at the Jenny Lind Childrens
Department, Norwich for reading much of the text. Sarah
Smith, Senior Nursing Editor at Baillière Tindall, de-
serves a special vote of thanks from us for steering us
so ably through the troughs and the heights of book
publishing.

December 1990   Barbara F. Weller
                                         Sheila Barlow

Part I
Principles of Child Health

1 The healthy child

An understanding of the development of the child, together with her own observations, will enable the nurse to provide care for sick children that recognizes and meets the child's individual needs. No two children are alike and the norms and milestones of average development must never be taken too literally. Each child is a unique individual.

Children do not exist in isolation but have parents (or parent substitutes) and are members of families with their own differing social and cultural influences. The nurse's assessment also needs to recognize that the environment, previous life experiences, family and home will all have important implications for the individual child's development and growth, both physical, mental and emotional.

The average standards are known as norms or milestones. They should be familiar to those who deal with children both in health and sickness, but it is important to realize that variations of up to 10 or 15% below or above any of these standards may still be considered within normal limits. For this reason, many paediatricians now refer to developmental progress as a percentile of the average, rather than using rigid figures.

ANTENATAL CARE

Good antenatal care is important to the future development of the child. Attendance by the mother at the maternity clinic at regular intervals during pregnancy will ensure that any problems which may influence fetal development are recognized promptly, as well as providing an opportunity for the mother (and father) to attend parentcraft sessions, e.g. in breast-feeding, in order to help the parents rear their baby happily and successfully (Short Committee Report, 1980).

FETAL DEVELOPMENT

Development of the fetus during pregnancy is a time of rapid growth. After fertilization, when the spermatozoon meets an ovum usually in the outer third of the Fallopian tube, the cells multiply rapidly into a morula which passes into the uterine cavity and embeds in the endometrium.

After 4 weeks the fetal shape resembles a mammal and is about 1 cm long. By about 8 weeks limbs have developed. At 12 weeks the fetus is obviously human. The length is now about 9 cm. All essential organs have formed before the twelfth week. After this the fetus continues to grow, peaking at about the 34th week of pregnancy. About the 27/28th week the fetus is said to be viable. i.e. if born the fetus attempts to breathe. After 28 weeks the fetal muscles develop and fat is laid down. The fetus is coated with a greasy substance known as vernix. The fetus is now able to move quite freely within the amniotic cavity. End of pregnancy occurs after a gestation period of about 40 weeks.

THE CHILD AT BIRTH

The average newborn infant may be expected to weigh approximately 3.5 kg (7½ lb) and to be about 50 cm (20 in.) long. The head circumference is approximately

33 cm (13 in.) with a cranium which is disproportionately large compared with the face.

Anterior and posterior fontanelles are open, moulding may be present and the sutures can be felt. The limbs seem short in comparison with the body, and the head and abdomen large in comparison with the thorax. Subcutaneous fat is sparse, the skin looks red and elastic and the hair is, as a rule, merely a fine down-like growth. The nails are soft and are inclined to peel off. The eyes lack pigment and usually appear blue. Reaction to light is merely reflex. Hearing is present. The infant is sensitive to hot and cold and responds to pain and hunger. Movements are mostly reflex. The respiratory rate is rapid at 40 breaths/minute and is frequently irregular in rhythm. The heat regulating centre is immature and variations in the body temperature may be sudden and considerable.

At birth, the newborn infant is utterly dependent on the adults around him. He is aware of changes in temperature, of being touched and of being handled, of sounds and of bright lights. He sleeps for long periods, cries, sucks and can make discriminating sounds.

Various reflexes are present. The main ones are:

1. Pupil reflexes—the newborn infant will turn his head towards the source of light providing it is not too bright. In pre-term babies the light may need to be shone for a longer period before this reflex is obtained.

2. Moro reflex—response to sudden sound causing the infant's body to stiffen, the arms to go up and out, then forward and towards each other. This reflex usually disappears at about the age of 3–4 months and may be difficult to elicit in the pre-term infant.

3. The grasp reflex—this may be obtained in the hand or foot by either introducing a finger into the palm of the hand which the infant grasps quite strongly or by gently stroking the sole of the foot behind the toes.

4. Placing and walking reflexes—obtained by holding the infant upright over the edge of a table, so that the sole of the foot presses against the edge. The infant will bend his hips and knees, putting the foot on the table. The opposite foot 'steps' forward.

5. Withdrawal reflex—pricking the sole of the foot will result in the infant's leg being flexed at the hip, knee and ankle.

6. Babinski's sign—stroking the sole of the foot causes the great toe to flex and the toes to fan out.

7. Rooting reflex—when the corner of the mouth is touched with a finger which moves towards the cheek, the infant will turn his head towards the object and open his mouth.

8. Asymmetrical tonic neck reflex—when the infant is lying quietly supine, the head may be turned to one side with the arm extended on the same side. The opposite knee is often flexed. This reflex usually disappears at about 2–3 months of age, but may persist longer and be more marked in spastic babies.

Developmental Considerations for Health Promotion, Care and Play Activities

Mothers and fathers should be encouraged to spend as much time as possible with their newborn infants, particularly during the first few hours after delivery. Research (Klaus and Kennell, 1976) has shown this to be the optimal period for 'bonding' or parent/child attachment. Bonding enhances the behavioural development of the child whilst helping to ensure that the parents are able to provide the care necessary for the infant's future. Facilities should always be available for the mother/father to be resident with their newborn infant.

Parents not able to have extensive close contact with

their newborn infant in these early days should be encouraged to visit, handle, fondle and care for their infants as soon as they are able to do so. In the Intensive Care situation it would be necessary to support and guide the parents in doing this. By acting as the 'role model' the nurse will be able to show the parents how to make physical contact with their baby, e.g. by placing their hands through the incubator portholes. This increases the parents' self-confidence and skill at care-giving before the infant is discharged from hospital.

Always ensure that, providing the infant's condition allows it, the baby is held during feeding so that he can watch his mother's (or nurse's) face. Talk, rock, touch, kiss, sing and call him by name during his waking hours in the 'en face' position (when the eyes of the infant and of the care-giver are on the same visual plane). Place a bright attractive but simple mobile within 30–45 cm (12–18 in.) of the line of vision.

As the newborn infant's temperature regulating system is not yet fully efficient, care should be taken to ensure that the environmental temperature is kept reasonably consistent at 21–24°C (70–75°F). Clothing should be light but adequate.

AT 3 MONTHS

Weight 5 kg (11¼ lb). Head now normal shape and growing rapidly in circumference. Posterior fontanelle closed. Begins to balance head when held in the sitting position. Limbs now well covered, the face round and the skin elastic. Second growth of hair replaces the initial down. The eyes have their permanent colour. Has achieved some coordination of eye movements and fixes on objects and may notice new surroundings.

Recognizes his mother, responds to her smile and

smiles with pleasure. Plays with own hands and feet. Attempts to grasp rattles and soft toys. Sleeps 18–20 hours/24 hours. Babbles in a socially responsive manner. Enjoys sucking for its own pleasure and will purposely place hand in mouth to suck. Has a well demonstrated sense of smell and taste (MacFarlane, 1977).

Developmental Considerations for Health Promotion, Care and Play Activities

Opportunities for the infant to experience new sensations and textures should be provided by changing the position of the cot or moving the infant from a 'baby chair' to a mat on the floor to allow full freedom of limb movements. Bathing time can provide immense pleasure for the infant to enjoy floating and splashing in the warm water.

High contrast moving (Muller *et al.*, 1986) toys should be suspended from the cot or pram, within easy reach of

FIG. 1 Resident mother sharing care of sick infant.

the child's grasp. They should be bright, of differing shades and textures, safely 'suckable' and of a good hand size, yet easy to clean and sterilize as necessary. They should also be changed frequently to give variety. Provide the infant with a rattle or other suitable toy to hold in the hand, which is strong enough to sustain dropping over the cot side.

The importance of the mother's presence to the infant should be recognized and facilities provided for her (or for a mother substitute) to be resident in hospital with her child if this should be necessary.

AT 6 MONTHS

Weight 7.5 kg (16½ lb). Eyes can follow people round; turns head to increase visual field. Can determine direction of sound. Enjoys new tastes and takes solid food. Begins to masticate and drink from a cup.

First teeth erupt (usually lower central incisors); carries everything to the mouth. Can hold objects in both hands. Grasps things deliberately. Sits up, if supported. Has pleasure in rocking his body. Spine is now very straight. Will smile at familiar faces and is capable of real laughter. Makes sounds involving the use of lips and tongue. Prepares for speech.

Becomes fretful if his mother disappears and may show fear and apprehension if strangers approach him.

Developmental Considerations for Health Promotion, Care and Play Activities

Opportunities for outings in pram and for change of position from cot to high chair should be provided. Let the child participate in self-feeding at mealtimes with an extra spoon, finger held foods, etc.

The child enjoys repetitive games, e.g. 'Hide and Seek'. He enjoys, too, opportunities to bang and rattle objects which he is now able to transfer from one hand to the other, and will look for dropped toys if they fall over the side of the cot or pram. Nesting toys, cubes and squeezy toys are all suitable at this age. As everything still goes directly to the mouth, all toys should be small and easy to grasp, but not small enough to swallow.

Involve mother/father actively in care of the sick child. Always provide facilities for them to live in if they are able

FIG. 2   Growth and motor development in the average child during the first 18 months. The figures indicate age in months.

to do so. In the parents' absence, care should be provided by one or two nurses on an assignment basis. Consideration may be needed to adapt duty rosters to meet developmental needs.

AT THE END OF THE 1st YEAR

By this time the weight will be about 10.5 kg (23 lb), the length 73 cm (29 in.) and the head circumference 46 cm (18 in.). The face and the limbs are well covered with subcutaneous fat and there are dimples over the knuckles, elbows and knees. The skin is firm and elastic and no longer hangs in loose folds as in the newly born.

The toddler looks around freely. Lachrymation is now fully established and crying is accompanied by tears. The toddler is now able to eat most foods with the family, masticates well and is beginning to feed himself. He has between 10 and 12 teeth (central incisors, 4; lateral incisors, 4; premolars, 2−4). The hair may need its first cut and the nails are now strong and hard.

He sits up on his own, can move from one place to another and becomes expert in rolling from back to front and creeping, rolling and pushing himself along on his feet. He can pull himself up with the help of the bars of the cot or of a chair and makes ready for the first steps which he is likely to achieve some time between the ages of 10 and 16 months.

During the latter part of the first year, the child enjoys movement skills of many kinds by constant experimenting. He can bring thumb and forefinger together and can pick up tiny objects. He loves tearing up paper. Most children can say several monosyllabic words, two or three proper words and may imitate a variety of sounds.

The toddler goes through a negative stage and may be quite difficult with diet for a time. When awake, the one-year-old is incredibly active but still needs 12–16 hours of sleep every day. He is filled with curiosity and anxious to make contacts with others, provided strangers allow him to make their acquaintance slowly and approach him quietly. He still needs cuddling and close physical contact with his mother or other familiar person. The majority of children at this age have a precious 'cuddly', comforter, teddy-bear or a soft doll.

Developmental Considerations for Health Promotion, Care and Play Activities

The toddler is still very reliant upon his mother (or mother substitute) and actively seeks her cooperation in play and other social activities. Enjoys pull-along and push toys as well as post-boxes and building bricks. Play is essentially self-directed, and attention span remains limited.

Allow every opportunity for movement but take care to provide a safe environment for the active inquisitive toddler in order to avoid accident.

He will enjoy being with other children, e.g. at meal-times. Diet can now be more varied and he should be offered drinks from a cup. He may continue to suck from a bottle, especially on going to sleep or at times of stress.

Health promotion during the first 12 months of life is primarily directed towards providing support for the parents, with nutritional and immunization guidance, for disease prevention, together with information regarding growth, development and the provision of a safe environment.

AT 2 YEARS

Weight 11–12 kg. Height approximately half the anticipated adult height. First set of teeth is almost complete,

20 in all (central incisors, 4; lateral incisors, 4; premolars, 4, canines, 4; second molars, 4).

He has developed bladder control during the day and is beginning to for the night. Beginning to show signs of independence and emancipation. He is no longer wholly dependent on his mother and at this stage develops and exhibits a will of his own. Temper tantrums in response to frustration are common and, unless the child is wisely handled, this can prove a trying period for the family. The 2-year-old can usually say phrases of 3–4 words and has a vocabulary of approximately 900 words. He lives entirely in the present and mothering and affection are still very important. Family rituals are very important to him for his security, e.g. on going to bed at night or for his bathtime. The use of certain words, e.g. 'wee-wee' for micturition, are also important to him. He continues to resent separation from his parents but is also showing an ability to handle separation for short periods at a time.

Developmental Considerations for Health Promotion, Care and Play Activities

Recognize that the child is still very dependent on his mother for security, but allow him opportunities to express his independence if able to do so. Encourage and support his parents to participate in nursing care and treatment.

All toys should be strong and suitable for the child's age. Such toys should include ordinary boxes, building-bricks, strong wooden engines and trucks, soft animals and glove-puppets. Sand, water and equipment which allows the child to imitate adult activities such as 'cooking', washing up, playing at 'doctors and nurses' and dressing up are all particularly popular. If any of the toys used can be taken apart, no part should be small enough for the child to swallow, inhale or to push into the nostrils or ears. He is now beginning to play simple games with other children and will enjoy the opportunity of being able to ride bicycles, trucks etc if able to do so. He will also enjoy quiet moments when he can have simple story-books read to him.

AT 3 YEARS

Not growing at the same rapid rate. Physical shape changing from 'toddler chubbiness to school-age slender-ness'. Incredibly active, he can jump off bottom steps and hop on one foot. Able to dress and undress himself if helped with buttons. Can brush his own teeth and wash face and hands if given some assistance. Able to build a tower of bricks.

Constantly asking questions and has a large vocabulary of approximately 1500 words. During this time, particu-larly if an only child, he may develop an imaginary companion or friend and tell 'tall stories' about their activities together.

Developmental Considerations for Health Promotion, Care and Play Activities

Recognize the child's abilities and provide opportunities for these skills to continue and develop, e.g. allow him to wash himself with some 'sideline' supervision. The pres-ence of mother is still important to him but he is now able to accept separation for short periods. Place in peer group in the ward. The child's 'imaginary friend' is part of normal development, and should be accepted without entering into the detail of the fantasy. Developing a keen sense of dramatic play, enjoys dressing up and acting out stories. Enjoys more 'co-operative play' and creative projects, e.g. making a collage mural for the ward notice-board. Still likes a story-time, especially on going to bed. Facilities for parents to be resident are still required should the child require admission to hospital.

The maintenance and promotion of health for the toddler involves updating immunization and nutritional advice, together with further information regarding dental health, accident prevention, sleep and activity patterns.

AT 5–7 YEARS

Starting school. Growth is slower and steadier, with considerable variation between one child and another. The first teeth begin to disappear; permanent set commence erupting usually in the seventh year and proceed erupting at a rate of '4' a year until about the age of 14 years.

Very active, developing considerable coordination of fine muscle movements both in sports and manual dexterity.

Elementary reading/writing skills achieved at about the age of 6 years. Has a well-developed sense of time and of personal responsibility.

The family unit continues to be his main security, providing support and acceptance as he learns to cope with new major experiences. Many children experience 'negative phases', e.g. nail-biting, quarrelling, peevishness etc.; these episodes are, however, usually short-lived.

Developmental Considerations for Health Promotion, Care and Play Activities

Play activities should include group games as well as individual play. It may be necessary, sometimes, to gather the more mobile children around the bedside of a child

confined to bed for activities such as 'story-time' or a game
of 'pass the parcel'. Both boys and girls enjoy home-like
activities: cooking, washing dolls' clothes, woodwork etc.

Recognize that the child's apparent 'maturity' may break
down during hospitalization. Reassure the child that he is
not being babyish if he cries. Reassure the parents, too,
that regression during times of sickness is normal. Encourage them to participate in care yet to recognize the
child's growing need for independence.

Health promotional education now needs to actively involve the participation of the child to ensure cooperation
and to promote the concept of self-care.

AT 8–11 YEARS

The slowed but gradual rate of growth is maintained
during this period with progress towards future adult body
shape. With the eruption of the permanent set of teeth,
prophylactic dental care continues to be of importance.

A time of great energy in which the child pursues many
physical activities and hobbies. Also a period of social-
emotional growth which takes the child's experiences
beyond that of his family. It is a time when the peer group
which has its own norms (rules) outside the family is all
important.

Developmental Considerations for Health Promotion,
Care and Play Activities

Group activities gain importance in play and the child
should be given opportunities for organizing these. Acting
out activities are less important whilst model building and
group games such as 'Ludo' are much more popular.

Television viewing is especially popular with this age
group and will need some monitoring and supervision.

Whenever possible see that the child in hospital is grouped with children of his own age and interests. Encourage his participation in treatment but recognize that there may be times/situations when the child needs to regress or 'divest' his apparent maturity. Always ensure that the parents are kept well-informed about treatment and progress. All the child's questions should be answered honestly and at a level which is appropriate to his understanding and language.

EARLY ADOLESCENCE

A period of transition leading up to puberty. Females attain puberty (in girls signalled by the menarche or the first period) about 1–2 years before the male. Both sexes are undergoing physical and emotional changes. The rate of growth shows considerable increase and it has been established that the timing of this growth spurt is related to the onset of puberty. Bodily changes and the appearance of secondary sex characteristics stimulate self-consciousness. Any deviations from members of the peer group will create anxiety and embarrassment to the individual child.

The pre-adolescent has enormous physical energy and a correspondingly healthy appetite with a consequent need for increased kilojoule (calorie) intake.

ADOLESCENCE

The rapid growth in height and weight commences in early adolescence and continues until the adult body size is reached. Bone growth is completed in the female at about 18 years and in the male at about 20 years, marking the end of adolescence when biologically the body has reached maturity.

Of utmost importance to the adolescent are peer friendships which provide emotional support as well as assistance in the adolescent's search for personal identity. Family relationships may be strained at this time when parents often feel overwhelmed by their loss of authority and control of their child. The adolescent in turn may see his parents as being 'conservative or reactionary' representing the so-called 'generation gap'.

Developmental Considerations for Health Promotion, Care and Play Activities

The adolescent in hospital should be nursed in a separate ward for adolescents, or failing this in a cubicle or side room where the privacy is respected as far as is practical by the ward staff. Unless specifically requested it should always be out of bounds to the younger children in the ward.

Care should be taken to involve the adolescent in all discussions concerning him and his opinions should be listened to and considered; questions should be answered honestly and factually. Information relevant to the priorities of adolescence should be offered (Muller *et al.*, 1986). The effects and implications of any treatment should be anticipated and the adolescent helped to understand the changes that may be introduced by either puberty or the medical condition. Where possible fact sheets should be given, with an extra copy for the parents.

THE FAMILY

The family is a social grouping that is found throughout the world, although its structure varies from society to society. Geraghty (1988) has described the family as a collection of individuals living together, each with strengths and weaknesses; a small group in constant interaction with each other which may or may not result in disharmony and imbalance.

Family Structures

The nuclear family

The family as it is commonly presented in the United Kingdom, and other industrialized nations is a nuclear unit consisting of mother, father and children (average size 2.4 children). Relatives do not play a major role in the maintenance of the nuclear family and may live some distance away, which may pose problems should an emergency arise in the family, i.e. illness of one of the children. The nuclear family tends to be child centred, which may sometimes mean that the parental expectations for their children are unrealistic.

The extended family

This type of family is less common in our society. Geraghty (1988) has described the extended family as a 'group of relatives who live in one, two or more households, usually in a similar locality and who see each other every day or nearly every day'. First and second generation families who originate from the West Indies or the Indian subcontinent tend to live near relatives and may in some instances share the same house. In these families Mother-in-law or Grandmother usually has a matriarchal role in the household, advising on health and related issues.

The one-parent family

The one-parent family may arise as a result of divorce, desertion or death of a parent or with single unmarried mothers, foster parents or guardians. Single parents may find it difficult to lead a social life in a society that is geared to couples and often find it difficult to obtain day care or creche facilities for their children if they want to work. Financial and housing difficulties are common amongst one-parent families.

The blended family
The blended family is one composed of parents and the children each of the parents brings from a previous marriage. This type of family is increasing with the rising rate of divorce and subsequent remarriage. Many more children now live with a step-parent which may lead to stress in personal relationships between and with parents and step-parents due to confusion, guilt and anxiety about personal events. A study by the National Children's Bureau (1987) showed that there was little difference in the material circumstances of children with step-mothers and those with both natural parents.

Transcultural Aspects

We live in a multiracial society and culture and ethnicity have an important influence on family life. Patterns of migration and settlement of differing ethnic minority groups vary considerably throughout the United Kingdom with new arrivals often settling with established relatives or members from their home village or community.

The culture of the family in which a child is reared will influence dietary patterns, language, dress, social roles, behaviour and beliefs related to health and care. Sub-cultural aspects such as religious beliefs and practices may also influence health practices and attitudes towards therapeutic interventions.

EDUCATION

An important element of continuity in the life of all children is that of 'going to school' and thus becoming a member of the community outside his home and family. In the United Kingdom there is a statutory obligation for all children to be educated according to 'age, ability and aptitude'; local education authorities also have the power to provide facilities for home tuition and schooling in hospital.

The Warnock Report (1978) recommended that children with special needs, i.e. those with long-term disease or handicapping condition should not attend special schools but wherever possible be integrated in normal schools.

Education in Hospital

According to his condition, age and abilities, education should be continued for the sick child in hospital wherever possible. Crocker (1980) suggests:

1. That going to school is a normal activity and provides a bridge between the normal school life at home and the hospital ward environment which is welcomed both by the parents and the children.

2. Schoolwork and related activities give the child a chance to succeed.

3. That doing schoolwork means 'You will be going home, it is important to keep up with your classmates.'

How this service is provided varies with each education authority. Some local education authorities provide education for children from the age of 2 years onwards and others may only appoint teachers on a part-time basis, whilst in hospitals where there is a large child population, a hospital school employing several teachers with its own head teacher may have been established.

In order to provide appropriately for the individual child, the schoolteacher should receive regular reports on the child's condition and have access to the nursing care plans.

The provision of nursing care will need to take into account the school programme, to avoid interruption as far as possible. The child's own school will usually co-operate to provide appropriate books, work and projects. Parents will often provide a willing 'ferrying service' between the child's own school and the hospital school-teacher. This is particularly important for the older child worried about forthcoming examinations.

THE CHILDREN ACT 1989

The Children Act 1989 is the most comprehensive piece of legislation regarding the rights, affairs and welfare of children to be enacted in the United Kingdom. The Act draws together existing legislation to produce a practical code integrating the law regarding private individuals with the responsibilities of public authorities. The Act, which is divided into several parts, brings about a balance between the rights of children and the responsibilities of parents, the rights of the family and the intervention of professionals, and between the prevention of child abuse and the protection of children who are at risk from abuse.

In the Act, parental responsibility means all the rights, duties, powers, responsibilities and authority which by law a parent of a child has in relation to the child. This responsibility is retained by both parents after divorce and can be acquired by fathers who are not married to their child's mother. The principle of non-intervention in family life is only to be breached if absolutely essential. The child's welfare must always be the paramount consideration of the court (Department of Health, 1989).

IMMUNIZATION AND VACCINATION

In the United Kingdom all immunization is voluntary and the Government relies on health education and personal contacts with family doctors, practice nurses and health

TABLE 1 Immunization against infectious disease (From Department of Health, 1990)

Vaccine		Age	Notes
D/T/P and polio	1st dose	2 months	⎫
	2nd dose	3 months	⎬ Primary Course
	3rd dose	4 months	⎭
Measles/mumps/rubella (MMR)		12–18 months	Can be given at any age over 12 months
Booster D/T and polio		4–5 years	
Rubella		10–14 years	Girls only
BCG		10–14 years or infancy	Interval of 3 weeks beween BCG and rubella
Booster tetanus and polio		15–18 years	

Children should therefore have received the following vaccines:

> By 6 months: 3 doses of DTP and polio, or DT and polio.
> By 18 months: measles/mumps/rubella.
> By school entry: 4th DT and polio; measles/mumps/rubella if missed earlier.

Between 10 and 14 years: BCG; rubella for girls.
Before leaving school: 5th polio and tetanus.

visitors for the uptake of this service. Good knowledge of the advantages and possible dangers of immunization and vaccination will set the minds of most parents at rest and convince them of the value of these protective measures to the health of their children.

It is possible to offer children substantive measures of protection against measles, mumps, rubella, diphtheria, whooping cough, tetanus and poliomyelitis. The necessary injections can be given in the local Child Health Clinic, general practitioner's health centre and occasionally in the home by the family doctor or health visitor. It is useful to issue to every child a card which can be easily produced in case of accident, showing an up-to-date record of tetanus immunization and reinforcing injections.

BCG vaccination against tuberculosis is not a routine procedure in the United Kingdom, but BCG (Bacillus Calmette-Guérin) is available to infants exposed to tuberculosis and to the infant who is to reside in or travel to any area where the risk of tuberculosis is judged to be high. It is also available to children who remain negative to tuberculosis testing at the age of 10–13 years.

REFERENCES

Crocker, E. (1980). Reactions of children to health care encounters. In *The Hospital Care of Children*. New York: Oxford University Press.

Department of Health (1990). *Immunisation Against Infectious Disease*. London: HMSO.

Department of Health (1989). *An Introduction to the Children Act 1989*. London: HMSO.

Geraghty, P. (1988). *Caring for Children*. London: Baillière Tindall.

Klaus M.H. and Kennell, J.H. (1976). *Maternal and Infant Bonding*. St Louis, MO: C.V. Mosby.

MacFarlane, A. (1977). *The Psychology of Childbirth*. London: Fontana/Open Books.

Muller, D., Harris, P. and Wattley, L. (1986) *Nursing Children: Psychology, Research and Practice*. London: Harper and Row.

National Children's Bureau (1987). Investing in the Future: Child Health Ten Years after the Court Report.

Short Committee Report (1980). *Second Report from the Social Services Committee: Perinatal and Infant Mortality*. London: HMSO.

Warnock Report (1978). *Special Educational Needs Committee of Enquiry into the Education of Handicapped Children and Young Children and Young People* (H.M. Warnock, Chairman). London: HMSO.

FURTHER READING

Baxter, C. (1987). *Hair Care of African, Afro-Caribbean and Asian Hair Types*. Cambridge: National Extension College.

Black, J. (1989). *Childhealth in a Multicultural Society*. London: British Medical Journal.

Elkind, D. and Weiner, I.B. (1978). *Development of the Child*. New York: Wiley.

Fuller, J. and Toon, P. (1988). *Medical Practice in a Multiracial Society*. London: Heinemann.

General Nursing Council (1982). *Aspects of Sick Children's Nursing*, Section 1. London: General Nursing Council for England and Wales.

Holt, K.S. (1977). *Developmental Paediatrics*. London: Butterworth.

Illingworth, R.S. (1980). *The Development of the Infant and Young Child*, 7th edn. London: Churchill Livingstone.

Jenkins, G.C. (1981). *The First Year of Life*. London: Churchill Livingstone.

Mares, P. Henley, A. and Baxter, C. (1985). *Health Care in Multiracial Britain*. Cambridge: National Extension College.

Open University (1979). *The First Years of Life*. London: Ward Lock.

2 The newborn

This chapter is concerned with the first year of life, a period of rapid growth physically, mentally and socially that will never again be equalled. The infant is completely dependent on his parents or substitutes for survival.

Nursing care of an infant needs to be planned in relation to his clinical needs, his development and also his family situation. Family centred or shared care with parents enables the nurse to recognize the infant/parent special relationship and gives her an opportunity to provide the parental health education vital to the promotion of good health for the child's future.

Nursing newborn infants is a great responsibility at all times but even more so when they are pre-term, weak or sick. Changes in the infant's condition may be extremely sudden and of urgent importance, and the nurse must be observant and capable of fine judgement and swift action when caring for these babies.

General points

For the nursing of sick babies, the cot should be large enough to allow for all procedures to be carried out with ease and for adequate observation of the infant.

The majority of babies are best nursed lying flat. At the head end, the bottom sheet can be protected by a piece of plastic sheeting covered by a small pillow-case. This allows for easy and frequent change of linen if it becomes soiled by mucous secretions or vomit.

No baby under the age of one year should be given ordinary pillows because of the possible danger of suffocation. In babies with dyspnoea or orthopnoea, or when it is necessary to nurse the baby in a recumbent position, small firm pillows may be built up in an armchair position or the head of the mattress can be raised by placing a pillow underneath it. Alternatively a baby 'Sitta' may be used to nurse the baby comfortably and conveniently in the sitting position. Babies who have to be nursed sitting upright, can be held in position if a rolled up napkin is placed underneath their thighs, under the draw sheet. It should always be remembered that young babies should be allowed as much freedom to move around and kick as is compatible with their condition. They also like the stimulation of a change in position whenever this is possible, e.g. if the infant is nursed in the centre of a cubicle it may be a good idea to move the cot adjacent to the window from time to time. The opportunity to lie on a mat or rug on the floor to kick and exercise will often be enjoyed.

Temperature control
The heat regulating mechanism in the newborn is inefficient and the baby may sustain a significant drop in body temperature unless great care is taken to avoid chilling (Sweet, 1988). The newborn infant is unable to shiver and to increase body temperature by this method. Brown fat is stored in the full-term infant and can be utilized for heat production if needed. An adequate intake of food is also essential for heat production. If the infant's temperature falls more energy (calories) from the diet will have to be used for heat production and will therefore be unavailable for growth, and the consumption of oxygen and metabolic rate will be increased. Every effort should be made to avoid unnecessary heat loss in the infant.

Temperature recording
The safest and most accurate method for measuring an infant's temperature is to take it rectally. Each infant should have his own rectal thermometer which has a short rounded bob usually coloured blue. Alternatively, an electronic temperature probe or thermistor can be used, which may be inserted into the rectum or oesophagus. Low-reading thermometers should be used for all new-born, pre-term, low birthweight and sick infants in order to ensure the early recognition of hypothermia. A rectal temperature is usually taken in all children up to the age of one year unless otherwise indicated.

Recording pulse and respirations
Both pulse and respirations are taken while the infant is asleep or resting and before he is disturbed or the cot side lowered. In small infants it is often difficult to feel the radial pulse. Alternative methods include listening to the apex beat, or feeling the pulse over the temporal artery immediately in front of the ear.

Record all temperature, pulse and respiration readings immediately onto the child's chart. Any sudden change, and all low/high temperatures should be reported to the nurse-in-charge.

Bathing a sick baby
In the United Kingdom most babies are bathed on the mother's or nurse's lap. Everything should be prepared and conveniently arranged before the baby is disturbed. The cubicle should be warm (21°C) and the windows closed. The nurse should wash her hands and follow the unit's protective policies. The temperature of the bath water should be checked to feel comfortable to the nurse's elbow.

After taking the pulse and respirations the baby is lifted from his cot, his clothes taken off (but leaving his nappy on) and a bath towel securely wrapped around him. The nurse swabs his eyes with sterile cotton cool and water from within outwards, using each swab once only, dipped in a gallipot of tapwater. The nostrils and ears are cleaned and the face washed and dried. The temperature of the bath water is rechecked. Holding the baby in the crook of the arm and supporting his head, the hair is washed and then dried. The nappy is removed and the buttocks cleaned—using wool swabs if necessary. If required, the temperature is taken. With a well-soaped hand, a lather is applied to the trunk and limbs. The baby is turned towards the nurse to lather the back. The baby is held securely and the head supported with the nurse's arm, then he is placed in the bath whilst retaining support. On

FIG. 3 A good way of holding a baby while lowering him into his bath.

lifting the baby out of the bath he is thoroughly dried, weighed if necessary and dressed. The cot is re-made and toys replaced. Hands are finally washed after completion.

When discharging a baby home, the mother can be told that a daily bath is desirable but not essential and that it might well be omitted at her discretion.

Care of the umbilical cord

Following delivery, the cord is ligated to prevent haemorrhage. It separates by a process of dry gangrene usually between the 5th and 7th day. The cord should be placed outside the napkin to promote drying. The cord and ligature should be observed frequently for bleeding, stickiness, oozing or foul smell, all of which indicate infection and should be reported. The cord should be kept dry at all times.

If the cord becomes contaminated with faeces or urine it should be cleansed with water only and dried with cotton wool swabs (Salariya, 1988). The application of spirit and powder or antiseptic sprays has been shown to delay separation of the cord (Barr, 1984).

Application of napkins

Increasingly, disposable napkins are being used; with some types special pants are worn. If the napkin requires to be secured with a safety pin this should lie horizontally in order to minimize any risk of injury should it accidentally become undone (Fig. 4).

Sore buttocks in the newborn may originate from a variety of causes, the most common of which are frequent loose stools, 'strong' ammoniacal urine, excessive fat in the feeds, careless or infrequent toilet and changes of napkins, inadequate rinsing of napkins after washing them in detergent, and unduly sensitive skin. Frequently the distribution of the rash gives a clue to the cause. A urine-

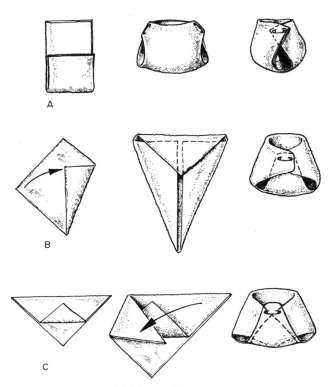

FIG. 4 Various ways of folding napkins.

soaked napkin will cause a widely distributed rash not only over the genitalia but spreading up to the abdomen and the sacrum and down to the thighs, while the skin folds and the natal cleft may be left unaffected. On the other hand, loose or fermented stools cause soreness of the perineum, around the anus and the back of the scrotum.

Intertrigo is a variant of napkin rash, which causes much soreness particularly in the groins and flexures. Intertrigo may also appear in the folds of the neck and is as a rule seen in fat and ill-kept babies. The soreness is caused by contact of two moist skin surfaces which are cut off from the air and gradually infected.

Treatment of sore buttocks varies according to the cause of the soreness. Dietary errors should be investigated and corrected. Ammonia dermatitis may be due either to a low fluid intake, which is readily put right, or to decomposition of urine when in contact with stools and intestinal bacteria. Frequent changing and careful toilet is the best remedy.

In many cases it is a good idea to expose the infant's buttocks to warm air to promote healing. Plastic pants should be avoided as they prevent evaporation and thus increase skin damage from urine breakdown (Foster *et al.*, 1989).

The stools of the infant
The stools of the newborn infant are at first dark green to black in colour with a shiny appearance and viscid consistency, and are known as meconium. After 1–2 days they gradually change to lighter ones and are then called 'changing stools'. The stools of breast-fed babies are a golden mustard colour and of soft consistency. They have a characteristic, slightly sour smell. From one to six stools are passed each day.

The stools of infants fed on any type of infant formulae tend to be pale yellow, larger in bulk and more formed than those of breast-fed babies. From one to three stools are passed daily. The stools of infants should always be carefully observed, for much can be learned from their colour, odour, frequency and consistency. Changes occur readily and may be caused by slight deviation from health, change of the usual feed or amount of fluid intake, or by medicines.

It sometimes happens that a newborn baby fails to pass meconium in the first 24–36 hours. This is an important abnormality and must be reported at once as it may be due to a variety of serious causes such as imperforate anus, meconium ileus and atresia of the bowel.

PREVENTION OF INFECTION

Nursing procedures to prevent cross-infection vary from unit to unit but the following principles will apply wherever infants are nursed.

1. Careful hand washing techniques by all members of the staff before touching an infant. This has been shown to be the single most important factor in reducing the spread of infection (Taylor, 1987; Christensen *et al.*, 1982; Reybrough, 1986). Parents will need instruction in the techniques to be followed.

2. The correct technique in the use of gowns and plastic aprons when used for infant care.

3. All staff should be free of respiratory, gastrointestinal or skin infections. If parents have an active infection they may need to be advised not to visit for a day or so. It might be suggested that a grandparent or aunt comes in their place whilst they are ill to avoid the risk of cross-infection.

4. Each baby should have his own individual equipment including baby bath/basin.

5. All linen bins should have well-fitting seals/lids and be emptied at frequent and regular intervals.

6. All potential sources of infection, e.g. suction bottles, vaporizers etc., should be disinfected and changed regularly.

7. Liaison with the Infection Control Nurse and regular surveillance to monitor any reported infection.

8. Isolation procedures should be instigated immediately with any sign or suspicion of infection. Preferably, the nurse caring for these infants would not be involved in the care of others. Parents will need support and guidance in the protocols to be followed in the isolation of their infants.

INFANT FEEDING

The normal infant approximately doubles his weight in the first 5 months of life and trebles his weight in the first year. In order to meet the demand for this rapid growth rate, the nutritional requirements of protein, carbohydrate, fats, vitamins, minerals and fluids must be met either by breast-feeding or by artificial feeding.

Breast-feeding

The best food for babies is undoubtedly human milk (Committee on Medical Aspects of Food, 1988). All mothers should be encouraged to breast-feed their babies for a minimum of 2 weeks and preferably for the first 4–6 months.

Good reasons for breast-feeding

1. Protection against infection and allergies. Colostrum secreted in the first few days after birth is a rich source of antibodies. Breast-fed babies are less liable to gastrointestinal infections.

2. Human milk is rich in polyunsaturated fatty acids which are better absorbed by the infant than the fats in cows' milk.

3. There is no risk of giving an overconcentrated feed to the infant.

4. If sufficient breast milk is given the infant will not develop protein malnutrition. In developing countries, breast-feeding offers the only chance of survival for many infants.

In order for breast-feeding to be a success it is important that the details of breast-feeding are discussed with the parents antenatally. Good teaching and patience on the part of midwives and health visitors will also be required during pregnancy and postnatally for breast-feeding to become well-established. This may take as long as 14 days, during which time the mother may become anxious and so worried as to give up the attempt.

Undue stress on the importance of breast-feeding may, however, cause feelings of guilt if the mother is unable to manage this for any reason. The nurse, midwife or health visitor advising the mother should know the family circumstances and whatever the mother's choice for feeding she should be well-supported with advice and guidance.

Management of breast-feeding
Immediately after birth, the mother should cuddle her newborn infant to her breasts for about 15 min and allow the baby to suckle for 1 or 2 min at each breast if she intends to breast-feed. Suckling and cuddling the baby at this early stage is valuable psychologically, allowing mother and father to 'get to know their baby'. Early suckling also releases the hormones prolactin and oxytocin which stimulate milk secretion and help the uterus to contract.

For the continued management of successful breast-feeding it is important for both the mother and the nurses to feel relaxed and at ease. Privacy must always be provided. The mother's position needs to be completely comfortable, and a low or easy chair with a suitable footstool

FIG. 5   The correct position for breast-feeding.

can be of great assistance in achieving this. The mother
should hold the baby comfortably in her arm but support
from a pillow may be necessary to avoid fatigue. The baby
must be allowed to play at the breast and nipple before
starting to suck as this acts as an excellent stimulus for the
milk flow. A little milk squeezed from the nipple may
cause a baby who is slow to realize that he is expected to
suck, to take the nipple into his mouth and start to feed.
He should always be allowed to take the whole nipple and
areola into his mouth (Ardran, 1958; Fisher, 1981) or
sucking may give the mother pain and cause sore nipples.
The baby will also obtain less milk if he takes only the tip
of the nipple into his mouth.

'On demand' rather than regular feeding allows frequent stimulation of the breast and nipple, reducing the
time taken for lactation to become established. The infant
should be allowed to feed until satiated (i.e. for an un-

restricted period of time) (Royal College of Midwives, 1988).

Management of problems associated with breast-feeding
For mothers with poor lactation, the flow of milk can be stimulated by hot and cold bathing before starting to feed, by breast massage, by adequate support from a good brassière and by drinking of fluids. Mothers should be encouraged to express surplus milk after each feed, as this helps towards a better supply at the next feed.

Adequate washing and drying of the nipples will prevent them from cracking, a very painful condition for the mother and one which will interfere with successful breast-feeding.

The mother's general nutrition and state of health may need some attention as conditions such as anaemia or inadequate protein or kilojoule (Calorie) intake will produce poor lactation.

Complementary feeds. Complementary feeds of either water, glucose/dextrose or infant formula are those offered after breast-feeds and have been shown by research trials not to be of any benefit to healthy, term breast-fed infants (Royal College of Midwives, 1988).

Supplementary feeds. Supplementary feeds are given to replace one or several entire breast-feeds per day. This may be done to rest the mother's nipples or because the mother is temporarily absent or indisposed.

The success of infant feeding. The success of infant feeding is assessed by the rate of growth. During the first few days of life the infant loses weight owing to passage of meconium and urine, the drying of the umbilical cord and the poor feed intake during this period. But, by the end of a fortnight, birthweight is regained. For the next 3 months the infant gains on average 170 g/week.

Infant Formula Feeding

When breast-feeding is not possible, infant formula feeds given to the baby should approximate to the composition of breast milk as nearly as is possible.

For the purpose of estimating the average feed requirements of the baby, it is necessary to know his expected weight, i.e. the weight he should be. It is useless to feed an underweight baby according to his actual weight as in this way he will never achieve his expected weight.

To calculate expected weight of infant

1. Take infant's birthweight.
2. After initial loss this should be regained by 10–14 days.
3. From 2 weeks to 3 months infant should gain 170 g/ week.

Calorie* requirements in 24 hours

	Per kilogram of body weight in 24 hours
Pre-term infants (up to 2.5 kg)	130–150
Underweight infants	130–140
Normal infants	110–120

* Instead of measuring the energy value of foods in calories there is a tendency to be correctly scientific and measure it in joules. Conversion is relatively easy if one remembers that approximately 4.2 joules = 1 calorie and 4.2 kilojoules = 1 kilocalorie (which is the large calorie used in dietetics).

Fluid requirements in 24 hours

Premature infants (up to 1.4 kg)	250 ml
1.4–2.5 kg	220 ml
Infants over 2.5 kg	150–200 ml

Number of feeds in 24 hours

Up to 1.4 g	2-hourly feeds × 10
Up to 2.5 kg	3-hourly feeds × 7
2.5–3 kg	4-hourly feeds × 6
3 kg upwards	4-hourly feeds × 5

Example to calculate feed for baby John

John's age	3 months
Birthweight	3.4 kg
170 g gain for (12 minus 2) weeks = 170 g × 10 =	1.7 kg
Expected weight is	5.1 kg

N.B. John's actual weight is 4.95 kg and so he is a little underweight.

(Remember that the aim is to feed to the expected weight for age.)

Calorie requirements for baby John

5.1 kg × 115 ml = 586 calories in 24 hours

Fluid requirements for baby John

5.1 kg × 175 ml = 893 ml in 24 hours

Number of feeds in 24 hours

4-hourly × 5 = 180 ml per feed
Each feed contains 120 calories
30 ml contains 20 calories
(Calculations taken to the nearest whole number.)

Choice of infant food formulae

In the United Kingdom, artificial feeds intended to replace breast milk are manufactured as infant formulae. These may be powders or concentrated liquids which require reconstituting with water, or alternatively are sold already reconstituted in a 'ready-to-feed' form. Because breast milk is variable in composition, the composition of infant food formula cannot be exactly the same as every sample of human breast milk, but when reconstituted according to the manufacturer's instructions it is usually comparable as regards most nutrients with the average mature human milk from the healthy well-nourished mother.

The ready-to-feed concept

Many hospitals have found the use of pre-packed feeds economical, much more convenient and labour saving as their use avoids the need for manufacturing bulk artificial feeds. The possible risk of infection is reduced also.

Most hospitals using this method use one brand of feed only, to avoid confusion and to achieve economy in purchase. The pre-packed feed is available usually in disposable 120-ml bottles. Sterile, screw tight teat units are provided to fit the top of each bottle. Although these teat units can be disposed of after each feed, in practice it is more economical for each infant to keep his own teat unit. Between feeds the teat is placed in a sterilizing solution, e.g. hypochlorite or one of the other sterilizing preparations using potassium monopersulphate or sodium dichloroisocyanurate, then rinsed in sterile water before use. The teat can then be replaced as necessary or disposed of when the infant is discharged home.

The feed of one or two bottles, according to the infant's requirements, is taken to the cot-side along with a special bottle-opener. The bottle-top is removed and the teat unit screwed on to the bottle and the correct volume fed to the infant as ordered. The teat unit is then removed, rinsed with cold water and returned to the ward kitchen where it can be disposed of appropriately. Sterile pre-packed feeds can be fed at room temperature or can be warmed up before the top is removed. Sterile pre-packed feeds may be kept for 3–6 months at room temperature.

Feeding the infant
Whenever possible the baby should be taken out of the cot for feeding, and held, comfortably wrapped, in the nurse's arms. He should have been changed recently and the hands should be washed again before feeding commences.

Feeding time should be used as an opportunity for cuddling and physical contact which play an important part in any infant's development but is particularly important for the baby deprived of his mother if she is unable to be with him.

The bottle should be held at a sufficiently steep angle to keep the teat constantly filled with milk and so prevent the baby from sucking in air. He should be allowed to bring up wind at least once during a feed, but babies who are sick may need to bring up wind very frequently, often before starting as well as during the feed.

The teat should, if possible, be the one the baby is accustomed to, and the hole should be of a size which allows him to take his feed without much effort, and yet does not deliver the milk so quickly that he chokes. Inadequate holes can cause a baby to tire before completing the feed and so he refuses the last few millilitres, or swallows air by sucking hard without effect. A teat with too small a hole is the commonest cause of wind (Downing and Howkins, 1984). Colic, vomiting and restlessness result.

When using an upright bottle it may be necessary to

twist the bottle and teat while the baby is sucking, in order to allow air to enter and replace the milk, though many babies will let go from time to time and so prevent a vacuum forming, thus solving the problem for themselves.

Babies who are too eager or are underfed tend to gulp the first 60 ml or so, a habit which is likely to result in vomiting. A feed of 30 ml of boiled water before the milk formula is given, or an increase in the milk-feed are two ways of solving this problem. Failure to bring up wind, and excess crying due to hunger or discomfort between feeds may cause air swallowing with distension which may in turn cause vomiting.

A blocked nose can cause quite serious difficulty in feeding and can be one of the most commonly missed reasons for refusal of feeds. The nasal passages may be cleaned by inserting a wisp of cotton wool in the anterior nares, so inducing sneezing; alternatively nasal drops may be prescribed for a short time. Any baby with a blocked nose will take feeds more easily by spoon, as he is unable to breathe adequately with a teat in his mouth.

Bringing up wind
It is important to help the baby to bring up his wind, if unnecessary regurgitations, vomiting and colic are to be avoided. The baby should be sat on the nurse's lap, his head and body well supported, or alternatively laid over the nurse's shoulder and his back either rubbed or gently patted. This is comforting to the baby and appears to help in obtaining the desired effect. The principle is of course that of the air bubble which rises in a bottle. All babies swallow air when crying or feeding, and the nurse should not be satisfied until the baby has had at least one good eructation. Babies who cry a lot should be allowed to bring up wind before starting to feed.

Equipment

Bottles. There are many types of bottle obtainable but the most commonly used is the upright, wide-necked heat-resistant glass or polypropylene bottle. The wide neck of the upright bottle makes it easy to fill, and easy to clean, so that the risk of contamination is reduced.

Teats. It is often a good idea to experiment with teats to find the one to suit the particular infant's needs best. A strong rubber teat is good for babies who suck strongly and is obtainable in three sizes of hole. The softer teat with airflow is helpful for babies with a poor sucking reflex. Long-lasting silicone teats are also available.

Sterilization

The sterilization of equipment can be carried out by boiling, autoclaving or immersion in a chemical solution, e.g. hypochlorite liquid according to the manufacturer's instructions.

The success of any of these methods is entirely dependent upon thorough cleanliness before sterilization in order to remove completely all traces of milk curd and fat.

Bottles will be easier to clean if each one is rinsed after use and filled with cold water. The use of hot water for this purpose will congeal the milk protein and make the bottle very difficult to clean; teats should also be rinsed immediately after use and some cold water squeezed through the holes.

Later the bottles can be washed using a soapless or detergent cleaner, hot water and a bottle brush and then sterilized. Teats should be rubbed inside and out with salt to remove any milk deposits, and thoroughly rinsed in cold water before sterilizing.

If the hypochlorite method of sterilizing is used, the

solution must be changed every 24 hours. It is important to ensure that all air bubbles are excluded from the feeding equipment and that it is all totally immersed in the sterilizing solution for the required length of time.

Preparation of an individual feed
Thorough cleanliness is essential. After setting out the materials required, the nurse should again wash her hands. The mixing instructions on the packet or formula container should be followed implicitly. Accuracy is essential.

To dilute infant formula made in the United Kingdom use:

1 level scoop of powder with each 30 ml (1 oz) measured volume of boiled water.

Scoops should be measured accurately and levelled with the edge of a knife.

Discharge home
Mothers and others who may need to make up feeds in the home should be carefully taught to follow the manufacturer's instructions. Research has shown that many serious errors may occur (Jones and Belsey, 1978). These include

- Adding too little or too much water.
- Measuring a scoop by pressing against the inside of the packet or tin.
- Compressing milk powder in the scoop.
- Adding sugar or solids to the bottle.
- Adding or subtracting an extra measure of powder.
- Using a scoop measure made for one brand of milk powder with another.

If necessary demonstrate home method in the ward kitchen to the mother and always give written instructions before she leaves the ward. Ensure the mother has adequate supplies of infant formula at home prior to discharge.

Some feeding difficulties

Vomiting. There are some babies who vomit more readily than others and this must always be investigated as the small baby can very quickly lose essential water and minerals and become dehydrated.

When describing a vomit, the nurse should always state whether it was forcible or effortless, and when it occurred in relation to the feeds. She should describe the appearance of the vomit, the presence of curds, blood or mucus and the apparent stage of digestion.

There are very many causes for vomiting in infancy, some of which are directly related to feeding including: failure to bring up wind adequately, sucking from a teat with too small a hole, gulping a feed too quickly and finger sucking associated with air swallowing.

Regurgitation and posseting. This should not be confused with vomiting. In these babies a small amount of the feed is returned on bringing up wind or between feeds. It is rarely of importance, but is ofen a sign that a little too much feed is being offered.

Principles of Weaning

The introduction of solid foods should be commenced somewhere between the ages of 4–6 months. Weaning is a gradual process which may take several weeks to achieve. This allows the infant time to adapt to new tastes, textures and a new method of feeding.

Gradually, the infant becomes less dependent on milk. By the age of 1 year, although milk is still an important food source, the infant will now be able to partake of a variety of other foods which provide good dietary sources of iron with differing tastes and textures.

Introducing solid foods

Additions to the diet should be tried 2–3 days before a further addition is tried, and if the baby obviously dislikes the taste after a few days then the addition should be omitted and tried again later.

Baby cereals mixed with milk are commonly the first foods introduced. A rice-based (gluten-free) one should be chosen initially. The additions to the diet should be given with a spoon. As the amount of solid food increases, feed volume should be reduced to prevent obesity. Extra fluids such as water or fruit juice should be offered to quench the thirst.

A large choice of commercially prepared weaning foods is available, and although they are convenient they are also expensive. Home-cooked puréed foods are cheaper and nutritionally suitable, providing salt or salty gravy has been avoided. Sugar should be used sparingly as a sweetener. Because of the poor iron content of milk, iron-containing foods such as red meat and liver should be included in the diet. As the baby becomes accustomed to the mixed diet the times of the feeds can be altered to fit in with the household mealtimes if these are the most convenient for the mother.

Vitamins

Young infants who are breast-fed by a well-nourished mother already receive an adequate supply of vitamins. Infants fed with an approved infant food formula will also receive sufficient for their growth needs.

When mixed feeding is introduced, however, there is a

risk that vitamin deficiency can occur. The DHSS report (1988) on *Present Day Practice in Infant Feeding* recommends that all infants from the age of six months should receive supplementary vitamins—available nationally under the Welfare Food Scheme. This should be continued until the infant is at least 2 years old or preferably 5 years old. The single daily dose of 5 drops contains approximately:

Vitamin A—200 µg
Vitamin C—20 µg
Vitamin D—7 µg

These vitamins for infants and young childen are available to parents under the Welfare Food Scheme either free of charge or at reduced cost.

PLANNING FOR DISCHARGE HOME

This should begin early and involve all members of the caring team. The following is a basic check list to ensure that the parents are adequately prepared for the discharge home of their baby.

1. Environment. As the baby may have arrived earlier than expected, have the parents had time to obtain all the necessary essentials, e.g. clothing, nappies and cot? Are they aware of the need for the room temperature to be comfortably warm to protect their infant against hypothermia?

2. Infant feeding. If the baby is artificially fed, does the mother understand fully the making up of feeds? Does she have all the necessary utensils? Does she know of how/ where to obtain further supplies of the milk formula? A written list of details is helpful for her to take home and refer to.

3. Equipment/supplies and drugs medication. Does the infant require any of these? Are the parents familiar with their use/reasons for these? Have adequate supplies been given to the parents until the next appointment? Do the parents appreciate the significance of ensuring that all drugs are kept within a locked cupboard?

4. Bathing. Is the mother confident and happy with this procedure? Has it needed modifying to fit in with her home conditions?

5. Has the mother been given an out-patient appointment for her infant? Provide her with written details of time, etc. Ensure that she is happy with the time and date provided. Are they convenient for her to keep?

6. The nurse should inform the health visitor before the discharge home, at least 48 hours beforehand. Do the parents know her name and that of the nearest child health clinic? Ensure that the health visitor receives a summary of the infant's nursing care whilst in hospital and any notes for future care.

REFERENCES

Ardran, G.M., Kemp, F.H. and Lind J. (1958). A cineradiographic study of breast feeding. *British Journal of Radiology* **31**, 156–162.

Barr, R.J. (1984). The umbilical cord: to treat or not to treat? *Midwives Chronicle Nursing Notes*, July, 224–226.

Christensen, G.D., Korones, S.B., Reed, L. *et al.* (1982). Epidemic *Serratia marcescens* in a neonatal intensive care unit. *Infection Control* **3**(2), 127–133.

Downing, L.J. and Howkins, E.J. (1984). Infant feeding in practice. *Nursing Times* **80**(5), 57–60.

Fisher, C. (1981). Breastfeeding: a midwife's view. *Maternal and Child Health*, February, 52–57.

Foster, R.L., Hunsberger, M.M. and Anderson, J. (1989). *Family-Centered Nursing Care of Children*. Philadelphia: Saunders.

DHSS (1988). Committee on Medical Aspects of Food (1988).

Third Report: *Present Day Practice in Infant Feeding*. London: HMSO.

Jones, R. and Belsey, E. (1978). Common mistakes in infant feeding. *British Medical Journal* **2**, 112–114.

Reybrough, G. (1986). Handwashing and hand disinfection. *Journal of Hospital Infection* **8**(1), 5–23.

Royal College of Midwives (1988). *Successful Breast Feeding. A Practical Guide for Midwives*. London: Royal College of Midwives.

Salariya, E. (1988). *Midwifery Journal* **4**, 70–76.

Sweet, B.R. (1988). *Mayes Midwifery*. London: Baillière Tindall.

Taylor, L.J. (1987). An evaluation of handwashing techniques. 1 & 2. *Nursing Times* **74**(2), 54–74; (3), 108–110.

FURTHER READING

Brunner, L.S. and Suddarth, D.S. (1991). *The Lippincott Manual of Paediatric Nursing*, 3rd edn (adapted by B.F. Weller). London: Harper and Row.

Cockburn, F. and Drillien. C.M. (1974). *Neonatal Medicine*. Oxford: Blackwell Scientific.

Kelnar, C.J.H. and Harvey, D. (1981). *The Sick Newborn Baby*. London: Baillière Tindall.

King, E.M., Wieck, L. and Dyer, M. (1985). *Paediatric Nursing Practice and Techniques*. London: Harper and Row.

Rickman, P.P. and Johnston, J.H. (1978). *Neonatal Surgery*, 2nd edn. London: Butterworth.

Vulliamy, D.G. (1977). *Newborn Child*, 4th edn. Edinburgh: Churchill Livingstone.

3 The infant at risk

The parents of infants who are born either before term, of low birthweight, or with abnormalities will need help in coping with this stressful situation. Inevitably, the shock of learning that their baby is small and immature or is suffering from a physical or mental handicap will be very great. Much time, sympathy and understanding is needed to help the parents come to terms with their situation. They will need to ask many questions from a variety of people. In hospital, the doctor and the senior nurse or midwife should be the ones to discuss the parents' concerns. The paediatric liaison health visitor, medical social worker and others will also be able to offer support and counsel the parents.

Babies who have undergone a difficult birth, have suffered from an infection in the perinatal period, those with a history of genetic disorder, low birthweight infants, those with respiratory distress and other infants with an acute perinatal problem are amongst those who will need particularly careful observation and nursing care. This is best given in the Neonatal Units which provide intensive care by nurses and midwives especially trained and interested in this branch of nursing. Prompt recognition, treatment and specialized nursing care can be assured in this way together with the most modern equipment and technology.

Close liaison with the pediatric health visitor will not only ensure continuity in the care of these infants and their families, but may also mean the detection of other problems which may present in the first few weeks of life. Certain tests are now carried out routinely within this early period, e.g. the Guthrie test to detect phenylketonuria, an inherited metabolic disorder.

ATTACHMENT OR MOTHER/INFANT BONDING

Klaus and Kennell (1982) define attachment 'as a unique emotional relationship between two people which is specific and endures through time'. This attachment has been shown to commence with delivery of the infant to the mother.

It is important for paediatric nurses to have insight and knowledge of this special relationship in order that they can promote the relationship despite the adverse situation of the infant requiring prolonged hospital care and treatment.

Physical Contact

The mother should have the opportunity to hold her baby quietly, to fondle and to suckle the infant unless this is specifically excluded for any clinical reason. For the infant who has to be removed immediately from the delivery room the mother should, at the earliest opportunity, be given a polaroid or 'instant' photograph of her baby and allowed to visit her baby; fathers, too, should be included.

Participation in Care

The opportunity for the mother to be involved in care is important for the development of attachment. The mother at first may feel a reluctance to do this, especially if her infant is pre-term, very low birthweight or obviously handicapped. The parents will be finding it difficult to adjust to the 'less than perfect child' when expectations were for a perfect baby to take home soon after delivery.

The nurse will need to show the mother how to hold and fondle her baby in an environment which must seem very bewildering and strange.

The 'role model' of the nurse is particularly important. The nurse should show by her actions that she sees the child as an individual by using the child's first name and talking to it gently as she provides care. This will give the parents confidence and courage to take on the caring opportunities that the nurse is able to provide for them to do, e.g. changing a nappy even though the infant is in an incubator.

The nurse should take great care also to explain to the parents 'unit policies', e.g. hand washing protocols and why they are important to the well-being of her infant. Every effort should be made to keep the parents informed of all developments and changes in their baby's condition.

Siblings and grandparents can also play an important role in visiting the unit and thus providing support for the parents.

A record should be kept of parental visiting and of their progress in caring for their infant. In this way, the possibility of any rejection can be foreseen early. When planning for discharge, it is helpful for the family health visitor to be provided with a summary of this information.

DEFINITIONS

Traditionally, infants under 2500 g (2.5 kg) were called 'premature'. It is now recognized that weight alone is not sufficient for estimating gestational age or for planning nursing care.

The infant at 'term' is one who is born after 37 weeks' gestation and before 42 weeks' gestation and weighing 2.5 kg or more.

FIG. 6 The normal posture of the premature infant.

Pre-term Infants

These infants are small and of less than 37 weeks' gestation. Nursing care is directly related to the degree of immaturity.

Low Birthweight Infants, or Small-for-gestational-age Infants

These infants are small due to poor intrauterine nutrition, often due to maternal health problems. Birthweight is below the tenth centile for gestational age.

Some babies are both pre-term and small for gestational age. The terms 'small for dates' or 'light for gestational age' may be used.

Characteristics of these small infants

1. Their heads appear large in comparison to the rest of the body.
2. They have a feeble cry, but often appear most alert.
3. Marked lack of subcutaneous tissue, dry loose red

skin with absence of skin creases. Lanugo (soft body hair) covers parts of the body.

4. Scalp hair is sparse, nails soft and external genitalia immature.

5. Irregular respiration.

6. Muscle tone is poor and the sucking reflex may be poor or absent.

Post-mature Infants

These infants born after 42 weeks' gestation vary considerably in birthweight. Due to placental deterioration *in utero*, these babies often tolerate the stress of delivery poorly and may suffer from hypoxia, meconium aspiration and jaundice. The body appears thin and long due to wasting of subcutaneous fat. The nails are often long and the hair profuse.

THE NURSING ENVIRONMENT

Temperature

These infants all need to be protected against heat loss as they are vulnerable to hypothermia. This results in increased oxygen consumption and metabolic rate, dehydration, lethargy and may result in death. The methods used to achieve and sustain a stable body temperature must depend upon the infant's age, maturity and size. Care must also be taken to avoid increasing the infant's temperature rapidly as this places considerable stress on the infant's metabolic requirements (see p. 38).

The nursery ambient temperature needs to be over 25°C for infants weighing about 2000 g and up to 30°C for those infants weighing less than 2000 g. The nursery environmental temperature should be regularly recorded.

Radiant warmer

An overhead radiant warmer maintained by 'Servo Control' over an open base or cot provides the nursing staff with good access to the infant for care and observations.

Incubator

As an enclosed box-like environment, the incubator can be set at a particular environmental temperature or the

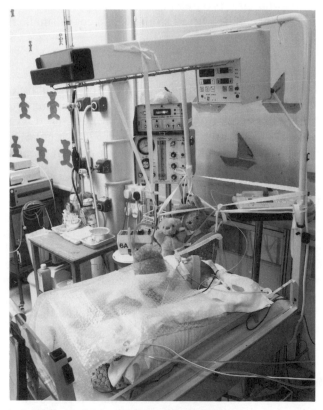

FIG. 7 Baby receiving artificial ventilation

infant can be attached to a temperature probe and the incubator maintained on 'Servo Control'. Oxygen and humidity can be delivered into the incubator at pre-set levels. Care needs to be taken that the incubator is not placed in direct sunlight to avoid creating the 'greenhouse' effect and thus increasing the ambient temperature.

Cot
Infants who are progressing and maintaining a stable temperature can be nursed clothed, in a cot or small crib.

Respiratory Assistance—Oxygen Therapy

Oxygen is essential to the body for the production of energy. Oxygen therapy may be needed in the treatment of respiratory failure and to relieve hypoxia. Oxygen levels should be monitored frequently and regularly by blood gas analysis and transcutaneous oxygen measurements. Maintenance levels of administered oxygen should be ordered by the paediatrician according to clinical need and maturity of the infant.

Excessive oxygen above 30% of the inspired air has been shown to have an adverse effect upon the retina of the eye producing 'retrolental fibroplasia' or retinopathy of prematurity. Other complications include central nervous system haemorrhage, apnoea and bronchopulmonary dysplasia (Phelps, 1982).

Oxygen may be administered through an incubator, head box, oxygen hood, croupette, oxygen tent, or a paediatric face mask.

Mechanical ventilation
The decision to use mechanical ventilation for the infant will be made on the following criteria:

Cyanosis unrelieved by high oxygen levels.
Apnoea with depressed respiratory rate.
Blood oxygen levels below 50 mm Hg in 100%.
P_{CO_2} between 60–70 mm Hg in 100%.
pH below 7.2.

The nursing management considerations of an infant requiring mechanical ventilation are basically the same as
for the older child, with the following exceptions. As the
risk of infection is very great, due to the immature immunological systems of the 'infant at risk', sterile precautions should always be used for changing the ventilator
tubing every 12–24 hours and suctioning of the airway.

N.B. Routine cultures should be taken daily after intubation.

Chest physiotherapy
Consultation with physiotherapist colleagues will be required in the presence of atelectasis and excessive mucous
secretions. In some instances this treatment will be carried
out by the nurse.
    Chest physiotherapy should never be performed till 30–
45 min after the last feed. Care should be taken not to
exhaust the infant and vital signs should be monitored
frequently. As 'cupped hands' are too large for the chest
vibration in these small neonates, a vibrator or padded
battery-operated toothbrush may be used most effectively.

NUTRITION

Adequate kilojoule (calorie) intake is essential for optimal
brain growth, to meet metabolic needs and to provide for
normal growth development; the low birthweight infant
requires at least 130 calories/kg/24 h.

Breast-feeding

Every effort should be made to support and assist the mother to produce her own milk if she wishes to breast-feed, even though at this stage the baby may be too weak or sick to suck at her breast.

The midwife will instruct the mother in the use of either an electric or hand pump (these may be borrowed or hired at low cost from the Health Authority or voluntary organizations, e.g. National Childbirth Trust) or to express her milk manually.

It is important that the mother understands the need to express her milk regularly at 3–4-hourly intervals to avoid engorgement of her breasts. At first, the milk supply may be poor, but if the breasts have been regularly expressed the supply will increase once the infant begins sucking at the breast.

Ideally, the milk should be collected, labelled and delivered daily to the ward so that it can be given to her baby without being frozen. Plastic bottles or bags are better for collection as leucocytes in the milk adhere to glass surfaces.

Infant Formula Feeding

There are many suitable infant food formulae available. The final choice must depend on the special needs of the infant, the mother's preference and unit policy.

GENERAL CARE

Observation
This is the most important tool of the nurse caring for the 'infant at risk'. Continued, intelligent observation of appearance, posture, activity and elimination will provide

TABLE 2   Methods of feeding

Route	Indications
Nasogastric Allow to flow in by gravity. Too rapid a feed may cause abdominal distension or regurgitation	Employed for infants unable to suck
Duodenal/jejunal Feed given by slow drip or continuous infusion. N.B. Gastric catheter may also be *in situ* to reduce abdominal distension and check gastric aspirate	For infants requiring mechanical ventilation and for those who are very small or ill
Gastrostomy Feed given by gravity	Usually used postoperatively and for infants requiring prolonged artificial feeding
Bottle and teat/breast May be introduced initially to alternate with nasogastric feeding to avoid exhaustion of the infant	For the infant who is vigorous and able to suck well
Total parenteral nutrition An infusion to provide protein, carbohydrate and fats can be given either through a peripheral or central venous line	Most often used post-operatively or for those infants unable to feed orally for prolonged periods

information for assessing progress and planning future care.

Cleanliness

The nature and frequency of bathing the infant would depend upon unit policy and the particular condition of the infant. The napkin area is cleansed at each nappy change.

Eye care
These should be cleaned daily with a single cotton wool ball soaked in sterile warm water, then wiped dry. A separate swab should be used for each eye and each movement.

Nostril care
Leave untouched but if blocked with secretions, wipe external nares gently; this will often stimulate sneezing and clear the obstruction.

Cord care
See p. 30.

PRINCIPLES OF NURSING CARE

1. Carefully planned and minimal nursing intervention. A basic principle of neonatal care is that the sick or small infant should be handled as little as possible and excessive repositioning avoided (Horsley, 1990). The infant is likely to become hypoxaemic and deteriorate if interventions and care are not planned and co-ordinated. A fall in oxygen tension may occur and may be prolonged (Murdoch and Darlow, 1984).

2. Control and monitoring of oxygen administration.

3. Protection of infant against heat loss or excessive heat gain.

4. Correction of abnormal blood chemistry.

5. Careful, adequate feeding to meet requirements for growth and metabolism.

6. Maintenance of respiration possibly with mechanical assistance.

7. Prevention of infection.

8. Maintenance of parental and family links.

SOME NEONATAL PROBLEMS

Haemorrhagic Disease of the Newborn

Occasionally a baby may suddenly vomit blood or pass a melaena stool or blood-stained urine, or may be found to be bleeding from the nose, vagina or umbilicus. The bleeding occurs without warning and is most common between the third and sixth day of life. The cause is lack of vitamin K, which in turn causes hypoprothrombinaemia. Those most at risk of bleeding are pre-term infants or those who have had a traumatic delivery.

Treatment is by giving vitamin K (0.5–1 mg either orally or intramuscularly).

Haemolytic Disease of the Newborn
(Rhesus Incompatibility)

Neither Rh-positive or Rh-negative individuals normally have anti-Rh antibodies in their serum, but if a Rh-negative woman bears a Rh-positive child or fetus she may develop anti-Rh antibodies. With future pregnancies these antibodies can pass via the placenta into the fetal circulation causing the red cells to haemolize, resulting in anaemia and jaundice of the newborn infant.

All Rh-negative mothers of Rh-position babies are now given anti-D immunoglobulin within 60 hours of delivery to prevent rhesus incompatibility problems with future pregnancies.

However, if rhesus incompatibility does occur the principal manifestations are:

1. Stillbirth or death within a few hours, associated with hydrops fetalis.
2. Icterus gravis.
3. Congenital anaemia.

Newborn infants with anaemia and jaundice resulting from rhesus incompatibility must be treated as soon as possible after birth with an exchange transfusion.

Sclerema

Sclerema is a thickening of the subcutaneous tissues, most noticeably in the back, buttocks and legs. The skin is cold and hard to touch. The exact cause is unknown, but implicated factors have been found to be:

Hypothermia.
Reduced peripheral circulation.
Staphylococcal or streptococcal infection.

Principles of care and treatment
This is planned to:

1. Monitor body temperature and gradually re-warm the infant.
2. Correct any metabolic problem, e.g. acidosis with intravenous therapy.
3. To provide for energy requirements and to avoid undue exertion of the infant by tube feeding, if possible with mother's own milk.
4. Combat infection. Commence antibiotics. Exchange transfusion is sometimes helpful by providing factors to aid the infant's own immunity system.

Respiratory Distress Syndrome

This syndrome carries a high mortality and is due to a deficiency of surfactant (an enzyme which lowers the surface tension of the alveoli). This leads to alveolar collapse, dilated alveolar ducts and pulmonary congestion. The blood supply to the kidneys and the gastro-intestinal tract is impaired. Oedema is often marked. Respiratory acidosis is present with consequent electrolyte disturbances.

The syndrome may occur immediately after birth or within a few hours of delivery. Most commonly affects pre-term infants, those born by caesarian section, males and those with a sibling history of respiratory distress. Maternal diabetes and rhesus isoimmunization increases the incidence.

Principles of care and treatment

This is planned to:

1(a). Decrease energy requirements and therefore oxygen consumption. Place infant under radiant warmer or in an incubator with less than 30% oxygen. Blood gases and pH monitored frequently. Mechanical ventilation may become necessary if respiratory failure occurs.

1(b). Nursing intervention reduced to a minimum to decrease stress.

Monitor continuously: heart rate; respiratory rate; transcutaneous P_{O_2}; temperature.

Monitor frequently: Dextrostix for hypoglycaemia; blood pressure.

Measure urine output and specific gravity.

2. Meet fluid and nutrition requirements initially by feeding intravenously with 5% dextrose. As improvement occurs nasogastric feeding is slowly introduced.

3. Antibiotics may be ordered either to treat infection or as prophylaxis.

4. Various studies are in progress using surfactant, either synthetically produced or of animal origin, with variable sucess.

Jaundice

This is a yellow discolouration of the skin due to the accumulation of bilirubin. Bilirubin is the product of the breakdown of the 'haem' portion of haemoglobin, and exists in two forms, albumin-bound and free. Bilirubin is normally excreted in the bile into the duodenum.

Physiological jaundice

Usually first noticed about the third day after birth, reaching a peak about 5–7 days later. This condition results from the increased breakdown of red blood cells and immature liver function: usually more severe in pre-term infants. Serum bilirubin levels may be increased by dehydration and poor feeding.

Treatment. Close monitoring of serum bilirubin levels. No active treatment indicated unless bilirubin levels rise above 140–170 mmol/litre for infants weighing 2000–2500 g, when phototherapy may be indicated.

Kernicterus

Kernicterus is the development of brain damage secondary to the deposition of bilirubin in the brain cells.

Initially the infant may appear yellow and lethargic, with poor sucking and a high pitched cry. Hypotonia or hypertonia with downward rolling of the eyes may be present. Apnoea and fits may also occur. Without recognition and treatment, permanent spasticity with mental handicap will result.

Treatment. Exchange transfusion after initial infusion of albumin 1 g/kg.

Necrotizing Enterocolitis

Disease of the bowel resulting in patches of necrotic mucosa and intramural gas, leading to severe abdominal distension, bleeding in the bowel and collapse. Precise cause unknown, but associated factors include prematurity, asphyxia, hypothermia, hypoglycaemia, and acidosis.

Onset is sudden, between 1–14 days after birth, but most commonly between 4–7 days.

Principles of care and treatment

Care and treatment depend upon the stage of disease when a diagnosis is made.

Early diagnosis.

Gastric decompression with nasogastric tube.

Total parenteral nutrition.

Broad spectrum antibiotics after specimen cultures have been made of blood, gastric aspirate and faeces.

Late diagnosis. As above, but proceeds to surgery for resection of any perforated, gangrenous bowel.

N.B. Prevention. Be alert to signs; note and report in vulnerable infants:

Increased amounts of gastric aspirate.

Abdominal distension—measure every 2–4 hours. Report any increase over 1 cm.

Test stools for occult blood.

Ophthalmia Neonatorum

Any prudent discharge from the eye within 21 days of birth is notifiable in England and Wales irrespective of the cause. The commonest causative organisms are staphylococcus and gonococcus.

Qphthalmia neonatorum once accounted for a high proportion of blindness in children, but nowadays owing to adequate prophylaxis and treatment with antibiotics, eye infections rarely have serious consequences. Symptoms vary from slight oedema of the eyelids, inability to open the eyes and presence of frank pus, to changes in the eye itself.

Principles of care and treatment

Infants with 'sticky eyes' should be nursed with strict precautions against spread of infection and should be carefully isolated from other babies with a special nurse attending them.

Appropriate antibiotic ophthalmic ointment or eye drops are prescribed. If one eye only is affected, the infant should be nursed on the affected side to prevent discharge from running over the bridge of the nose into the healthy eye. The baby's arms must be effectively restrained to prevent him from touching his eyes and so spreading the infection.

If the infection persists blockage of the lacrimal duct should be suspected.

Naevi or Birth Marks

Naevi (singular: naevus) consist of a localized cluster of dilated blood vessels. There are various types of naevi, some of which are present at birth, others appear some months later. Of the different types most disappear spontaneously but others persist. Some naevi are very extensive and may disfigure an entire side of the face or cause enlargement of the tongue associated with difficulty of speech, eating and breathing.

CHILD ABUSE/NON-ACCIDENTAL INJURY

Unfortunately, some young children suffer repeated injury at the hands of their parents or other carers. The nurse should always remember that the reasons are very complex. Young parents in an overcrowded home and short of money may feel it to be the last straw when faced with a constantly crying child and give vent to their feelings. The nurse should never judge but attempt to understand and support the parents whilst at the same time protecting the child.

Many such children appear well cared for and loved, and the assault by one or other of the parents may be due to momentary loss of control. Other children present with profound physical and/or sexual abuse and emotional neglect. Often the bruising and haematoma are obvious but occasionally rib and other fractures are detected only by radiographs, taken for other reasons; and the parents may give no history of previous injury.

Protection of the child suspected of being abused, or who has been abused and is admitted to the ward or is in the accident and emergency department is of paramount importance. The Department of Health (1988) document 'Child Protection: Guidance for Senior Nurses, Health Visitors and Midwives' makes the following recommendations that in Accident and Emergency departments:

1. The agreed health authority procedures and guidelines are readily available and staff are familar with them.
2. There is a senior nurse available to give advice and

support to staff particularly where there is a difference of opinion with others or conflict with parents.

3. The agreed procedures for obtaining advice as necessary from the paediatrician whenever children are brought to the department are followed.

4. There is access to the 'child protection register' and staff are familiar with the procedure for making enquiries from it.

5. There is a proper recording and reporting system of all cases of suspected or actual abuse admitted to the department.

6. There is a system for notifying community nursing services about all visits made to the department by children.

7. Staff know how to obtain advice from the social services department.

For the child admitted to the paediatric ward care must be taken that all conversations with the parents, care-givers and child remain private and that information is kept confidential. The senior paediatric nurse has a responsibility to ensure that:

1. There is an agreed procedure for obtaining and recording information about the child and its family from other agencies including full details about decisions on the future care of the child, who has access, whether there is a 'place of safety' order, as well as the names of the social worker and health visitor for the family.

2. She/he is informed when a child is thought to have been or has been abused is admitted to the ward.

3. She/he is kept informed about the level of knowledge or experience of all the staff on the ward so that appropriate support and advice can be given to them.

4. There is a proper recording and reporting system of

all cases of suspected or actual child abuse admitted to the ward that is well known to all staff.

5. Staff attend multi-disciplinary training events.

Role of the Social Services Department

Statutory powers for the protection of children rest with social services but health authorities and their staff have a duty to support them to carry out this function. There should be an efficient communication system through the nursing staff with social workers and the Social Services Department to ensure that the documentation of formal and informal referrals is satisfactory.

Police

Most police authorities now have named officers for child abuse. These officers receive specialist training and regularly attend conferences in accordance with Home Office Regulations. The named officer will be known to the social worker and is readily available to nursing staff. The police authority retain the right to pursue their investigations into allegations of child abuse taking into account the recommendations of case conferences.

Voluntary Sector

Voluntary organizations offer a range of services to children but this will vary from district to district. The paediatric nurse should be familiar with the services available in the local area and how to make contact with them if necessary. The National Society for the Prevention of Cruelty to Children (NSPCC) has a statutory duty to protect children. The society has a national overview of child abuse and there are 61 Child Protection Teams pioneering protection of children jointly with social workers, police and health authority staff. The NSPCC Child Protection Teams aim to prevent child abuse and neglect and where there has been abuse to rehabilitate families and help parents improve their parenting skills.

Prevention of Child Abuse

Midwives have a significant role to play in the prevention of child abuse because of their involvement in the ante-natal and post-natal care of women and their partners. Frequently there are clues that point to potentially abusive parents before the birth of the baby (Whaley and Wong, 1987). The midwife is in an ideal position to observe and report unusual attitudes and behaviour in pregnancy and early parenthood which may be the first indication of future difficulties.

PAEDIATRIC PROCEDURES

Intravenous Infusions

General nursing responsibilities

Nursing action	Explanation
1. Prepare equipment. Check intravenous fluid with doctor and check for any sediment/ contaminant. Prepare infusion.	To ensure that the correct solution is given. If sediment is observed the fluid should not be used.
2. Explain the procedure to a child old enough to understand in simple words. Ensure the parents understand the need for the infusion. Ask them to hold and comfort the child during the procedure.	This will help to allay fear and anxiety for the child and assist in co-operation.

Nursing action

3. Once the infusion is established check the child at regular intervals for:

- any leakage from the infusion site.
- any swelling of the site. It may be helpful to compare with the opposite limb.

Report and record occurrence.

4. If an infusion pump at a constant pre-set rate is being used the site should be checked hourly to ensure that extravasation has not occurred.

Explanation

This will indicate that infiltration of the tissues is occurring and therefore the child is not receiving correct quantities of fluid intravenously.

This helps to maintain patency of the vein. As the pump is designed to function against resistance, leakage may occur through a dislodged cannula.

N.B. The serial number of the intravenous fluid should be noted on the child's records.

Blood Transfusions

The main indications for a blood transfusion to a child are:

To restore circulating volume, e.g. after haemorrhage.
To provide blood components which may be deficient in the child, e.g. platelets.

If blood is to be given, it will have to be cross-matched and grouped in the laboratory, but the doctor and nurse should check the label against the patient's record sheet. The amounts to be given in a specified time will be ordered by the doctor but will rarely exceed 10–15 ml per 600 g of body weight.

Equipment required is the same as for intravenous infusions.

Scalp vein infusion
For a scalp vein infusion, the infant's head is shaved over the parietal bone and an assistant holds the head securely. Once the needle is in position, it may be secured by strapping or by plaster of Paris approximately 7.5 cm (3 in.) in width (Fig. 8).

Splinting for intravenous therapy
When a limb is used adequate splinting is essential and this is a highly skilled procedure, as immobility must be achieved without compressing important blood vessels. The splint should be well padded and covered. For an infant, the splint need be only about 7.5 cm (3 in.) wide but the length should be sufficient to allow for it to support a loop of tubing. This takes the weight off the tubing and makes it possible to adjust the position of the needle in the vein by suitable padding. This method also minimizes the vibrations caused by restlessness or movement of the bottle which in turn helps to cut down inflammation within the vein. If the internal saphenous vein is used, the splint should reach from the fold of the buttock to about 25 cm (10 in.) beyond the toes or if a vein in the arm is used, from the head of the humerus to about 25 cm (10 in.) beyond the fingers. The foot and ankle are rotated externally and immobilized on the splint by lengths of 2.5 cm (1 in.) adhesive strapping passing across the heel just below the knee. In this way pressure on important blood vessels is avoided. If the antecubital vein is used, the arm is rotated externally and three lengths of strapping applied; one across the palm of the hand, one just below the antecubital fossa and the third high up on the arm and across the bony prominence of the shoulder. In either case a firm bandage and cotton wool are applied to give added immobility, but a space of about 5–7.5 cm (2 to 3 in.) is left uncovered so that the condition of the

FIG. 8 Infant receiving intravenous therapy. (Note paediatric giving set.)

TABLE 3   Blood transfusions

Specific observations	Explanation
Immediately flow starts:	*For incompatibility reactions*
Record ¼-hourly pulse and hourly temperature	i.e. Rising pulse rate
	Sudden elevation of temperature (normal—36.4°C)
Observe colour and feel of skin and any respiratory distress	Twitching to convulsions
	Skin of face flushed
	May shiver
Estimate urinary output and concentration	Urinary output diminished
Throughout transfusion continue to:	*For allergic reaction to blood*
Record ¼-hourly pulse (rate/volume)	i.e. Appearance of shocked state
	Respirations fluttering (very shallow and rapid)
Observe respirations, colour and feel of skin and general appearance of infant	Where history in family (asthma, eczema or hay fever)
As for all infusions:	*To avoid overloading (also i.v.)*
Hourly recordings on i.v. chart	of circulation with possible heart failure or pulmonary oedema
Rate of flow—drops per min	
Amount given in that hour (1 drop = approx. ¹⁄₂₀th millilitre)	Maximum rate of intake 2 ml/kg/h
Frequently listen for bubbly sounds on respiration	
Note any cough or dyspnoea	
Any engorgement of neck veins	
Maintenance of rate of flow	*Difficulty of flow (also i.v.)*
If slowing down:	Rate ordered frequently very slow
Apply warmth to limb	
Check and adjust temperature of room	Also muscles around vein liable to go into spasm
Check splint and entry site of infusion	Easy to occlude circulation in newborn

FIG. 9 (A) Correct splinting of leg for intravenous therapy. Note that any strapping used must be taken over a bony prominence to prevent constriction of blood vessels. (B) Correct splinting of arm for intravenous therapy into a vein of the dorsum of the hand. Note roll of foam sponge to prevent wrist drop.

limb can be watched. A pad of foam sponge can be used to prevent foot-drop or an over-extension of the elbow. The splint should be firmly tied to the bed to ensure immobility.

Good splinting is essential, not only for the successful running of the intravenous drip infusion, but also because it enables the child to move up and down the cot or for his parents or nurse to lift him out for feeding or weighing. In order to make this possible an extra length of sterile tubing should always be attached to the adult giving set. Moving the child at regular intervals is one way of preventing hypostatic pneumonia.

Care should be taken to see that the limb and splint are not twisted and that neither groin nor tubing are kinked or constricted. It is a good plan to have a bed cradle over the limb, to facilitate inspection and to support the weight of the bedclothes.

Replacement transfusion

Indications for replacement transfusion:
   Hyperbilirubinaemia.
   Anaemia in rhesus incompatibility.
   Polycythaemia—partial exchange with saline or plasma.
   Severe sepsis.

Dangers: air embolism, thrombosis, sepsis, acidosis, hypoglycaemia, hypocalcaemia, bleeding, heart failure and necrotizing enterocolitis.

Nursing action	Explanation
1. Ensure that the environmental temperature is sufficient to maintain the infant's body temperature.	Apnoea, with an increased need for oxygen and calories can occur as a result of chilling during the procedure. Acidosis may also occur as a result of stress and chilling.
2. Attach the infant to a cardiac monitor to record immediately any apnoea or bradycardia; if noted the procedure should be halted until condition stabilizes.	
3. Check temperature, apex beat and respiration.	
4. Aspirate stomach. Urine-collecting bag may be applied.	To prevent aspiration. A urine bag is applied to avoid contamination of the site.
5. Secure the baby comfortably.	To prevent the infant moving and dislodging the exchange catheter.
6. Check the blood with the paediatrician and record the serial number on the appropriate chart.	Freshly donated blood—group O Rhesus negative or the ABO group of the infant and compatible with the mother's serum is used to avoid incompatibility problems.

Nursing action

7. Note time of commencement and time of withdrawal and replacement of the blood. It should take approximately 1 min to remove and replace 10 ml of blood.

Explanation

Blood is exchanged slowly. Rapid exchange can aggravate cardiovascular changes.

8. Check Dextrostix before commencement of procedure, half-way through procedure, and at the end of the exchange transfusion.

Rebound hypoglycaemia may occur after the exchange transfusion as a result of the anticoagulant in the donated blood containing dextrose.

9. Make frequent recordings of heart rate, respiratory rate and pattern; also note the infant's colour.

10. At completion of the exchange transfusion closely observe the infant. Check temperature, apex beat and respirations immediately and then at frequent intervals for at least 4 hours post-exchange transfusion. Observe the umbilicus for any bleeding.

To detect at an early stage the development of complications.

REFERENCES

Department of Health (1988). *Child Protection: Guidance for Senior Nurses, Health Visitors and Midwives*. London: HMSO.

Horsley, A. (1990). The neonatal environment. *Paediatric Nursing*, February, 17–19.

Klaus, M.H. and Kennell, J.H. (1982). *Parent–Infant Bonding*. St Louis, MO: C.V. Mosby.

Murdoch, D. and Darlow, B. (1984). Handling during neonatal care. *Archives of Disease in Childhood* **59**, 957–961.

Phelps, D.L. (1982). Neonatal oxygen toxicity—is it preventable? *Pediatric Clinics of North America* **29**, 1233–1240.

Whaley, L.F. and Wong, D.L. (1987). *Nursing Care of Infants and Children*. St Louis, MO: C.V. Mosby.

FURTHER READING

Cross, V.M. (1975). *The Preterm Baby*. London: Churchill Livingstone.

Neligen, G.A., Kolvin, L., Scott, D. McL. and Garside, K. (1976). *Born too Soon and Born too Small*. London: Spac International Medical.

Young, D. and Weller, B.F. (1979). *Baby Surgery*. London: Harvey, Miller & Medcalf.

King, E.M., Wieck, L. and Dyer, M. (1985). *Paediatric Nursing Practice and Techniques*. London: Harper Row.

4 The sick child: home and hospital

The sick child is a member of a family unit. The family is very important to the child until adulthood, providing carers and role models. Over the past 30 years the importance of reducing the periods of separation between children and their significant care-givers has been acknowledged (Bowlby, 1953). A parent or other close member of the family may choose to be resident with the sick child or be present visiting for several hours each day. The carer present will be able to participate in the provision of care given to the child. The degree of participation will depend on the level of sickness of the child and the confidence of the carer.

Parents will need help in coping with the stressful situation of seeing their child sick or suffering pain. They may also be unfamiliar with hospital routine and even simple procedures they see carried out may, to them, seem traumatic or repulsive. It is also not easy for a mother, used to being in full charge of her child, to share this care and her authority with that of a nurse who to both of them is a stranger and who may, inadvertently, make the mother feel inadequate or embarrassed in the hospital surrounding. Fear of the outcome of an operation may change the parents' manner temporarily. They may withdraw or alternatively become very demanding. On the other hand, nurses may feel observed and criticized by experienced mothers and either avoid them and their children, or become officious and aggressive.

All these emotions add greatly to the stresses of caring for sick children but if understood, make paediatric nursing all the more challenging and interesting.

Nurses caring for children for the first time may well be puzzled by the problems arising from their behaviour. They will understand them far better if they consider them in relation to the child's family and social background. Children, in the same way as adults, are the product of their country, their district, their educational and social environment, and their daily pursuits and contacts. The younger the child, the more dependent he will be on his mother or his mother substitute. It is important to realize that in some families a childminder or nanny means as much to the young child as his mother, and that she often looks after him during the mother's absence at work. This should never be forgotten when offering residential facilities to be with the child in hospital. In addition, the pre-school child is defenceless and immature both in body and mind. He cannot express himself clearly. He has not yet learned to be adaptable and to make easy social contacts, and he misses his usual routine, his diet, familiar streets and familiar faces.

His emotional development is still immature and he lives in the present, incapable of understanding a to-morrow. He has a lively imagination and readily interprets what he sees and hears into frightening fantasies. Although language comprehension may not yet be fully developed the child is very sensitive to the tone of people's voices, to their gestures and to the expressions on their faces and may read fearful and alarming things into them (MacNamara, 1977). Doctors and nurses should always bear this in mind when talking about a child to others in a ward or outpatient department whilst the child is nearby.

ADOLESCENCE

The adolescent is in a period of physical and emotional transition—moving from the child to the adult (see p. 17). This usually occurs between about 10 and 20 years of age and is associated with the process of individual identity change (Marcia, 1982). On the one hand, the teenager is seeking independence from parents and those in authority, and on the other continues to need guidance, support and acceptance. It is a time when peer group values are most important. Belonging to 'a crowd' and sharing in the group's identity, e.g. in dress, hair styles, language, behaviour, etc., enables the teenager to be self-assertive whilst rejecting parental values. At this time any health problem that differentiates the young person from his peers is considered as a major tragedy, although these fears may not be expressed overtly.

Physical growth and sexual development occur so rapidly during adolescence that young people often have difficulty in adjusting to their new body image. Physical examinations, treatments and maintaining hygiene can all provoke embarrassment for the teenager; illness and surgical interventions can further increase anxiety regarding normality.

Friends from school/club/college should be encouraged to visit and join in any social activities. A record/cassette player should be provided (headphones may be necessary in view of the 'noise' of some modern 'pop' music). Whenever possible, snacks and drinks should be provided as a social activity for the adolescent and his friends, particularly if the adolescent is in hospital for some time. Opportunities, too, for hobbies to be pursued should be considered.

Some scheduling of visiting may be needed in order to avoid conflict of the young person's interests and of situations which may create stress and unnecessary anxiety, e.g. too many visitors at the same time. Care should be taken to keep parents informed about their child's treatment and progress.

Acceptance by the nursing staff of the young person's interests/clothes/appearance is important, although overt approval need not be given. Cigarette smoking may cause some conflict for the nursing staff in view of its health hazard. However, particularly if the young person has been smoking for some time, hospital is not the best place to forbid it. It would be better to provide set smoking times in private, and when the opportunities arise set a good example by refusing to smoke and also discussing with the adolescent the problems associated with smoking as a matter of health education.

Summary

1. Independence should be fostered by encouraging the young person to participate in the decision-making process regarding health care needs.

2. Health promotion and education—adolescents as a group are eager to learn about themselves (Whaley and Wong, 1987) and opportunities should be provided for discussion of relevant health care issues which may be associated with growth and sexual development. It may also be helpful to provide fact sheets and other health promotion material (Muller *et al.*, 1986).

3. Privacy should be provided, together with the opportunity for social interaction with peers (Weller, 1980). Encourage them to set their own parameters for daily living which do not infringe the rights of others, and ensure that these rules are known and respected by others.

4. Promote continuity of school/college work and of special interests.

THE NURSING PROCESS AND SICK CHILDREN

The Nursing Process is essentially a problem-solving approach to the provision of nursing care. Duberly, a paediatric nurse, has written 'Nursing care is also influenced by the dependence of the patient upon others for his continuing care.' The Nursing Process therefore has a particular relevance to paediatric nursing as it allows for the recognition and integration of the child's dependence, developmental needs and those of his family unit.

The framework of the Nursing Process is classified in four stages:

1. Assessment

This stage of collecting information should review four main areas:

(i) *Child*—presentation of physical, psychological and developmental state; knowledge about illness/reasons for admission and previous hospital experience; language and use of family expressions.

(ii) *Family care*—usual routines and who does what when; alterations due to illness.

(iii) *Family*—structure; understanding of child's illness/ admission; if parents wish to be resident and/or participate in giving care; support and instruction needs.

(iv) *Reason for admission*—medical instructions or medications.

Part of the assessment will be to identify the desire, willingness and ability of parents, or other care-giver, to participate in the provision of care for the child.

2. Planning

Using the information obtained during the assessment, goals of nursing care should be formulated into a nursing care plan. The care plan should be developed with the help of the child's main care-giver(s). Care that can be safely delivered by this carer should be clearly identified to enable a participating role to be established and responsibilities to be clearly evident. The teaching of carers should also be included in the plan.

3. Implementation

Continual support and assistance to the child and family will be required during the giving of nursing care. Participating care-givers will become increasingly more confident. Any instruction given should be stated on the nursing care plan with the expectation of the role and responsibility involved.

4. Evaluation

The assessment of change and the effectiveness of care should be done in partnership with parents or other care-giver. There will be the need to continually re-assess the child and family's coping and stress, identifying the need for further teaching and support.

PAEDIATRIC NURSING MODELS

Attempts have been made to adapt published nursing models to meet the needs of sick children. Most of the nursing models have been developed for use in adult nursing and do not address the full range of needs presented by the sick child. The role and responsibility of a participant care-giver other than the self-carer or the nurse is not really considered in the models available and is of importance to the sick child. The Roper model (1980) based on the psycho-social-physical 'needs' of the individual is widely used but does not include parental involvement in the provision of the care. The Orem model can be adapted for use with children (Cheetham, 1988).

At the Hospital for Sick Children, London, an attempt has been made to define the concepts which form the essential parts of nursing sick children and then by identifying the relationship between them, have produced a 'partnership in care model' (Casey, 1988). The child is recognized as a developing individual moving along a spectrum from almost total dependence of the infant to independence of the adult. For the child to reach his full potential he needs to be healthy and well cared for. It is recognized it is the child's family who assist in meeting these needs and mediate between the child and the environment. The model of care identifies those aspects of care which can continue to be safely provided for by the family, those which the family may give with supervision, and those which require the skills of the paediatric nurse. The boundaries between these aspects of care will differ for each child depending on the level of illness, complexity of care and the confidence of the family participant. The model of care is therefore formed out of a relationship between child, family and nurse (see Fig. 10).

For many years parents have carried out aspects of care with which they are familiar whilst a child is in hospital, washing and feeding being two common areas. Webb (1985) identified that parents were more keen to participate than nursing staff considered them capable of. Participating in a child's care should be discussed with the family when the child is admitted to enable the family to function at their best. It is important that where a parent has been instructed in carrying out a procedure, however small, there should be recorded evidence of what has been taught. The nurse then makes an assessment based on

PLANNING

During the planning of care, the following areas should be discussed and recorded:

1. When family care will be carried out and by whom;

2. Goals of nursing care and methods of evaluation;

3. Plan for parent/child teaching;

4. Who will carry out nursing care and when.

ASSESSMENT

The assessment profile should review:

1. CHILD—presentation (physical, developmental, psychological status); previous hospital experience; knowledge about illness/ reasons for admission.

2. FAMILY CARE—who does what and when; usual routines; alterations to these due to illness/admission.

3. FAMILY—structure; understanding of child's condition/reasons for admission; if parent(s) wish to be resident and participate in 'family' or 'nursing' care.

4. REASON FOR ADMISSION—medical instructions which affect nursing care.

And also identify: child and family's learning and support needs; problems requiring nursing care; need for referral to other team members.

IMPLEMENT-ATION

During this stage of the process, the following should occur:

1. Continual support and assistance to the child/family whilst they are performing care;

2. Perform family/nursing care as agreed with the child and family;

3. Carry out teaching programmes as planned. Refer to and consult with other members of the team as planned.

EVALUATION

During this phase the nurse should:

1. Continuously re-assess the child and family's coping—further need for teaching and support;

2. Identify and record the outcomes and plan changes with the child and family.

FIG. 10 The partnership model and the nursing process. The nursing model dictates the way the nursing process is carried out. It provides the background knowledge about the nature of the child, the family and nursing to guide nursing practice. Reproduced by kind permission of Ann Casey.

professional judgement whether the parent or child is able to carry out the care safely. The ward requires to develop a policy concerning the teaching of family care-givers, and for the accountability for the care given.

The partnership model identifies the care which the child normally gives himself, the care carried out by the family and the extra care required due to the health problem. The process of nursing then organizes these aspects of care into a plan to deliver the care, identifying who is responsible for each part.

For some parents being able to participate in the nursing care of their child will reduce tension and give great pleasure even when the child is very sick. Parents may be able to develop and undertake some very complex nursing skills with the appropriate support and supervision. It must be recognized that for other parents the emotional involvement may make this approach too demanding even to participate in seemingly simple aspect of the child's care.

PRIMARY NURSING

The partnership in care model lends itself to 'primary nursing'. The 'primary nurse' assesses the needs of the child, identifying, in consultation with the family, the most appropriate care-giver for satisfactorily meeting the needs of the sick child, whether child, family or nurse. When assessing the daily needs of the child the primary nurse will take into consideration the changes taking place in both the child and the family. The revised daily nursing care plan will reflect those changes, allowing child and parent to participate in the provision of care which the child's condition, together with the parent's presence, confidence, ability and desire allow.

The primary nurse will build a relationship with the

TABLE 4 Example of a nursing care plan

Victoria Fisher   Age 3 years

Date	Nursing problem	Objective	Nursing action and its rationale	Care by Child/Family/Nurse	Signature
3/8/90	Hot, flushed and pyrexial (temperature 38.8°C)	To relieve fever and promote comfort	Cool bathing and frequent changes of clothing Frequent cool drinks Monitor temperature 4-hourly	Mother will sponge as needed. Will give and record drinks Mother doesn't feel confident to monitor temperature along—needs further instruction and support	
	Runny, sore nose	To promote healing of skin around nose	Apply cream to skin. Provide soft tissues to mop nasal discharge	Mother will do this as needed. Knows how to dispose of soiled tissues	
	Mucosy cough	To encourage expectoration to clear chest	Continue with tipping and tapping of chest as agreed with physiotherapist	Taught by physiotherapist. Mother will give physiotherapy at 2.00 p.m.	
4/8/90	Anorexic and lethargic	To promote appetite and return of energy	Provide small helpings of favourite foods: tomato soup baked beans crisps chips ice cream	Mother will give	
			Encourage play activities which will stimulate and encourage social interaction	Play worker has discussed with parents suitable toys and ideas	

family who visit and share their anxieties. This will allow the correct level of appropriate support to be provided.

PREPARATION FOR A HOSPITAL STAY

Sometimes the sick child at home will need to be admitted to hospital and the nurse's advice will often be sought by the parents as to how their child should be prepared for this stay. Children should be told about hospitals, doctors and nurses from an early age, just as they are prepared for other experiences in life such as going to school (Hales-Tooke, 1973). Rodin (1983) stated that children prepared in any way cope better than children who are not prepared at all.

For the emergency admission it may be too late for detailed preparation, but the nurse will remember the child's need for comfort and security and that all questions should be answered honestly and directly without giving more detail than the child can understand.

For the child on the waiting list to be admitted, the time can be usefully spent in preparing for his admission. Some paediatric departments produce their own admission booklets which give helpful details about the ward routine and the facilities available. Often a comic or colouring section is included which helps the child to feel that this is really for him. A further advantage of this type of material for preparation for hospital is that the parents too can be involved, providing that sufficient information is given to them by the medical or nursing staff. There are also several books about hospital written for children that can be bought or borrowed from the local library.

Increasing numbers of children's departments and hospitals organize preparation programmes for those children to be admitted within a short time (Petrillo and Sanger, 1980). Parents and siblings are also invited. Depending upon local circumstances, the preparation programme may take a variety of formats but most essentially should include active participation by the children (not just simply listening) and their parents. Information should be presented using a variety of methods—visual, spoken and written. Puppet shows to tell a story have also been used. A tour of the ward and the opportunity to see various items of hospital furniture and equipment is usually welcomed, especially if the children are given the opportunity to listen with stethoscopes and bounce on beds. A tour of the theatre complex may also be included where parents can ascertain their role in the anaesthetic room (Glasper, 1988).

Accurate information is an important factor in reducing stress for children admitted to hospital (Muller *et al.*, 1988). Written information should be provided for the parents to take home at the end of the programme as a reference or to serve as a reinforcement of the information given.

The Hospital Stay

The hospital experience may be deeply disturbing to children. To many of them being put to bed in the daytime implies punishment. This should be considered, particularly with children admitted from a waiting list or merely for investigations. They do not feel ill and to put them to bed on admission can only add insult to injury.

Nurses' uniform

The newly admitted child may never have seen people dressed in nurses' uniform and to some, hospital doctors and nurses have in the past been used as threats. It frequently happens that children are drawn to the ward domestic staff, presumably because they wear less unfamiliar clothes and, in the case of a local hospital, talk the dialect to which the child is used.

As part of a policy to create a more attractive, less clinical environment, on some paediatric wards the nurse is provided with a colourful attractive tabard or apron over her uniform.

Routine

Children are very dependent on a familiar routine, and no other person can imitate precisely the way in which the mother would set about the daily toilet or the dressing and undressing routine. This may lead to distress as well as protest. Children are readily labelled as having food fads. But the child is used to certain foods, cooked and served in the way favoured by his mother at home. Family menus are very repetitive and only rarely will hospital diet be anything like the meals to which the child has been used.

Using a pot may be a worrying experience to a child who at home is used to going to the lavatory, but it is necessary for collection of urine and stool specimens. Occasionally children fail to use the pot when given one, only to wet or soil themselves a few moments after it has been taken away. This should be treated with understanding. It is often helpful to place the pot on the floor where it is easier to balance than in bed, and where the child may feel more secure.

Visiting

Where neither a parent is able to be resident unrestricted visiting can make separation of mother and child more bearable. Some parents are reluctant to visit because they think their child will cry when they have to leave. The nurse can explain to them that this is only to be expected, and that it is quite natural and far less harmful for the child that he should cry and be comforted than to feel abandoned because the parents do not visit.

Unrestricted visiting means that parents are welcomed to be with their child at any time. This allows parents to be there at times when the child particularly needs them, e.g. at bedtime, and participate in the care. It also means that the non-resident parent can choose to stay all day or to pop in and out according to their family needs.

Contact with home
Occasionally children cannot be visited, perhaps because they have come from a considerable distance. Arrangements should be made to keep up contact with home in every possible way. Examples of this are: daily postcards or parcels from home; telephone calls between mother and child; photographs of members of the family to be kept on the child's locker; school and evening prayers. Any such link with home will make the stay in hospital less traumatic.

Play
Play is a fundamental part of every child's inheritance through which he develops physically, emotionally and intellectually. It is through play that the child explores his environment, communicates and learns; there is no dividing line between work and play. Toys are the tools of play. Throughout childhood the child plays, at first through contact with his mother, then on his own and later with other children of his own age. Play is a natural activity which allows the child to learn about the things about him. It is also an activity in which the child has control and make decisions about (Poster, 1983). With play, the child expresses his feelings and fantasies and thereby learns to cope with the reality of everyday life.

Play has these same values for the sick child and the

need increases with being in hospital away from his home and family. Bolig (1984) concluded that there appear to be four main functions to planned hospital play:

1. To provide diversion, that is some kind of simple occupation to take the child's mind off what is going on about him.
2. 'Playing out' problems and anxieties.
3. Restoring normal aspects of life.
4. Aids understanding so that through play a child can become more aware of hospital events and communicate fears.

During illness the child regresses, becoming emotionally a little younger than his normal self, only able to concentrate for short periods and will play happily with easier toys than usual.

Often parents will ask for some guidance about suitable toys to buy as gifts. The nurse can remind them of their 'odds and ends' at home, the button box, the box of old keys, magazines, the rag bag, all of which will provide a link with home and are of occupational value. Other ideas that are inexpensive include providing a special companion for the sick child with a hand puppet or rag doll, which not only provides friendship but enables the child to use the toy in dramatizing his situation. Toys that are too complicated or too involved should be avoided. Instead there should be things provided for the child to do, as well as visual stimulation, e.g. mobiles to hang on extension frames, snowstorm pictures or a felt board and scraps to make adjustable pictures. Children also need facilities for play apart from toys, e.g. a firm surface such as a bed table or tray, a 'play wall' for pinning up pictures, 'pop star' posters or drawings. Play containers for holding a child's precious toys may be a basket, box or bag, and for some children 'play arms' are useful, such as the aids used by the elderly to pick up objects from the floor or bed. Mirrors can be used to reflect activities in the ward and elastic bands to project paper messages or pellets to companions. If the ward has a play area the child should always be taken there, providing that his condition allows it, for set periods each day.

An increasing number of children's units now have playgroups with qualified playleaders as part of the ward team. Hospital play specialists are trained to provide suitable play equipment and activities for all ages of child confined to bed, wheelchair, or up and about, with a wide range of disabilities and disorders. The nurse needs to work closely with the playleader, who should receive regular ward reports of each child's progress in order to ensure that individual needs are met.

For those working in wards where there is not a playleader, the nurse should attempt to provide as much organized play as possible, involving parents and volunteers. The following guidelines will provide a general framework for the nurse to use:

1. Supply materials which stimulate play and allow expression.
2. Playtime should be given priority in the ward routine and should be without interruption.
3. Allow the child to play at his own pace.
4. Play for and with the child who cannot play for himself.
5. Relate play to knowledge of each child's development.

The equipment provided should include simple creative craft materials, puppets, books, building bricks, both board and card games as well as facilities for playing with sand, water, clay or dough. Children in hospital enjoy playing with ordinary household items and also hospital

FIG. 11 Children playing in the ward setting.

equipment such as stethoscopes, syringes (without needles), bandages and tubing, which allow them to act out their feelings about hospitalizaton. Wearing nurse's caps and face masks in bed as well as other dressing-up gear can be great fun for the child as well as being therapeutic, as an ill child who is happily occupied is likely to get well far more quickly than one who is not.

Giving medicines

The keynote to the administration of medications should always be a matter-of-fact attitude on the part of the nurse giving the medicine. Avoid evaluative statements such as 'this medicine has a nasty smell'—to approach a child with an attitude of apology and a look of disgust is likely to court disaster. The child will feel that he is expected to dislike the taste and to make a fuss. Utilize the power of positive suggestion by saying 'I am going to give you some

TABLE 5   Benefits of planned play programmes in hospital. (From Sweet, 1988.)

1. Children can pursue activities to continue normal growth and development.

2. The strangeness of the environment can be reduced through familiar toys and activities (particularly so in an emergency).

3. Concerns, confusions and fear can be expressed unsuspectingly through role-play and puppets; problems can therefore be dealt with (important for all health care encounters).

4. Incidents and injuries can be reduced (because of safe outlets for energies, and supervision).

5. Waiting time does not seem as long to children when they are playing (especially important in clinics).

6. Children can have some satisfaction in doing something themselves, instead of always having things done to them.

7. Play can provide opportunities for meeting other children; children tend to give each other a great deal of companionship and support.

8. Children can prepare themselves for treatments or procedures by 'practising' through play.

9. Parents tend to feel more comfortable and less anxious when they see their children playing; parents can learn from observing their children at play.

10. Children playing can provide medical staff with opportunities to observe their normal behaviour when they are doing familiar things and not frightened; such observations might aid diagnosis and/or treatment approaches.

11. Play can be an antidote for both boredom and pain.

12. Children can do things that will foster their physical health and recovery, without realizing what they are doing, for example, blowing bubbles after cardiac surgery is fun, or riding a tricycle in a hospital playground does not seem like physiotherapy.

medicine to take your hurt away' (Whaley and Wong, 1987).

Medicines for children should be camouflaged to make them palatable. This is often done in the pharmacy where brightly coloured syrups of various kinds are available. Medicines are usually taken better in solution than in tablet form. Both should be placed as far back on the tongue as possible and followed by a favourite drink. Sometimes it is necessary to mix a drug with a drink or some semi-solid food such as a mashed banana or jam, but even if this is done, the child should be told that the medicine is there. In these cases it is important that the food chosen is not an essential one, in case the child becomes permanently suspicious of its taste. Pre-operative drugs are often bitter. If they have to be camouflaged, syrup or honey are best, as they are quickly digested and the danger of vomiting and inhalation during anaesthesia does not arise.

Some children co-operate best if they are allowed to take the medicine from a coloured spoon, through a straw or polythene tube or from a doll's tea set. The nurse should be adaptable and use her imagination to the full.

On the occasions where there is difficulty every effort should be made to determine why the child is uncooperative and an appropriate remedy sought. If despite explanation and encouragement mild physical coercion is needed, this should be carried out quickly and carefully. It is best to take the child out of his cot and sit him on the lap safely wrapped in a small blanket. The nurse may have to shape his mouth with one hand and pour the medicine in, but it should be remembered that this method is not without danger as a screaming, struggling child may well inhale some of the medicine thus forced into his mouth. Some medicines are best given by placing the spoon at the back of the tongue and letting the medicine go down by gravity. At all times, care must be taken to see that the whole dose is taken and that none is spat out or allowed to run down the chin or bib.

The effect of the drug given should be watched and recorded carefully and signs of intolerance recorded and reported at once (UKCC Administration of Medicines, 1986). Punctuality in the giving is essential, as in many cases the efficacy depends on the concentration reached in the blood and a certain level may have to be maintained throughout the 24 hours. Children also get used to a certain routine and co-operate more readily if the medicine times follow a familiar pattern.

Dosage of drugs. Children's tolerance of drugs differs from that of adults; large dosages are often well tolerated. The dosage of drugs is often based on the child's body weight. Accurate weight charts and the checking of weights by a qualified nurse are consequently important.

Body weight formula for calculating paediatric drug dosage:

$$\frac{\text{Child's weight (kg)}}{70} \times \text{adult dose}$$

$$\frac{\text{Child's weight (lb)}}{150} \times \text{adult dose}$$

Children require a higher dose per kilogram body weight than adults, since they have a higher metabolic rate.

Body surface measurements are more accurate for calculation of paediatric doses.

The following formulae are used to estimate the paediatric dosage based on the child's body surface area.

1. $\dfrac{\text{Surface area of child (m}^2)}{1.75} \times \text{adult dose} = \text{child dose}$

2. $\dfrac{\text{Surface area of child}}{\text{Surface area of adult}} \times$ dose of adult

$\qquad\qquad\qquad\qquad$ = approximate child dose

3. Surface area (m^2) $\times$ dose/m^2 = approximate child dose

Resuscitation

Complete apnoea requires prompt and effective action to prevent cardiac arrest.

In this situation one nurse will usually begin resuscitation of the child, while another calls for medical aid and fetches the resuscitation box or trolley. If the nurse is alone with the child perform cardiopulmonary resuscitation for one minute before calling for help. As the emergency procedure varies from hospital to hospital, all nurses must acquaint themselves with the set procedure within their own hospital. As with the adult patient, success depends on team work. The aim of emergency resuscitation is the restoration of an effective circulation of oxygenated blood by means of artificial ventilation and external cardiac massage. Speed is essential to ensure survival of the brain cells which can only survive undamaged without oxygen for approximately 3 min. Neurologically intact survival has been only in those children who receive immediate resuscitation and respond quickly (Torphy *et al.*, 1984).

Artificial ventilation. The first essential is to establish and maintain a clear airway by hyperextending the head and pulling the chin forward, as obstruction will prevent adequate ventilation. A quick check should be made that vomit is not present in the mouth, by placing a finger in the mouth. If the child has vomited, the vomit should be allowed to drain away by tilting the head and chest downwards.

Mouth to mouth breathing must be started if a re-breathing bag (e.g. Ambu type) is not available. The nurse, using her own lungs as a positive respirator, can ventilate the patient's lungs. If the child is small enough the nurse places her mouth over both the patient's nose and mouth. In the older child she places her mouth over the patient's mouth and pinches the nose. She blows until the patient's chest is seen to expand; she then releases her mouth from the patient while expiration takes place. This procedure is repeated 16–18 times/min.

External cardiac massage. The nurse places the heel of one hand over the lower half of the sternum, the other hand is placed on top of it (see Fig. 12). In infants this technique may be modified by placing one hand behind the infant's chest in order to give a firm base. Keeping the arms straight the nurse will depress the sternum approximately 2.5 cm (1 in.) with a firm rocking movement 70–90 times/min. This action compresses the heart causing blood contained within to be ejected; when pressure is released, the heart refills.

Ideally external cardiac massage and artificial ventilation should be combined. However, if only one nurse is available three or four good ventilations of the lungs should be performed initially, followed by one respiratory ventilation and six cardiac compressions.

Once medical aid arrives, cardiac massage and ventilation will be taken over by the resuscitation team. If possible the head of the bed or cot will be removed to allow free access and a fracture board placed underneath the mattress. An intravenous infusion will also be set up to enable the following drugs to be given.

Sodium bicarbonate 8.4% to counteract metabolic acidosis, calcium gluconate 2%, adrenaline 1:10000.

Isoprenaline (vasopressor) to sustain the blood pressure.

Infant

Young child

Older child/adolescent

FIG. 12 Cardiopulmonary resuscitation (CPR) in children. In the young child, the heel of the hand is placed over the lower sternum. In older children and adolescents, both hands are used.

Effective resuscitation produces a palpable pulse in the carotid and femoral arteries. A pink colour returns to the face and spontaneous respiration and consciousness will return.

Safety measures in hospital

Restrainers and cot sides. In hospital special precautions have to be taken for the child's safety. This is not only for the child's sake, but also because the health authority can be held responsible for any accident.

Cot sides. These should never be left down, not only to stop a child falling out, but also to prevent an active toddler from climbing back in and falling out later. When making the bed of a young child he is best lifted out or else a nurse should be on either side of the cot while the sides are down, or only one side let down at a time. A toddler can roll over with amazing rapidity and fall out on the far side. Bed trays left in position invite the child to climb on to them and make an otherwise adequate cot side low enough for him to fall over. The vertical bars on cot sides should be no more than 8 cm (3 in.) apart.

Restrainers. The use of restrainers for children at whatever time of the day or night should seldom be necessary and they should only be applied when there is no other method of managing the child while he is undergoing some form of investigation or treatment, or occasionally as a protective measure to prevent the child from injuring himself. The presence of a parent often helps eliminate the need for restrainers but it is very important to ensure that the parent does not leave without the staff knowing. Restrainers should never be used routinely and should only be used as the result of a deliberate decision of the primary nurse and of the consultant or member of the medical staff to whom he has delegated this responsibility. If used, restrainers should be put on with the child's co-operation as part of the process of being dressed. When put on for the first time, the mother may be asked to be present and the cooperation of both mother and child enlisted. The right approach will allay feelings of anger and frustration and will avoid psychological trauma to the young patient. Improvised restrainers must never be used (e.g. a harness made from bandages).

Sometimes it is necessary to prevent children from touching their mouth or face as, for instance, after operation for cleft lip or strabismus. Simple splints can be made from a piece of foam latex rolled round the arm, alternatively a roll of corrugated cardboard can be used. These restrainers are known as elbow splints and are applied with light, open-woven bandages. The bandage should first be carried round the child's arm, preferably over a sleeve, and then the well-padded splint is incorporated in the following turns of the bandage. It this is not done, bandage and splint are liable to slip off like a cylinder. For wrists and ankles special restrainers can be made. Alternatively a crêpe bandage tied with a clove hitch may be used. Tubular gauze is another simple alternative. Infants are sometimes wrapped firmly in a blanket to avoid movement during procedures such as subdural tap or taking of venous blood (Fig. 13). Whatever restraint is used, it must be released at least at 4-hourly intervals to allow free movement under supervision.

Prevention of accidents in hospital
Whenever possible children should be allowed to be up and about, rather than kept in bed. This places an extra burden of responsibility on the hospital staff.

The child who presents the greatest problem is the

toddler. No equipment left standing about is safe from their urge for adventure. They enjoy opening and closing doors, and easily get their fingers caught. Any unguarded electrical point lends itself to investigation, and milk and other drinks are upset for the mere fun of it.

Children's wards should be as homely as possible and untidiness will be accepted by the nursing staff. But danger should be anticipated and accidents prevented by wise precautions.

FIG. 13 Restraining the patient.

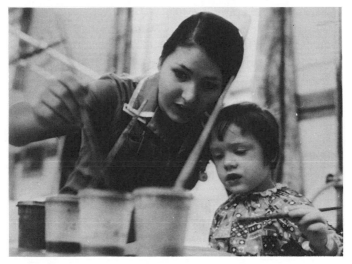

FIG. 14 Painting whilst confined to bed can be fun and absorbing for the young patient.

Very young children should never be allowed out of sight, and objects which may cause accidents should be removed or suitably guarded. Children should never be left unaccompanied in the bathroom and neither bathrooms nor lavatories should have bolts or keys. Drinking glasses and sharp feeding utensils are unsuitable for the very young. Drinks should be just the right temperature, for a toddler will not wait to test a drink set before him but will eagerly immerse his entire face in a cup. Infants under a year should never be given a soft pillow and are usually best left without any pillows at all. If pillows have to be used they should be small, firm ones or the mattress should be raised by placing a pillow underneath it.

Electrical equipment should never be used unless a nurse can remain with the child for the entire time or it can be kept out of the child's reach. Toys should be chosen for their safety, and sharp, protruding corners or wires removed. *Mechanical toys which give off sparks are as dangerous in an oxygen tent as the striking of a match*, and watch must be kept on the type of toy given to children nursed in a tent.

Before taking a rectal temperature the bulb of the thermometer should be inspected and the nurse should keep a firm, restraining hand on the child to avoid sudden movement. Safety pins should be used only where absolutely necessary and should always be left closed when not in use. In many instances a piece of strapping or a tape can replace safety pins very satisfactorily. Finally, two nurses must always be present when injections are given, as even an apparently reliable 10-year-old may suddenly lose control of himself and move, or grasp a nurse's hand, thus breaking the needle.

Any accident should be reported at once and all details recorded. The parents should be told about it when they next visit, even if the accident was a trivial one.

Care by Parent Schemes

North America pioneered the concept of 'Care by Parents Units' in the late 1960s and early 1970s. The movement was inspired partly by the feeling that families were the proper people to look after their own sick children and partly by the need to cut the escalating charges of American hospitals which included high nurse staffing costs (Cleary *et al.*, 1986). Only few 'Care by Parent' units have since been established in the United Kingdom. The underlying philosophy of these units is that a paediatric nurse(s) is available for consultation and for parental education but that all nursing tasks are carried out and recorded by the parents. The benefits to child health and family well-being include: reduction in the length of inpatient stay; helping the parents feel more confident at managing their child's condition, a particular benefit for those children who are chronically or terminally ill. The children also suffer less psychological disturbance (Caldwell and Lockhart, 1981).

However, whilst many parents do provide excellent care for their sick children, it needs to be recognized that they may be incapable physically or emotionally of providing all the necessary care (Glasper *et al.*, 1989), either in hospital or at home. Even in those specially structured units, parents frequently feel increased anxiety related to their care-giving responsibilities. Those parents most involved in direct total care may feel increased anxiety over those less involved, and 24-hour care responsibility may be too much for some parents (Monahan and Schkade, 1985), who will need further assistance, relief and support from the nursing team.

SICK CHILDREN AT HOME

Community Paediatric Nursing

Some sick children have in the past been cared for at home by their parents. However, developments in the delivery of nursing care and medical, surgical and technological advances mean that many more sick children with complex health care problems of an acute or long-term nature can now be nursed at home. The care needs of these children have become increasingly sophisticated (Whiting, 1989); children being nursed at home include those discharged from hospital following surgery or inpatient medical care, and also those receiving total parenteral nutrition, those with a tracheostomy, the chronically ill child or one who is terminally ill. The composition of the community paediatric nursing team varies and not all health authorities have a distinct paediatric district nursing service. Essentially the role of the community paediatric district nurse is to facilitate individualized care for the sick child within his own home and family. This is achieved in collaboration with the primary health care team which includes the family general practitioner, practice nurse, health visitor, midwife and other district nurse colleagues. Close liaison with specialist nurse practitioners concerned with the care of children with specific health care problems, e.g. cystic fibrosis, diabetes, pre-term neonates, is maintained.

Wherever it is possible, children should be treated in their own homes under the care of the family doctor, with help from the services of the local authority, the community paediatric nursing team (where available) and attention at the hospital outpatient department if necessary.

Nursing the child at home may tax the parents considerably, particularly if they have more than one child to care for. Few children feel ill enough to want to be quiet and inactive for any length of time. Most will want to do things, see what is going on and demand constant company. The mother's work will probably be much reduced if she brings the sick child into the living-room adjoining the kitchen, where she herself has to spend a good deal of time. Often this also means a ground-floor room with a more interesting view out of the window, a saving in heating and far less expenditure of the mother's energy with fewer journeys up and down stairs.

When the sick child is being cared for at home the mother may require advice for certain situations. The following are very basic to the nurse used to working in the well-equipped children's ward, but will prove helpful to the mother seeking guidance.

When to seek medical advice
When to seek medical advice is a constant worry to parents since general practitioners are particularly busy people. Whenever possible it is best to call him before 10 a.m., and the mother should be able to give a brief description of the illnes. Advice should always be sought the same day for the drowsy, irritable child with a head-ache or earache. Also for the child with any breathing difficulty and for the child of any age with vomiting, pain and diarrhoea, when it is important that the mother should know not to give an aperient. If the child has unexplained bruising or any signs of bleeding the doctor's guidance should be sought. This also applies to the very young child under the age of 6 months whenever he is poorly, refusing feeds or showing any other unusual signs. A child can be very ill without a raised temperature—his health should always be considered in relation to how he looks, any change of behaviour, what he complains of and the appearance of his urine and stools. When a child is ill no observation is too minor to be reported to the doctor, indeed some small symptom noted by the mother will often be most helpful to the doctor in making a diagnosis. Every mother should get to know her family doctor, practice nurse, health visitor as well as the community nursing sisters who are often attached to group practices in order that she can feel able to seek advice whenever worried.

Medicine cabinets
Medicine cabinets should always be kept locked and well out of the child's reach. All tablets should be kept in child-resistant containers. All medications in current family use must be clearly labelled. Once a course of treatment is complete any medicines left over should be flushed away

down the sink, unless the doctor has particularly suggested that they be retained. There are now some medicine cabinets available with in-built lights—these are more expensive but are the safest, so that when medicines have to be given at night (and often in a hurry) the labels can be clearly read.

First-aid boxes
All homes should maintain a first-aid box that can also be taken with the family when they go on holiday. A basic list should include:

Small pair of scissors with rounded ends.
Tweezers for removing splinters.
Safety pins.
Small stock of sterile packed dressings in assorted sizes.
Roller bandages in 1″ and 2″ (2.5 and 5.0 cm) widths.
A triangular bandage.
Small roll of cotton wool.
Small roll of adhesive tape.
Box of adhesive strip dressings.
Jar of Vaseline.
Antihistamine cream for insect bites.
Antiseptic lotion.
Protective cream for minor burns.

Occupational play activities
There is no need to spend a great deal of extra money on toys or books. Here are a few suggestions, inexpensive, and yet perfectly capable of providing many hours of pleasurable play for the child.

Ages 9–18 months. Magazines and comics to tear up, as well as to look at; simple toys that can be taken apart; balloons, teddy-bears or dolls with various rags to dress and undress; simple rattles made from well-sealed tins filled with pieces of wood (this will make just enough noise without deafening the family).

18 months to 3 years. Old Christmas cards and magazines; large beads to string; crayons; hollow blocks and other building-bricks; a small aquarium or a budgerigar. A bird table just outside the window that can easily be seen by the patient; jigsaw puzzles or picture trays, bought or home made; conkers, daisies and other flowers to play with and examine; percussion instruments; radio, video and record players if available with children's music and stories.

3–5 years. Beads and conkers (through which father has made a hole); sewing cards with large, blunt needles and coloured thread; rags and bandages to dress and nurse dolls; a nurse's outfit; a doll's tea or cookery set; glove-puppets (home-made).

Dinkie toys; matchboxes with which to build; simple construction toys; interlocking bricks.

Blunt, round-ended scissors; coloured paper; gummed shapes; a scribbling pad; crayons.

5–8 years. Mother's button box to tidy (have a supply of matchboxes); cut-out dolls; dish-cloth yarn and thick needles for knitting dish-cloths for favourite aunts; loosely woven dish-cloths as a foundation for weaving with coloured wools and bodkin. Cotton-reels with four nails at one end for french knitting, coloured wool and a blunt knitting needle.

A book of trains and engines; old motoring and fishing magazines.

Tracing paper and pencils; a magnet; an old watch; a

kaleidoscope; milk bottle tops to make mosaic patterns, mould or string up into 'mobiles'.

Matchboxes to build with or to cover in coloured paper; paints and colouring books; bits of felt or dyed lint and scissors to cut out shapes and for picture making; Plasticine; letter and number cards; toy money. Small squares of lint stuck to figures cut out of magazines, fluffy side outwards, can be made to adhere to a board covered with lint or felt.

Pipe cleaners and large beads can be made into animals and other figures. A thick notebook can be used to make into a diary (words and drawings).

8–12 years. Scissors and thin paper for cutting out strips of people or animals and doilies by folding the paper before cutting and leaving a small piece of the contour uncut to form the link after unfolding; make-up to experiment with; making masks and puppets.

Marbles; packets of inexpensive stamps, a geographical atlas and a notebook for starting a stamp collection. A mirror to play with reflections of light or sunshine; playing cards; an encyclopaedia; 'hobby' books.

Portable T.V.; pop records/cassettes and a player. Suitable video recordings.

A few points to be remembered

1. Protective sheets may be necessary to prevent undue soiling of the top sheet and blankets.

2. Supply a good steady surface such as a tray.

3. Sick children tire quickly, and toys and occupations will need frequent changing.

4. Big or complex toys tire a child more easily than small, simple toys which can easily be changed.

5. A toy enjoyed today may be boring tomorrow.

6. Needless to say the toys given for the various age

groups will please older or younger children. It is usually possible to ask friends or neighbours for the loan of books, jigsaws or other toys no longer needed by their own children (some will be only too glad to pass them on for good). The same applies to magazines, scraps of material, gramophone records or cassettes and videos.

7. The charm of any of these toys and occupations will fade quickly if all are left lying around all the time. Their value is greatly enhanced and their interest doubled if they are tidied away regularly to be brought out again another time.

8. Toys from children who have had an infectious complaint should, of course, be disinfected or destroyed in due course.

Toy libraries
Advise parents to make contact with the nearest Toy Library by writing to:

Toy Libraries Association,
  Seabrook House,
    Wyllyotts Manor, Darkes Lane,
      Potters Bar,
        Herts. EN6 2HL

A Toy Library provides good quality toys which may be borrowed and taken home. See Appendix 2, p. 437.

PAEDIATRIC PAIN

In the past there has been considerable debate about the ability of infants and young children to feel pain. The main argument put forward for this view related to the immaturity of the nervous system and its ability to transmit sensation. In older children, behavioural signs indicating pain were often thought by health care workers to be due to fear, anxiety, sadness and separation from their parents (Abu-Saad, 1984). In some instances where the child did not complain of pain the assumption was made that they were pain-free and appropriate analgesia withheld.

Pain is an unpleasant sensation, made up of physiological, psychological, social, ethnic and cultural components. In most situations more than one of these factors contribute to the child's pain experience, while staff attitudes to assessment and treatment also affect the child. Fear and anxiety may also contribute towards the pain. For the hospitalized child feared or actual separation from their parents can add to the fear of medical and nursing procedures (Alder, 1990).

Pain may be classified as acute or chronic. Acute pain is characterized by its sudden onset and limited duration. Chronic pain is often considered to be pain that lasts for longer than six months (Escobar, 1985).

The Infant

There is now evidence which indicates that infants do feel pain (Anand and Hickey, 1987) and that the pain response is remembered with disruptive behaviour which may interfere with the infant's feeding patterns and mother/infant interactions (Fitzgerald and McIntosh, 1989). Behavioural and physiological indications that the infant is in pain will include:

Crying for an average of 3 minutes.

Facial expression, grimacing with lowered brows, eyes tightly closed with an angular squarish mouth.

Body movement, rigidity or stiffening of the body followed by thrashing movements. An attempt to withdraw a limb from a heel stab.

Increase in blood pressure, glucose levels and palmar sweating (after 37 weeks gestation) with decreased oxygenation levels.

The Child

The young child has only a limited vocabulary to describe pain and his initial reaction maybe similar to that of the infant. Other behaviours indicating pain include clenching of teeth and lips, rocking the body or rubbing a part, e.g. the ear when there is earache. Temper outbursts too are common with the child becoming restless and overactive, unlike the older child (or adult) who, as a result of cultural influences, may withdraw e.g. in the Anglo-Saxon culture where 'it is sissy for a boy to cry'.

Older children are usually able to indicate where the pain is and to describe and express their pain clearly, using a wide range of words or similes.

The Adolescent

Adolescents may react to the pain experience with considerable composure and self-control. Very often their main concerns are related to their peer group, i.e. 'am I going to be left behind by the trouble this pain is giving me'? and therefore may be reluctant to report any pain unless provided with the opportunity to do so. Adolescents are often able to use pain assessment methods devised for adults.

Pain Asessment and Management

In order for appropriate pain management to be provided some form of pain assessment is needed.

Pain assessment

Pain assessment involves:

1. Observational skills with recording of behavioural and physiological changes. This includes noting the position of the child, e.g. lying quietly with legs drawn up on his abdomen may indicate severe abdominal pain. Changes in sweating, blood pressure, pulse and respiration rates may also indicate pain. However, these physiological changes are short-lived and may also be due to anger, fear and anxiety (Johnson, 1977). These indicators are useful only as part of the total assessment.

2. Questioning of the child and the parents. Using a language that is readily understandable to them can provide important information about the pain and the child's previous experience of pain. Parents know their child and are sensitive to any change in behaviour. Care should be taken to avoid the use of jargon or words which the child may not understand. Most children can describe pain or 'the hurt' if asked the right questions, can point to where it hurts or mark the place on an outline drawing of the body (Eland, 1985).

3. Tools for pain assessment. Several methods have now been developed and can be used with children from the age of three to 15 years (Price, 1990). Local paediatric department policy will indicate the agreed tools to use, but in using any pain assessment scale or measure the nurse needs to be aware of influencing factors that may affect the assessment, e.g. familial, cultural and previous experience of pain and hospitalization. Figure 15 shows examples of pain rating scales.

Pain management

Management of effective pain relief for children may require a number of interventions. These will also include

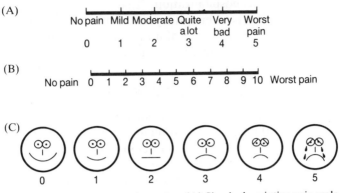

FIG. 15 Different pain rating scales. (A) Simple descriptive pain scale. (B) Numeric pain scale. (C) Faces pain scale.

preparation for the hospital stay, wherever possible. This helps the child to develop coping mechanisms for the experience (Rodin, 1983). Comfort measures such as ensuring that the child's favourite teddy or 'cuddly' is always there, or helping the child assume a comfortable position will be important. Complementary therapy methods that may also be of value include distraction, relaxation, guided imagery and cutaneous stimulation.

Pharmacological interventions. A wide variety of non-narcotic and narcotic analgesics are available. The aim of the administration of any medication should be *the prevention of pain*. Analgesia is most effective when it is administered either prophylactically or when the pain is minimal. It may be more appropriate to administer analgesics to a fixed regime to maintain blood levels, as the use of a 'when required' or 'prn' schedule leaves the decision to the assessment of the nurse. Wherever possible the oral form of the most appropriate drug is used as many children view 'needles' and injections as the most painful part of hospitalization (Eland and Anderson, 1977), although the preparatory use of a local anaesthetic cream, e.g. EMLA, or use of a skin coolant spray, helps to reduce the pain of injections and needle stabs.

CARE OF THE DYING CHILD

The care of children suffering from a terminal illness calls for some of the nurse's finest qualities and there is probably no situation which taxes her emotions more severely, nor any other groups of illnesses which she would more sincerely wish to give of her best, both in the care of the patient and by offering mental and spiritual help and comfort to the parents.

Once the child's condition has been recognized, the parents will want to ask innumerable questions of every person in the hope of getting some understandable information. These will often be repetitious and far seeking, as the parents will be wanting some explanation as to why this should happen to their child. Any information given should be consistent. Parents often sense what will have to be said and some will ask a direct question. An honest answer is the only right one in such a case but at the same time the parents can be assured that everything possible will be done to relieve pain and keep suffering to a minimum.

The child, too, will need to know something of his illness, although a great deal will depend upon his age (Gonda and Ruark, 1984) and understanding. In order to help maintain his trust in the medical and nursing staff it is important that information is not withheld from the child. Children rarely ask outright, 'Am I going to die?' but if the nurse finds herself in this situation she should first ascertain what the child means by dying. Children at different stages of development have different ideas, fantasies and experiences. One way of handling this sort of situation is to convey, gradually with honesty (Dominica, 1989), the idea of the long-term nature of the illness. That it is not an illness or disorder that can be treated straight away and finished with, but it has an up and down course that cannot be measured in a day or a week. This explanation will relieve the child's anxiety and enable him to anticipate and understand when he has bad days.

Children should also be told whenever there are changes in their medication or treatment. Pain should never be denied and the nurse should never say, 'It won't hurt' when it will, or, 'Don't be a cry baby' when an older child has recourse to tears. But, rather, when a child asks 'Will it hurt?' the nurse should say 'It does hurt a bit, but the little hurt will make your bigger hurt go away. I'll be very quick, and it will hurt as little as I can make it.' Whenever possible help the child to keep control, i.e. choosing the site for the injection. Encourage the child to count as the injection or treatment is carried out, 1 . . . 2 . . . 3, which will help the child to settle and to anticipate the end. Praise the child for his bravery at the end of the injection or procedure.

Parents should be with their child as much as they wish, and should be allowed and encouraged to do those things for the child which only a mother or father know how to do.

Children with malignant or terminal illnesses often develop curious fancies, one typical one is the desire to have 'A special meal in the middle of the night'. No nurse should be too busy or too rigid in her routine to grant such a request.

No child should be allowed to die alone. Anticipation of impending death is one of the nurse's primary duties and she should always ensure that members of the family are present if they wish to be. When all is over, those nearest to the child should be left alone by the bedside to hold their child if they wish and to say their goodbyes. Wright (1986) has suggested that a main reason for relatives to see the deceased is to 'say goodbye and reaffirm their love'.

Last Offices

With respect for the parent's religious wishes the general procedure of carrying out the last offices essentially differs little from that customary for adults. Dominica (1989) states: 'the choice of clothes is intensely personal. For some it will be a traditional white shroud, for others a jogging suit or jeans, for yet others the clothes worn for First Communion or for parties.'

If the jaw is inclined to drop, 2.5- to 3-cm bandage, still rolled up as supplied, can be used as a prop between chin and sternum and camouflaged by the gown. This is particularly easily done with infants whose necks are short. With young infants the knees may be drawn up, and they should be straightened by bandaging, some cotton wool being placed between the prominences of the knees to avoid marking the skin. The child's hands are placed together with the fingers interlaced, holding a little white flower. If the arms tend to sag, a roll of cotton wool or a rolled-up napkin can be placed underneath the elbows beside the body to support their weight. The face is covered with a square of gauze or an embroidered handkerchief reserved for the purpose. After securing the body in a sheet, a pall is placed over it and it is carried to the mortuary.

Personal belongings or toys are parcelled up in the usual way but occasionally the parents appreciate the suggestion that a beloved toy should be left with the child.

Meeting the Needs of Other Children

Answering the questions of other children in the ward about the sudden disappearance of a patient or the inevitable disturbance caused by a death may not be easy. No two children are likely to react in the same manner, though they will all sense that something unusual has taken place. It is always best to state the truth simply, as for instance 'Johnny was so weak he fell asleep and will not wake up again because God has taken him to heaven'. But the nurse should also add immediately—'this will not happen to you—you are not weak, are you?', or words to that effect. As a rule children will be satisfied with this straightforward, honest statement.

Talking about death with children, particularly with those who are terminally ill, is important. Spinetta (1974) shows that children as young as 6 years can appreciate the seriousness of an illness that they are facing, therefore to avoid any discussion may lead to a loss of trust and isolate them from comfort. Not to talk to them about the death of others hinders their development and curiosity.

It has been found that children know about and understand death early in life. They understand the concept much as in the way adults do, i.e. that dead persons disappear from daily life and that their body is elsewhere —a grave, coffin or cemetery. Usually they see death as an endless sort of sleep and as the end of thought. They also look for the reasons why death occurs: illness, handicap, wishes for death or despair.

Many hospitals have the service of a Chaplain available. Whether normally religious or not, most people find it helpful to talk to him at this time and he or the appropriate religious teacher or pastor should be called if the parents ask for contact to be made. A sympathetic nurse will soon sense what kind of comfort will be of best help to each individual parent. Often the parents have been so preoccupied with their dying child and their impending loss they have, for the time being, hardly given a thought to their other children at home. This is positive comfort and may be very helpful as it reminds the parents that their responsibilities have not come to an end and that there is much purpose left for them in life. In some instances it is possible to remind parents that children probably lack the apprehension and fear an adult may feel and that their passing is thus made a great deal easier for the parents to come to accept.

The parents' wishes as regards religious observances and orthodox rites should be ascertained and the necessary arrangements made in good time. The nurse should be familiar with the practice of other denominations as well as her own, and all children should be christened, confirmed or given the last rites or any other religious observances as may be wished by the child's family.

REFERENCES

Abu-Saad, H. (1984). Assessing children's responses to pain. *Pain* **19**, 163–171.

Alder, S. (1990). Taking children at their word. *Professional Nurse*, May, 398–402.

Anand, K.J.S. and Hickey, P.R. (1987). Pain and its effects in the human neonate and fetus. *New England Journal of Medicine* **317**, 1321–1329.

Bolig, R. (1984). Play in hospital settings. In *Child's Play: Developmental and Applied* (T.D. Yawkey and A.D. Pellegrini, eds). Hillsdale, NJ: Lawrence Erlbaum.

Bowlby, J. (1953). *Maternal Care and Mental Health*. Geneva: World Health Organisation (WHO).

Caldwell, B.S. and Lockhart, L.H. (1981). A care-by-parent unit: its planning, implementation and patient satisfaction. *Children's Health Care* **10**, 4–7.

Casey, A. (1988). A partnership with the child and family. *Senior Nurse* **8**(4), 8–9.

Cheetham, T. (1988). Model of care in the surgical ward. *Senior Nurse* **8**(4), 10–12.

Cleary, J., Gray, O.P., Hall, D.J. *et al.* (1986). Parental involvement in the lives of children in hospital. *Archives of Disease of Childhood* **61**, 779–787.

Crocker, E. (1980). Reactions of children to health care encounters. In *The Hospital Care of Children* (G.C. Robinson and H.F. Clark, eds). New York: Oxford University Press.

Dominica, F. (1989). Care for the dying child and family. In *Care for the Dying Patient and the Family* (J. Robins, ed.), Lippincott Nursing Series. London: Harper and Row.

Eland, J.M. (1985). The child who is hurting. *Seminars in Oncology Nursing* **1**(2), 116–122.

Eland, J.M. and Anderson, J.E. (1977). The experience of pain in children. In *Pain: A Sourcebook for Nurses and other Health Care Professionals* (A.K. Jacox, ed.). Boston: Little, Brown.

Escobar, P.L. (1985). Management of chronic pain. *Nurse Practitioner*, January, 24–32.

Fitzgerald, M. and McIntosh, N. (1989). Pain and analgesia in the newborn. *Archives of Disease in Childhood* **64**, 441–443.

Glasper, A. (1988). Parents in the anaesthetic room: a blessing or curse? *Professional Nurse* **3**, 4.

Glasper, A., Gow, M. and Yerrell, P. (1989). A Family Friend. *Nursing Times* **85**(4), 63–65.

Gonda, T.A. and Ruark, J.E. (1984). *Dying Dignified. The Health Professionals Guide to Care*. Englewood Cliffs, CA: Addison Wesley.

Hales-Tooke, A. (1973). *Children in Hospital: A Parent's View*. London: Priory Press.

Johnson, M. (1977). Assessment of clinical pain. In *Pain: A Sourcebook for Nurses and other Health Care Professionals* (A.K. Jacox, ed.). Boston: Little, Brown.

MacNamara, J. (1977). *From Sign to Language: Language Learning and Thought*. New York: Academic Press.

Marcia, J.E. (1982). Identity in adolescence. In *Handbook of Adolescent Psychology* (J. Anderson, ed.). Chichester: John Wiley.

Monahan, G.H. and Schkade, J.K. (1985). Comparing care by parent and traditional nursing units. *Paediatric Nursing* **11**, 463–648.

Muller, D.J., Harris, P.J. and Wattley, L. (1986). *Nursing*

Children: Psychology, Research and Practice, Lippincott Nursing Series. London: Harper and Row.

Petrillo, M. and Sanger, S. (1980). *Emotional Care of Hospitalized Children: An Environmental Approach*, 2nd edn. Philadelphia: Lippincott.

Poster, E.C. (1983). Stress immunization: techniques to help children cope with hospitalization. *Maternal and Child Nursing Journal* **12**, 119–134.

Price, S. (1990). Pain: its experience, assessment and management in children. *Nursing Times* **86**(9), 42–45.

Rodin, J. (1983). *Will this Hurt?* London: Royal College of Nursing.

Roper, N., Logan, W.W. and Tierney, A.J. (1980). *The Elements of Nursing*. London: Churchill Livingstone.

Spinetta, J.J. (1974). The dying child's awareness of death: a review. *Psychological Bulletin* **81**, 256–260.

Sweet, B.R. (1988). *Mayes' Midwifery: A Textbook for Midwives*. London: Baillière Tindall.

Torphy, D.E., Mutes, M.G. and Thompson, B.M. (1984). Cardiorespiratory arrest and resuscitation in children. *American Journal of Diseases of Childhood* **138**, 1099–1102.

UKCC Administration of Medicines (1986). *Administration of Medicines*. Advisory Paper.

Webb, N. (1985). Care by parents in hospital. *British Medical Journal* **291**, 176–177.

Weller, B.F. (1980). *Helping Sick Children Play*. London: Baillière Tindall.

Whaley, L.F. and Wong, D.L. (1987). *Nursing Care of Infants and Children*, 3rd edn. St Louis, MO: C.V. Mosby.

Whiting, M. (1989). Home truths. *Nursing Times 'Spotlight'* **85**(14), 74–75.

Wright, B. (1986). *Caring in Crisis*. London: Churchill Livingstone.

FURTHER READING

General Nursing Council (1982). *Aspects of Sick Children's Nursing: A Learning Package*, Sections 2 and 3.

Hatch, D. and Sumber, E. (1981). *Neonatal Anaesthesia*. London: Edward Arnold.

Kubler-Ross, E. (1973). *On Death and Dying*. London: Tavistock Publications.

McFarlane of Llandaff, J.K. (1982). *The Practice of Nursing using the Nursing Process*. London: C.V. Mosby.

Robertson, J. (1979). *Young Children in Hospital*. London: Tavistock Publications.

Weller, B.F. (1980). *Helping Sick Children Play*. London: Baillière Tindall.

Whaley, L.F. and Wong, D.L. (1987). *Nursing Care of Infants and Children*, 3rd edn. St Louis, MO: C.V. Mosby.

Part II
Principles of Care

5 The child with respiratory problems

Ear, nose and throat conditions are very common in childhood, and may account for much minor illness and frequent admissions to hospital or visits to the outpatient clinic. Repeated attacks of catarrh, otitis media, obstructed breathing and sinusitis may contribute to poor general development and diminish mental alertness; loss of schooling may affect the child psychologically as well as educationally.

For children prone to ear, nose and throat infections and congestion, there are some simple measures which are well worth trying in an attempt at improving the tendency to recurrent infections. Among these are simple but thorough education in nose blowing and encouragement to breathe through the nose. Occasionally simple practices such as allowing the child to sleep with the head lower than the rest of the body may encourage drainage and parents should realize that plenty of fresh air, particularly during the day, is as a rule more beneficial than keeping the child indoors for fear of his catching cold.

THE COMMON COLD

Owing to an infant's small air passages, a cold in infancy can be a serious illness. Nurses must always remember this and avoid going near babies when they themselves have a cold; they should realize that a day off duty may prove a greater degree of conscientiousness than being on duty while they are a source of danger. If a nurse herself has to use a handkerchief, this must be done away from the baby's cot and should be followed by hand-washing.

Very young babies breathe wholly through the nose and find mouth-breathing difficult. Nasal obstruction may therefore interfere considerably with feeding as sucking is made almost impossible.

Complications which may arise from a common cold in infancy include otitis media, pneumonia and gastro-enteritis.

CHOANAL ATRESIA

Choanal atresia is a congenital abnormality in which the openings at the back of the nose are blocked by plates of tissue. Since the newborn infant cannot adapt to breathing through the mouth, the condition has to be corrected as an urgent surgical measure or the baby will die. As the baby struggles to breathe the lips can be seen to move as in a flutter, a typical sign of this condition. An oral airway is introduced and the obstructing plates pierced by means of a probe. If the condition is unilateral treatment can be delayed until the baby is stronger and the structures involved are less minute. In this case babies should always lie on the affected side to ensure an adequate airway.

CONGENITAL LARYNGEAL STRIDOR

Congenital laryngeal stridor is not a dangerous condition and children usually outgrow it by the age of 1 year or 18 months. Parents, however, are concerned about the noise the child makes on inspiration and about the sucking in of the intercostal spaces. The condition is best observed when the child is crying or when asleep. Congenital abnormalities, such as laryngeal web or papilloma, must be excluded as both are dangerous forms of respiratory obstruction, but in the majority of cases the parents can be reassured and told that no treatment is needed although it may take several months for the condition to disappear.

CROUP

Laryngitis stridulosa, or croup, is an acute laryngeal spasm causing the patient to struggle for breath in a sudden attack of dyspnoea. The condition affects children of 3–5 years. The stridor usually occurs in connection with a cold. In a typical case the child awakens in the middle of the night, apparently struggling for air, sweating profusely and in a state of acute anxiety. The attack may last as long as an hour and is followed by normal sleep. Often the child has no recollection of the episode on waking in the morning although the attacks are very frightening to the parents. A warm drink may be helpful, and late, heavy meals should be avoided.

LARYNGOTRACHEITIS

Laryngotracheitis, inflammation of the larynx and trachea, is probably caused by a virus; *Haemophilus influenzae*, haemolytic streptococci and staphylococci are often isolated but are thought to be secondary bacterial invaders. Children most commonly affected are aged between 6 months and 2 years.

The chief manifestations of the disease are respiratory obstruction and inspiratory stridor caused by inflammation and congestion of the respiratory tract. The whole of the larynx and trachea is coated with thick, viscous secretions so that the air passages are narrowed. Adequate oxygen exchange becomes impossible and this leads to serious respiratory difficulties and general exhaustion.

Although pyrexia is occasionally absent, the temperature is usually 39.4°–40°C (103°–104°F). The child look anxious, grey and collapsed, the pulse rate is rapid and the volume poor. An almost incessant cough adds to the exhaustion and leads to extreme restlessness. Respirations rise to 60 or more per minute as the child struggles for air, and the intercostal spaces and supraclavicular region are drawn in and the stridor increases.

Treatment

Treatment is required urgently. A humidified atmosphere is beneficial as the moisture prevents the secretions from drying.

Occasionally an emergency tracheostomy may have to be performed as a life-saving measure, and fine judgement and careful observation are needed when caring for the patients as sudden deterioration is common. All necessary equipment for tracheostomy should be at hand, including an electric sucker for the extraction of the viscid mucus.

Principles of Care

To procure rest should be one of the prime concerns. Well-positioned pillows; frequently turned, loose, comfortable clothing (sometimes nothing beyond a napkin if the child is being nursed in a tent); sponging of hands and face; frequent, small sips of water or a glucose drink. Soothing stroking of the head by a parent may help to induce rest and so to preserve the strength of the child. The giving of oral fluids may be difficult, but small quantities should be offered if the child is able to take them.

Regular and careful observation of pulse and respirations should be maintained to detect any increasing signs of respiratory obstruction.

Sedatives should be used with caution and are rarely of much value in the acute stages. A course of intravenous benzylpenicillin and gentamycin is usually commenced pending the bacterial results of nose and throat swabs taken on admission. In exceptionally severe infections steroids may be given.

TRACHEOSTOMY

Tracheostomy has to be performed whenever the lumen of the larynx has been so narrowed by disease as to make adequate air entry impossible, or to reduce the 'dead space' within the respiratory tract to increase oxygen exchange.

The trachea is opened by a surgical incision and held open either by dilators or by insertion of a tracheostomy tube. This may happen for several reasons, including:

Congenital abnormalities such as papilloma, laryngeal web or cysts.
Trauma, e.g. oedema following intubation or scalding.
Infections such as diphtheria or laryngotracheitis.
Paralysis, e.g. in anterior poliomyelitis.

Signs of obstruction

Distressed respirations, wheezing inspiratory stridor.
Restlessness.
An anxious expression.
Sucking in of the intercostal spaces, the diaphragm, neck muscle, sternal notch and the lower end of the sternum.
An increasing pulse and respiratory rate.
Cyanosis in most, but not all, cases.

With the above signs in mind it should normally be possible to appreciate the impending need for this life-saving procedure and only rarely is an unprepared tracheostomy required. Occasionally a bronchoscopy is done before the tracheostomy and sometimes an endotracheal tube is also passed.

Principles of Care

The patient is received back into a warm room. At the conclusion of the operation the tube is fastened securely around the neck by means of tapes. The tapes should always be tied with the neck flexed, as in this position the neck is narrowest to prevent the tube slipping out when the head is brought forward. The knot is tied at the side/front of the neck. If white tape is used care must be taken not to confuse with the ties of the child's bib or nightgown: Plastic tubing threaded through the tape or a small pad of polyurethane foam will prevent the tape cutting into the skin.

Nursing action	Explanation
To maintain rest. As a rule best maintained by sitting the patient up, well supported with pillows.	Reduced exertion reduces oxygen consumption.
To maintain a clear airway. The chin should be kept off the opening of the tube by extending the neck. This may be achieved by placing a small pillow or pad under the infant's shoulders to allow the head to fall back slightly.	Infants and small children have very short necks.
Fluffy clothing and blankets should be avoided. Clothing worn should be prevented from covering the tube.	To prevent blockage of the tube and inhalation of wisps of fluffy material.

Nursing action	**Explanation**
Suction is applied through fine sterile catheters at regular intervals and when required.	To remove secretions. Paren⬤ may be taught to assist with suction.
0.5 ml of 0.9% saline solution may be ordered by the surgeon to be instilled into the tube. After insertion the saline is immediately sucked out. Disposable gloves should be used for this procedure.	To help clear secretions.
Administration of oxygen and humidified air. The patient may be nursed in a humidified environment.	To assist in preventing the secretions drying.
Observe for complications. At first the patient will require an individual nurse.	To ensure a patient airway.
Observation of the colour, the quality of the pulse, and respiratory distress with restlessness.	To ensure blood oxygen level is adequately maintained.
Listen for audible vocal noise. The obstruction in the tube should, if possible, be removed by suction. If this fails the tube should be removed and the tracheal dilators inserted.	The tube is obstructed and help should be sent for immediately.
Maintaining hydration and nutrition. Frequently small amounts of fluids should be given orally. A light diet as soon as condition permits. Care should be taken to avoid any fluid entering the tube. If swallowing is difficult a nasogastric may be used.	A tracheostomy ⬤es not interfere with f⬤ing.

sing action	Explanation
estraint. Wrist restrainers or elbow splints may be necessary.	To prevent the child handling the tube.
Communication. Speech is impossible and care should be taken to maintain communication by talking to the patient and providing a means whereby a child can indicate his needs, e.g. paper and pencil, or bell.	The tracheostomy tube bypasses the vocal cords and prevents the use of the voice. Parents should be encouraged to talk to the child.

Tracheostomy performed in acute illness, as in laryngo-tracheitis, can often be allowed to close after only a few days by plugging the tube for experimental periods. In cases of congenital abnormalities or neoplasm it may have to be permanent. Parents and children may learn to manage the tube at home with support of the community nursing services, although respite care may need to be provided, particularly for the children of single parents (Jennings, 1989).

The child with a long-term tracheostomy should be encouraged to make 'sounds' so that he experiences the sound of his own voice. Some children even learn to speak by placing a finger over the tracheostomy.

Removal of tube

After having had a tracheostomy for several days, children re rather apprehensive when the tube is to be removed t is often helpful to give a sedative before attempting do so.

TONSILLITIS

Tonsillitis is frequently caused by the haemolytic streptococcus, is common in children. The patient is ften ill, particu children under school age.

As children are not always capable of describing pai accurately, they may complain of abdominal pain. Vomiting may be present and it is not easy to exclude acute appendicitis. As the neck is frequently held stiffly, the condition may also be mistaken for meningitis. Often mesenteric adenitis develops simultaneously causing general rigidity and confusing diagnosis still further.

The child is generally ill and fractious. The face is flushed, the temperature perhaps as high as 39.4°C (103°F) and headache may cause him to turn away from the light. Saliva may dribble from the mouth or alternatively the lips are parched and cracked.

When any other conditions have been excluded, a throat swab is taken to determine the causative organism and its sensitivity to drugs. Penicillin, given by injection, is the drug most commonly used.

Principles of Care

If admitted to hospital, children suffering from tonsillitis may be isolated from other children for at least 24 hours after commencing treatment. If there is a high temperature the bedclothes should be light and supported by a bed cradle. An electric fan, well out of reach of the child, may be used, and tepid sponging may be carried out with the doctor's permission. Mouth toilet, including mouth washes with a mild antiseptic such as glycothymne or with saline, will help to keep the mouth clean are often

Paracetamol gargles may relieve the pair swallowing given about 20 min before meals to d food in the easier. As the child is likely to refuse encouraged to early stages of the illness, he shonds. Ice cream take frequent drinks of cool, blen other foods soothing and is often taken eaglate in many a refused. Parents will be able t of care.

Paediatric nursing

Antibiotics usually make tonsillitis a short illness and the child is greatly improved after 24 hours.

Special points
If nursed in an open ward, these children should never be placed next to others suffering from acute rheumatism, nephritis or congenital heart disease, as streptococcal infections are serious in patients suffering from these conditions.

TONSILLECTOMY AND ADENOIDECTOMY

Operation for the removal of tonsils and adenoids is among the more common surgical procedures in a children's unit. The removal of diseased tonsils and hypertrophied adenoids improves a child's general health, and other illnesses such as recurrent tonsillitis, otitis media, sinusitis and general development can be improved.

Frequently, tonsillectomy or adenoidectomy is performed on children under the age of 5 years. The presence of the mother during the stay in hospital is particularly beneficial to both child and mother and may be the best means to ensure that there are no psychological after effects.

Pre-operative Nursing Management

Nursing action	Explanation
Temperature, pulse and respiration rate are taken.	To identify any infection that would cause the operation to be postponed.
Long hair is tied back.	To prevent contamination of the operation site.
General preparation for anaesthesia.	Parents encouraged to assist in preparing the child and accompanying the child to the anaesthetic room.

Post-operative Nursing Management

Nursing action

Explanation

Position. Nursed on the side with the upper leg bent and upper arm flexed (tonsillectomy position). A pillow in the back assists in maintaining the position until the patient regains full consciousness.

This position prevents any blood trickling down the throat, ensuring it comes out of the mouth.

Observations. Restlessness and noisy respirations together with regular swallowing movements are indications of bleeding. If these symptoms go unnoticed the pulse rate rises and the pulse becomes weaker.

The complication of bleeding post-operatively is due to the highly vascular operation site. Serious haemorrhage necessitates a return to theatre.

Fresh blood in vomit may be an indication of bleeding.

The temperature is taken 4-hourly in the axilla.

The early signs of infection require identification. Mouth breathing post-operatively makes oral temperature recording unreliable.

Relief of pain. Observe for pain (p. 113). Analgesia is usually needed regularly during the first 12 hours. Paracetamol gargles before meals, will ease throat pain during the first few days.

Reduces the incidence of shock, restlessness and haemorrhage. Prevents stiffness of the throat, allowing movement and thus preventing infection.

Maintaining hydration and nutrition. Cool drinks of fruit juice and water should be encouraged in the first 12 hours. A normal diet may be given during the first few days.

Parents will encourage the child to take frequent drinks. Drinking prevents the throat from becoming stiff and painful.

Nursing action

Mobility. The child may be sat up after 12 hours, providing observations remain stable, and the hands and face are sponged.

After 24 hours the child should be gradually mobilized.

Discharge. The child may be discharged home after 1–3 days, providing the temperature is normal. The convalescence continues at home avoiding infection and crowded places.

Explanation

Parents will help keep the child amused and assist in sponging child.

DEAFNESS

Deafness in childhood may be temporary or permanent. Permanent deafness may be congenital nerve deafness caused, e.g. by an attack of rubella in the mother during the first 12 weeks of pregnancy or the result of meningitis. Cerebral palsy sufferers often also have an associated nerve deafness.

Among the acquired causes are repeated attacks of otitis media and perforation of the ear drum with subsequent scarring and adhesions. Transitory deafness may be caused by an accumulation of wax, a foreign body in the meatus, meatal boils and blocking of the Eustachian tube due to a cold, sinusitis or adenoids.

Total deafness is rare. Once any doubt about a child's hearing has arisen, no time must be lost in seeking expert advice—a 'wait and see' attitude may prejudice the entire future of the child. Tests to assess the degree of deafness can now be carried out on very young babies at special audiology centres staffed by specialists. Once the deafness has been confirmed a training and stimulation programme can be planned with the child's parents who will have a great part to play in developing any potential of hearing, speech and intelligence. They should therefore be encouraged to participate in the training from the start. Deaf children should be allowed to mix with those with normal hearing, and education will take place within ordinary schools, with special classes for the benefit of the deaf child.

OTITIS MEDIA

Otitis media is inflammation of the middle ear. In young children the structures of the ear, nose and throat are particularly closely related to one another, and their smallness easily accounts for frequent congestion and blocking and for the spread of infection. Otitis media is common as a secondary infection following a common cold or tonsillitis.

In babies, the short, straight and rather wide Eustachian tube may even become obstructed by vomit. Special care should be taken where possible to nurse the 'vomiting' infant in an upright position.

Signs and Symptoms

The onset of otitis media may be insidious and the first signs may be that the young child rolls his head on the pillow, pulls his ear and is abnormally irritable. Pain soon becomes severe and the temperature rises as high as 39.4°C (103°F). The child resents being touched and looks toxic.

Treatment

Antibiotics are usually prescribed. A careful explanation will need to be given to the parents to ensure that the full course of antibiotics is completed as often the child's symptoms improve within 2–3 days. On completion of treatment the child's condition should be reassessed to ensure that the infection is completely resolved.

Pain relief
The application of gentle heat, e.g. a warm compress, may help to alleviate pain and promote comfort. Analgesia is often needed, particularly at night.

Prevention of middle ear infection
To prevent middle ear infection parents should be taught always to feed their infant in the upright position in order to prevent inhalation into the Eustachian tube during swallowing.

Children should also be taught at early age whenever they have a 'cold' or upper respiratory tract infection to blow their noses properly, and not to hold one nostril closed whilst blowing (Foster *et al.*, 1989).

Grommet tubes
Tiny drainage tubes called Grommet tubes are placed in the ear to allow air to enter the middle ear. The tubes have small flanges at each end and they act as aerators as well as drains. They are left in situ until the Eustachian tubes, blocked by catarrh, have cleared. Sometimes the tubes come out on their own.

Advice for parents. Care at home for a child with a Grommet in position.

1. When washing your child's hair, it is a good idea to place a piece of cotton wool smeared with vaseline into your child's ear hole (entrance of the ear canal.) This will

prevent soapy water entering the canal which can cause irritation (Flood, 1989).

2. Your child may swim, but do not allow your child to swim under water, or dive (Flood, 1989).

3. If your child should develop a discharge from his ear, or severe pain, contact your family doctor.

4. You will be asked to attend the outpatient department for a follow-up. The surgeon will check whether the Grommet is functioning and, with the aid of a hearing test, will check that your child continues to hear normally.

OTORRHOEA

Serous or purulent discharge from the ear may be either acute or chronic. In either case, treatment will consist of three main factors:

Treatment by antibiotics.
Regular, thorough aural toilet by syringing or mopping.
Building up the patient's general health.

Ear Mopping

Ear mopping should be painless and is essentially the same in children as in adults. The auditory meatus in young children up to the age of approximately 18 months is of different anatomical shape and in order to straighten it sufficiently to reach the bottom of the meatus when mopping, the pinna should be gently pulled in a backward direction; in older patients hold in a backward and upward direction.

The delicate skin of children easily becomes excoriated by aural discharge. The area around the ear should be gently washed with cotton wool and saline, and zinc ointment or lanolin applied.

MYRINGOPLASTY

Occasionally a long-standing perforation of the ear drum is closed by skin graft. The necessary skin is taken from the upper arm, inner aspect of the thigh, a vein or from the ear. Working with the help of a microscope throughout the operation, the surgeon cleans the ear carefully and removes the upper skin of the tympanic membrane before applying the graft. The graft is kept in position by tiny plastic or nylon sponges, packed tightly into the auditory meatus and left undisturbed for at least 10 days. The operation is very delicate and only about half the cases are entirely successful. If the graft has taken discharges cease and the danger that infection might enter the middle ear is eliminated. Hearing is restored to a useful level.

CLEFT LIP AND CLEFT PALATE

Approximately one baby in every thousand is born with a cleft lip or cleft palate so that most nurses are likely to meet this abnormality in the course of their paediatric nursing experience. Cleft lip and cleft palate are often hereditary and are caused by a failure of development in the first 3 months of pregnancy. Many degrees of severity of this deformity occur and either condition can be present without the other. The cleft may be unilateral or bilateral, it may merely be a small notch in the upper lip, and incomplete or extend deep into the nostrils. Cleft palate may involve only the uvula or be a small hole in the soft or hard palate, but more often the cleft extends through both hard palate and soft palate. The cleft may be narrow or wide and may include the alveolar margin and if associated with a bad cleft lip causes an ugly protrusion of the premaxilla bone. In the majority of cases cleft lip is associated with an asymmetry and flattening of the nose.

Cleft Lip

General points

A mother who has a baby with a cleft lip is likely to be deeply distressed at the time of the birth. It is often helpful if the midwife can show the mother some photographs of similar babies before and after surgical repair. Parents may also find it helpful to be placed in touch with the Cleft Lip and Palate Association (CLAPA), a self-help group for parents and their children.

Closure of the cleft lip may help to push back the protruding premaxilla, improving the appearance and later producing a better dental arch and a more regular development of the teeth. A small prosthesis achieves the same thing. The operation is usually carried out when the baby is well established and thriving, which is often within a few days of birth.

Nutrition

Cleft lip without cleft of the palate does not often interfere with sucking and in many cases breast-feeding can be carried out successfully. Alternatively, special nipple shields and teats are available and only severe cases of cleft lip and cleft palate need to be spoon-fed from birth. Even then the breasts should be expressed and the milk given to the infant as long as lactation can be maintained. When the cleft is complete, feeding may be very difficult as regurgitation through the nose causes the baby to cough and sneeze. When spoon-feeding, the milk should be allowed to run on to the back of the tongue or into the cheek, as this reduces regurgitation through the nose and checks irritation.

Babies with cleft palates tend to swallow air during feeding and special care must be taken when 'bringing up the wind'. A little boiled water is often given after feeds to clean the mouth and prevent crusts of milk from forming around the edges of the cleft.

Pre-operative nursing management

Pre-operative examination. A photograph taken for record purposes.

For comparison post-operatively

Nursing action	Explanation
Nose and throat swabs for culture.	The baby should be free from infection.
Feeding. Feeds should be given by spoon, being careful not to injure the mucous membrane inside the mouth. A special spoon with the sides bent to form a trough is useful.	To prevent injury to the suture line feeds are administered post-operatively by spoon.
Boiled water should be given after all feeds.	To reduce the risk of infection of the surgical wound.
After feeds the chin should be well dried.	To prevent excoriation.
Estimation of haemoglobin.	To correct any anaemia and for estimation of blood loss during operation.
Parental involvement. Ideally the mother should be resident with her child and participate in the care.	The patient benefits from being handled by its own mother, who is able to carry out many aspects of child care as she would do at home.

Preparation for theatre. In the usual way.

Post-operative nursing management

Position. The infant is nursed on his side with the foot of the bed raised.

To assist the free drainage of secretions.

Nursing action	Explanation
	Oedema may obstruct the airway, particularly the nasal passages.
Pain relief. Analgesia will be required at least for the first 24 h when the child can be expected to be in most pain (Foster, 1989).	To promote comfort, relieve pain and prevent crying which places tension on the suture line.
Restrainers. Elbow splints are applied, particularly during the semi-conscious phase, or alternatively the child is held by the mother.	To prevent handling of the suture line and possible tissue damage by rubbing.
Wound care. Tension on the sutures should be prevented. Sometimes a Logan's bow is applied to prevent tension. Crying should be prevented by frequent picking up and handling.	Tension will cause a widening of the wound line when sutures are removed. Presence and handling by mother will reduce stress.
Toilet of the suture line is carried out regularly and after feeds. The wound is kept dry. Alternate sutures are removed on the 4th and 6th days if catgut sutures are not used.	To prevent infection. To reduce scarring.
Feeding. The first feed is given when the infant appears hungry. A normal feeding pattern is then resumed giving the feeds by spoon.	Post-operative feeding problems are unusual. Mother will wish to participate in feeding and other aspects of care.
The baby can be put to breast after the sutures have been removed.	

The child is ready for discharge once the suture line is healed.

Cleft Palate

Repair of cleft palate

The usual age for repair of cleft palate is 12–24 months, i.e. before the child begins to talk. Orthodontic treatment may have been started with the intention of moulding the maxilla into a well-shaped arch and to stimulate growth of the underdeveloped maxilla.

The preparation of the child with a cleft palate for operation differs little from that of preparing for repair of a cleft lip. The post-operative management is also principally the same as described under cleft lip.

Specific care

Post-operative analgesia will be needed for a longer period and elbow splints will be worn for variable period of time. Parents should be carefully instructed so that they can participate in all aspects of child's care.

For the first 10 days all foods should be liquid or semi-solid and meals should be followed by a drink of plain water to wash down any remains of food. Care should be taken during feeding not to insert the spoon into the mouth where it might damage the suture line but to feed the child from the side of the spoon.

The child is usually discharged on a soft diet and the parents should be advised not to give any hard foods to the child to avoid damage to healing of the suture line until advised by the surgeon.

Long-term care

The successful long-term outcome for these children depends upon a team approach to care. This will include the early involvement of the orthodonist and speech therapist. The parents will need advice and support to encourage early speech. Exercises to develop the throat and palatine muscles with games such as blowing bubbles, by encouraging chewing and practising the consonants 'K' and 'T' assist in the production of normal articulation.

Due to the increased risk of middle ear infection for these children, the parents should ensure that the ears are examined and the hearing tested at regular intervals. If the child develops an upper respiratory infection the family doctor should be informed for the introduction of early treatment.

PIERRE ROBIN SYNDROME

Sometimes babies are seen who have a series of abnormalities, referred to as Pierre Robin syndrome.

These babies have a small, receding mandible (retrognathia), a widely cleft palate and an abnormally small mouth (microstoma). The tongue seems to have insufficient anchorage so that it slips down the back of the throat (glossoptosis). It follows that the tongue obstructs the airway when the baby lies on his back; normal feeding is impossible.

The nursing care of these babies is all-important. The nurse must build up pillows or wedges of polyurethane which make it possible to nurse the baby face down so that the tongue falls forward by gravity. Sometimes a frame or plaster cast can be constructed. Tube feeding is usually necessary until the baby weighs about 2 kg (4 lb), but a plate made of acrylic resin may help to occlude the cleft palate during feeding. Sucking should be encouraged, as this strengthens the tongue and develops the mandible.

The surgeon may stitch the tongue to the mandible and cause adhesions to form—Douglas operation—or he may transfix the tongue with wire to prevent it from slipping back. As the baby grows bigger the difficulties resolve themselves sufficiently so as no longer to endanger the child's breathing and life.

Complications. These include aspiration pneumonia and cyanotic attacks which, if severe, lead to brain damage.

RESPIRATORY TRACT

Young children are very prone to diseases of the respiratory tract, mainly due to the small lumen of the air passages and to their poorly developed immunity to infection.

During infancy and early childhood, respirations are often shallow, rapid, and irregular in rhythm. At birth the baby breathes about 30–40 times/min, by the end of the first year the respiratory rate at rest decreases to approximately 24–30 respirations/min, by the age of two it is 20–24 and by the age of 5 years the respiratory rate is the same as that of an adult.

Respiration

Changes in the rate and depth of respiration occur easily in children and the cause is not always in the respiratory system. Abdominal pain may cause shallow breathing while any increase in the metabolic rate, such as fever, will send the respiration rate up. It is possible to learn much from careful observation of a child's breathing. In obstruction of the air passages, the neck and chest wall can be observed sucking in at the intercostal spaces or the suprasternal notch.

The respiratory rate is best taken when the child is asleep to gain the most accurate results.

Examination of the Child

It is usual for a nurse to assist the paediatrician in his examination. It is her duty to see that the patient is comfortable and well supported, with a small blanket at hand to avoid unnecessary exposure. The child who is old enough to understand should be told what is going to happen and it is usually beneficial to spend a few minutes gaining the child's confidence. He could handle the stethoscope or listen to his own or teddy's chest. The stethoscope should be warmed before use as the touch of a cold object may frighten or arouse protest.

The paediatrician will first watch the child's breathing for depth, regularity, complete and symmetrical expansion of the chest wall, any undue wasting and any drawing in of the intercostal spaces. He will note whether the respirations are abdominal or thoracic and determine the position of the apex beat. By now the child will have gained confidence and only then will the doctor use his stethoscope.

X-ray examination

It is often difficult to obtain good radiographs of young children, but it will help a great deal if someone with whom the patient is familiar can accompany him to the department. If possible arrange for the mother to be present and assist. It is well to remember the fear a child may feel when confronted with a dark, unknown room or with the enormous structure of the X-ray machinery. The X-ray plates and table should be covered with a soft warm material to prevent protesting screams which may make the procedure difficult and unsuccessful.

Positioning of babies and toddlers, particularly when they are feeble and limp or crying, may cause problems.

The child cannot be expected to hold his breath during exposure. Often, therefore, more than one picture has to be taken and both lateral and posterio-anterior pictures are required.

Special investigations

Laryngoscopy. When a doctor wants to inspect the larynx, trachea or the vocal cords, or if he wishes to remove secretions such as blood, mucus or vomit by suction, laryngoscopy is performed. With very young infants laryngoscopy can often be done without an anaesthetic; with older children, except in dire emergency, a general anaesthetic is given.

Bronchoscopy. Bronchoscopy may be done for various reasons. At times it may be performed in order to observe the interior and lining of the lung. Pus and viscous secretions may be sucked out and the cause of collapse of the lung may be observed or removed, as for instance a foreign body or a tuberculous gland. Tissue may be removed for biopsy examination.

The procedure is the same as for adults, but children are usually given an anaesthetic and preparation is carried out accordingly. The throat may be made insensitive by means of a cocaine or Decicain spray.

Bronchoscopy is not entirely without danger. The small air passages may go into spasm during the procedure causing asphyxia. A drink given before a good swallowing reflex has returned and the effect of the local anaesthetic has worn off will have serious consequences, as fluid may enter the lungs. Approximately 4 hours should elapse between spraying the throat and giving the first drink, 5 ml of water, followed by larger amounts if tolerated.

Bronchography. Preparation of the patient for broncho-graphy should include postural drainage being carried out at night and by a physiotherapist or nurse immediately before the child goes to the X-ray department. This will remove some of the stagnant mucus or pus.

Bronchograms are done in the X-ray department or operating theatre under a general anaesthetic. Premedication should ensure that the child is fast asleep before being moved to unfamiliar surroundings. Radio-opaque substance, usually iodized oil, is introduced into the main bronchus by the passage of a fine catheter over the back of the tongue into the trachea. The child is rotated to allow the dye to flow into the lobes and the radiograph will show the outline of the bronchial tree of selected lobes. Irregular filling will demonstrate abnormalities suspected on clinical grounds and from straight X-ray.

On return to the ward, postural drainage is started almost at once. Thus the danger of the iodized oil, pus or secretions spilling into the healthy parts of the lung is reduced. Frequently, the patient complains of a sore throat after a bronchogram and there may be a productive cough for some days.

The radio-opaque substance used for bronchography contains iodine which may set up sensitivity reactions. Sensitivity tests should be carried out before the procedure and the consent form is signed by the child's parents.

ACUTE BRONCHITIS

Upper respiratory tract infections are very common in childhood, and may occur in the prodromal period of measles or pertussis. They may be mild or severe. When the inflammation spreads down into the bronchial tree, the patient suffers from bronchitis.

Acute bronchitis most frequently attacks children from

overcrowded homes who are ill-nourished and debilitated. It is a common complication of measles or influenza, and children suffering from fibrocystic disease of the pancreas, Down's syndrome or congenital heart defects are particularly prone to this and other chest infections. Allergic bronchitis, a familial condition, may also occur. In younger children the illness remains a serious one.

Signs and Symptoms

The child suffering from acute bronchitis looks and feels ill. His cheeks are flushed and his skin and mouth are dry due to a fever of 39.4°–40.6°C (103°–105°F) or more. Respiratory difficulties make him restless and irritable. The accessory muscles of respiration come into play and the alae nasi may be working. The respiratory rate is increased and the respirations may be shallow due to pleural pain. A cough, harsh and dry at first but later productive, is present throughout the 24 hours and is both an early and an exhausting feature of the illness.

In young children the sputum is swallowed and this may at times lead to gastric irritation and vomiting. Occasionally the mucous secretions form a plug in one of the bronchial tubes causing collapse of a lobe or segment of the lung.

Specific Treatment

Oxygen therapy may be of use, provided the atmosphere is kept moist during the early, dry stage of the illness. Steam from a kettle may be used at home to warm and moisten the atmosphere of a room. Humidified oxygen which may be given into a tent is the method of choice in hospital.

Drugs
Appropriate antibiotics are given to combat the infection.
Drugs to relieve bronchial spasm are used selectively.
Cough mixtures and expectorants are rarely of value for
children. Nasal drops may be ordered to clear the upper
respiratory passages.

Complications
Collapse of one or more sections of the lung, anaemia,
and general debility may follow the acute stages of the
illness while in young babies diarrhoea and vomiting are
frequently associated with it.

Principles of Care

As children suffering from acute bronchitis may be incu-
bating measles, they should be isolated from the general
ward in a warm, well ventilated cubicle for the first few
days. Breathing may be difficult so several pillows should
be arranged to give maximum support in a sitting position
that the child finds comfortable. Alternatively, the child
may be nursed flat, the pillows removed and the foot of
the bed raised to promote drainage by gravity. Unless the
patient does so himself, the position should be changed
frequently so as to move secretions and avoid the formation of mucous plugs. When the secretions are profuse
and the patient too weak to cough nasopharyngeal suction
will be required.

Humidified air
The objective should be to maintain a circulation of
moistened air within an enclosed area, whilst being able to
observe the child without obstruction.

The most common method of administration is to release
air under pressure through a container of water with a

narrow outlet. This creates a vapour which is directed into a tent, incubator or cubicle. The moistened air causes the child's clothing and bedclothes to become damp, requiring them to be changed at intervals for dry ones. Frequent observation of the patient's body temperature and the incubator/tent temperature is required to observe for an increase in temperature that may result from a patient being in an enclosed space. The temperature may fall causing the patient to become cold in the moist atmosphere.

Someone should be available within the vicinity whilst therapy is in progress, preferably the mother. As the acute stage of the illness passes the child will require suitable play activities to maintain rest.

Oxygen therapy

Oxygen is given when prescribed by the doctor, unless being used in an emergency situation for resuscitation. It may be dangerous to give oxygen in excessive amounts or in too high a concentration (see p. 56). The oxygen concentration or amount to be given per minute should be ascertained from the doctor. An accurate flowmeter is required. The usual precautions when giving oxygen apply. The danger from striking a match and smoking does not apply with small children but remains a hazard with parents, visitors and older children. Explosions can result from sparks given off from mechanical toys or nylon clothing and visitors need to be warned of this.

Children soon show signs that they lack oxygen by being restless and looking anxious. The respirations become rapid and gasping and the lips and extremities cyanosed.

Methods of giving oxygen. Not all methods used for giving oxygen to adults are suitable for children. In newborn infants, oxygen given through an endotracheal tube or into an incubator are the most commonly used methods. There are various methods of oxygen tents for use at different ages.

Patients with a tracheostomy may have to be given oxygen. The humidified oxygen can be delivered directly into the tracheostomy tube by means of a polythene catheter or a specially designed collar and fitting. Alternatively, the patient may be nursed in an oxygen tent. Chest physiotherapy is given to assist coughing and the removal of secretions. Clothing should be light and warm.

Coughing may be troublesome; often warm milk and honey are enjoyed and very effective for relief. Fluids should be given freely, but sore throat, trachitis and cough may cause the patient to be reluctant and difficult. For bottle-fed babies spoon-feeding may prove less exhausting than sucking. The feeds should be small and frequent so as to avoid distension of the stomach and resulting pressure on the diaphragm.

The patient is observed for physiological signs of a deteriorating condition. Temperature, pulse and respirations are taken 4-hourly and any changes reported. The pulse volume and respiratory rate should be observed with special care to detect signs of oxygen shortage. The blood gases will be estimated at regular intervals. Intake and output charts should be kept as the intake may be small and renal output poor. As a rule the illness is acute and of short duration and mouth toilet, treatment of pressure areas and the care of bowels present few problems.

BRONCHIECTASIS

Bronchiectasis is a dilatation of the bronchi and bronchioles, resulting from the blockage of a bronchus, and may occur as a result of repeated chest infections, pertussis or measles. One or several sections of the lung may be involved. Additionally, a swallowed foreign body that has 'gone the wrong way', e.g. a peanut, resulting in bronchial obstruction will lead to bronchiectasis. It is inadvisable to give peanuts to young children in view of this danger.

Children so affected are pale, undernourished, under-developed and generally suffer from poor health. They usually have chronic upper respiratory tract infections and frequently the mother gives a history of several attacks of otitis media, sinusitis and chronic cough. In its severest form, which fortunately is now being seen far less than some years ago, clubbing of fingers may be present. The teeth may be carious and the tongue coated. Halitosis is common and these children usually breathe through their mouths on account of the chronic nasal obstruction which is present. Hearing is frequently impaired. The chest wall may be deformed, there is shortness of breath and often a low-grade fever. Sputum is profuse, greenish, purulent and very offensive in advanced cases. The younger children are inclined to swallow the sputum, which causes gastric irritation and loss of appetite. Interrupted schooling, the result of frequent admissions to hospital, adds to

FIG. 16   Breathing exercises can be made to be fun.

the impression of dullness so often seen in these children.

Straight radiographs and bronchograms are done to confirm the clinical diagnosis. The sputum is sent for culture and for tests to determine the sensitivity to various drugs of any organisms present. White blood counts, blood sedimentation rate, Mantoux or Tine test and sinus X-ray are performed and estimations of peak air flow and inspiratory–expiratory volumes are made. Antrum washout may be necessary for the frequently associated sinus infection, and dental treatment should be given when indicated.

The patient is treated with postural drainage of the lungs and intensive chest physiotherapy. Nose drops are sometimes useful for clearing phlegm before postural drainage is attempted.

Postural drainage of the lungs. When the internal passages become inflamed, the membranes lining the lungs produce mucus or phlegm. If the phlegm becomes too thick or too

FIG. 17 Postural drainage.

much, it may hinder recovery by blocking the passages. Usually phlegm is coughed up and spat out, though children often swallow it without very much harm. If the phlegm is very thick, it cannot be brought up so easily and may stagnate. Postural drainage is to remedy this. From the physiotherapist, nurses and parents can learn to understand the positions which allow for maximum drainage of the affected lobe.

LOBAR PNEUMONIA

Various organisms may be responsible for causing the lungs to become infected and setting up inflammation. In lobar pneumonia one or several lobes of the lung may be affected. Lobar pneumonia rarely affects young infants. The patients are, as a rule, otherwise healthy, active children who are taken ill with great suddenness. They appear very ill with little warning, though occasionally an attack of vomiting, abdominal pain or a convulsion may herald the illness.

(A)   (B)

FIG. 18   Use of pillows in upper respiratory tract infections. (A) *Wrong*: young children should never be given large, soft pillows as there is a danger of suffocation and overheating. (B) *Right*: the pillows are arranged to allow air to circulate, important in cases with pyrexia, and to allow for full expansion of the chest on inspiration.

Principles of Care

Nursing action	Explanation
The child's temperature will be measured 4-hourly, the bedclothes cradled and the room temperature controlled. An electric fan can assist in bringing down the body temperature.	The temperature rises rapidly to 39.4°C.
Sponging of face and hands will be soothing and can be done by a parent.	Will promote patient comfort.
Nursed sitting up, supported by firm pillows, or alternatively a baby chair may be used for small children.	Breathing is shallow and rapid.
Deep breathing exercises with encouragement to bring up sputum when cough becomes productive.	Painful cough may cause cough to be suppressed and prevent good expansion of lungs. May have referred abdominal pain.
Administration of oxygen may be required.	If cyanosis present and respiration laboured.
Copious oral fluids monitored on a fluid balance chart.	The high fever will cause urinary output to be low and urine concentrated.
Mouth, lips and pressure areas treated as regular intervals.	The fever causes the mouth and skin to be hot and dry.
Administration of antibiotics as prescribed according to sensitivity of the organisms.	Bacterial infections respond well to broad spectrum antibiotics.
Parents can be taught to carry out some aspects of nursing care.	By participating anxiety is reduced and parents feel needed.

BRONCHOPNEUMONIA

In contrast to lobar pneumonia, bronchopneumonia most commonly affects babies and children who are already weak and debilitated and this is one of the reasons why it is by far the more severe of the two illnesses. It often affects very young infants and is a fairly common complication of whooping cough, measles, severe burns and fibrocystic disease of the pancreas.

Occasionally the onset is acute but more often there is a history of an apparently harmless cold for 2 or 3 days. Then cough and fever develop and the child soon appears to be severely ill. Convulsions are common at the onset.

Principles of Care

Most of the nursing points applicable to lobar pneumonia are the same for bronchopneumonia. It is important that all treatment and nursing management are planned to make any disturbance of the patient as infrequent and brief as possible.

In addition to the use of antibiotics the treatment may include digitalis preparations if there is evidence of cardiac failure.

Complications

In spite of modern therapy bronchopneumonia continues to be a serious illness. As large areas of the lung are congested, pulmonary circulation is restricted causing considerable strain on the infant's heart. One or more lung segments may collapse, later leading to bronchiectasis. Other complications include convulsions, diarrhoea and vomiting, and pleurisy.

Convalescence

Following discharge the child may not be quite ready to return to school but will need to rest at home until back to normal. Medical supervision should continue until the doctor is satisfied that the lungs are once more fully expanded.

The family health visitor and/or school nurse should be informed prior to discharge.

PLEURISY

When the pleura become inflamed, as may happen as a complication of pneumonia, the condition is known as pleurisy.

As the inflammation spreads from the lungs, the two layrs of pleura rub against each other and cause severe pain. The child restricts both breathing and coughing to a minimum on account of the pain, and this causes both rapid and shallow respirations. He may also lean towards the affected side in an attempt to splint and immobilize it. Sometimes the pain is referred to the iliac fossa and may cause the doctor to suspect acute appendicitis. As an effusion forms, the inflamed surfaces are separated and the pain subsides.

A Mantoux or Tine test and a radiograph of the chest must be taken to exclude tuberculosis and, if an effusion is present, some fluid should be sent for examination and culture.

Treatment

Treatment and analagesia for the underlying cause is often all that is required. In mild cases the effusion is absorbed spontaneously but when it causes respiratory distress or displaces the heart and mediastinum, chest aspiration must be performed. In either case fibrous adhesions form and often show up on routine radiographs throughout the patient's life. Apart from this, recovery can be complete but a good follow-up and prolonged convalescence are desirable.

Principles of Care

Nursing care aims mainly at relieving symptoms and building up the child's strength and weight. A good general nursing routine is obviously called for as the illness may be a long and tedious one.

Any empyema will require to be drained. Chest aspirations may be used at daily intervals. Alternatively a drainage tube may be inserted into the pleural cavity at the site of the empyema and connected to an underwater seal drainage system or into a dressing. The drainage tube may require resiting to be effective. Intensive physiotherapy is important to achieve full expansion of the underlying lung and obliterate the empyema cavity. The nurse and parents should encourage the patient to cough and carry out deep breathing exercises to expand the lung.

Hand in hand with drainage, the empyema is treated by antibiotics given orally, by injection, or into the empyema cavity by instillation through the drainage tube.

The patient with empyema looks toxic, his colour is grey and he is apathetic. His appetite is poor and he is often anaemic. The tongue is coated and the temperature may swing at a high level. The diet should be nourishing and appetizing, and extra vitamins may be prescribed. Occupation with suitable play activities will also help to keep the patient happy and at rest.

ASTHMA

Asthma is a respiratory disorder which presents as bronchial spasms, expiratory difficulty, wheezing and a feeling of suffocation. Asthmatic children are very frequently seen in paediatric departments and, during the course of an attack, may present an alarming and pathetic picture.

One in five children suffer from the condition at some time (Milner, 1987). The first attack may occur as early as the first year of life, and occurs more often in boys than girls. Eczema may be replaced by asthma in the older child.

Common Causes of Asthma

An attack of asthma in the sensitive child may be precipitated by various factors.

Allergic factors

Allergies are thought to be inherited since other members of the family are commonly found to suffer from hay fever, eczema or migraine. In asthma, the allergic factor is most usually inhaled and can usually be traced to the environment. Sensitivity to the house mite, found in dust around the home, is the most important of this group and explains why these children commonly develop their attacks at nights as the house mite finds an ideal dwelling in bedding and mattresses. The house mite lives on shed human skin and prefers humid, warm and dark living conditions (Lane and Storr, 1987). If the child's attacks are noticed to be seasonal, pollen or moulds are most likely to be the causative factors. Occasionally, sensitivity to pets occurs and it may be necessary for the pet to be taken care of elsewhere. This is a difficult family decision, but much unnecessary illness can be avoided for the child and this should always be explained to him.

Emotional factors

These can often be observed in the child's relationship with his parents. Very commonly the child is described as being quiet and introspective and is often of above average intelligence. Times of acute excitement as well as anxiety can be the triggering factor (Lane and Storr, 1987).

Infection

Infection may trigger an attack in a child and this is usually of viral origin.

Exercise

Excessive exercise has been implicated in precipitating an attack in the sensitive child.

Principles of Care

The nursing care is planned to relieve symptoms, give prescribed treatment and reassure the child and his parents.

Nursing action	Explanation
Sit the child up, well supported with pillows. Comfort may be gained by leaning forward on a bedtable covered with a pillow, with an open window nearby.	Respirations are laboured, expiration appearing more difficult than inspiration. There is an audible wheeze.
Oxygen and suction may be required.	The child will appear grey and cyanosed.

Nursing action	Explanation
Encourage the child to rest.	The shortage of oxygen and laboured respiration cause the child to be restless and anxious.
Intravenous infusion may be set up for the administration of bronchodilators during the first 24 hours. In persistent attacks corticosteroid therapy may be ordered.	To prevent repeated intravenous injections for administration of drugs.
Parents should be encouraged to stay with the child and participate in aspects of nursing care as they feel able.	Helps to relieve anxiety of child and parents.
Diversional play therapy.	Helps to relieve anxiety. Encouragement should be firm and sympathetic.
Sips of cool drink will be soothing. A normal diet will be established fairly quickly.	The breathing difficulties can cause the child to feel nauseated.

Home Care

In the general management of asthma exposure to known precipitating factors must be avoided and is the most effective treatment (Sly, 1986). All pillows and quilts should be Terylene or other synthetic material and the mattress should be enclosed in a dust-proof cover. Other beds in the house should be treated in the same way. The mattresses and the house should be vacuumed once a week, with the windows open preferably when the child is out at school. Over-enthusiastic or more frequent vacuuming should be avoided as this only stirs up the dust. Bedroom blinds rather than curtains should be used, and

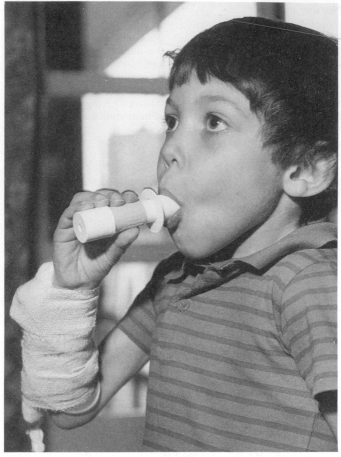

FIG. 19   Asthmatic child using spinhaler.

upholstered furniture avoided. The bedroom should be kept warm, dry and well ventilated.

Care should be taken to explain to the parents the nature of asthma, and that the treatment is aimed at reducing the number of attacks (Lane and Storr, 1987). It is important that the parents should not treat the child as an invalid, but encourage him to participate in all school activities. Psychotherapy may be required for the asthmatic child who is emotionally disturbed. Although the majority of children improve as they grow older, physiotherapy will be needed throughout childhood in order to prevent the development of a 'pigeon chest' which in itself leads to repeated chest infections in later life. Breathing and postural exercises can be taught to the child and his parents in order that they can be carried out regularly in the home.

Drug therapy
Sodium cromoglycate (Intal) or Intal Co is effective in preventing an asthmatic attack when inhaled through a spinhaler, nebulizer or aerosol. Parents and children will need careful instruction in the use of sodium cromoglycate and it should be emphasized that regular administration is required whether symptoms are present or not. Salbutamol nebulizer for use at the commencement of symptoms may also be prescribed.

Investigations

Attempts will be made to identify precipitating causes by means of sensitivity tests. Inspiratory, expiratory and peak flow volumes of air will be estimated.

STATUS ASTHMATICUS

When one attack of acute, spasmodic asthma virtually runs into the next attack, the patient is said to suffer from status asthmaticus.

Treatment and management initially are similar to that

in ordinary attacks but, as this state may persist for many hours, exhaustion may be extreme. Relaxation and rest must be achieved by any means available, and this may tax the parents' and nurse's ingenuity severely. As so much energy is expended on the act of breathing it is difficult to get the child to take sufficient fluids. Sponging the face and hands, changing and turning the pillows and gentle massage of the patient's scalp with a hair brush can be very soothing. Quiet reassurance by speaking to the child and the presence of a parent may do much to calm his fears. Hot drinks, given in small amounts as often as possible, help as much as drugs in getting the patient off to sleep.

, The child may develop respiratory acidosis, and require intravenous therapy to correct the pH balance and prevent dehydration. Unfortunately, death can no longer be regarded as rare in this condition, and the use of a respirator giving intermittent positive pressure may be life saving.

N.B. One of the reasons for the present increase in deaths of these children whilst in status asthmaticus, is due to the intensive usage of anti-spasmodics before admission to hospital. It is important that an accurate history of the drugs received by the child is known on admission to avoid a lethal dose. The greatest danger comes from aminophylline, which is very toxic in high doses and should not be repeated if there is no response to the initial full dose. Severe asthma may persist throughout life but mild cases may have cleared by the age of 15 years.

BRONCHIOLITIS

Bronchiolitis is most common in infants under 6 months and seldom seen in children over 2 years of age. It tends to occur in epidemics, particularly during the winter. The infecting organism is a virus of which the Respiratory Syncytial Virus (RSV) is the most common. Submucosal inflammation causes obstruction to the bronchioles.

Principles of Care

The partial obstruction of the airways in the infant causes difficulty in breathing with the use of accessory muscles of respiration. There is a high respiratory rate of 60–80/min and frequently cyanosis is present. The infant is immediately nursed in a humidified oxygen tent, well supported with pillows or placed in a baby sitta.

The rapid pulse and respiratory rates are frequently observed for signs of improvement or deterioration. Difficulty may be encountered identifying the apical heart beat in the acute stages. Precautions are taken to prevent the infant being exerted or becoming cyanosed by reducing the amount of disturbance to as little as possible with planned nursing care.

Antibiotics are seldom prescribed unless a secondary bacterial infection is diagnosed.

Difficulty is encountered in feeding due to the high respiratory rate. Tube feeding of small frequent amounts is often necessary to reduce exertion and maintain nutrition and hydration. The feed may be offered by mouth as the illness subsides.

As the condition improves, tolerance to handling improves. The infant can be picked up and fed as well as being taken out of oxygen for short periods. From being washed in the cot, gradually the infant can be bathed, care being taken not to exhaust the child.

During the early acute stages of the illness the care will require the skills of the nurse. However as the child improves the mother should be encouraged to participate in the care, handling and feeding of the child.

Recovery is slow and the infant is usually discharged during the convalescent period, when the parents feel they are able to manage the child at home and social conditions permit.

The family health visitor should be informed prior to discharge.

REFERENCES

Flood, J. (1989). Glue ear. *Nursing Times* **85**(36), 38–41.

Foster, R., Hunsberger, M. and Anderson, J. (1989). *Family-centered nursing care of children*. Philadelphia: Saunders.

Jennings, P. (1989). Tracheostomy care: learning to care at home. *Paediatric Nursing* **1**(7), 13–15.

Lane, D.J. and Storr, A. (1987). *Asthma. The Facts*, 2nd edn, pp. 65, 76, 169. Oxford: Oxford University Press.

Milner, A.D. (1987). Recent advances in childhood asthma. *Update* **34**, 398–403.

Sly, R.M. (1986). Asthma. In *Current Pediatric Therapy* (S.S. Gellis and B.M. Kagan, eds), Ch. 12. Philadelphia: Saunders.

FURTHER READING

Ballantyne, J.V. and Groves, J. (1978). *Otolaryngology*. Bristol: Wright.

Blodgett, D. (1982). *Manual of Paediatric Respiratory Care Procedures*. Philadelphia: J.B. Lippincott Co.

Chanmed, H. (1988). *Choosing a Model*. London: Edward Arnold.

Cooke, R.W.I. (1979). *A Guide to Ventilator Care of Infants*. London: Vickers Medical.

Gregory, G.A. (1981). *Respiratory Failure in the Child*. London: Churchill Livingstone.

Kuzembo, J.A. (1980). *Asthma in Children*, 2nd edn. London: Pitman Medical.

Norther, J.L. and Downs, M.P. (1978). *Hearing in Children*, 2nd edn. Baltimore: Williams & Wilkins.

Office of Health Economics (1986). *Asthma*, No. 79. Series of

Papers on Current Health Problems. London: Office of Health Economics.

Sutherland, S. (1987). *Help Me, Mummy, I Can't Breathe*. London: Condor Book Souvenir Press (A&E) Ltd.

Williams, H.E. and Phelan, P.D. (1975). *Respiratory Illness in Children*. London: Blackwell Scientific.

Williams, H.E. and Phelan, P.D. (1982). *Respiratory Disease in Children*, 2nd edn. London: Blackwell Scientific.

6 The child with cardiovascular problems

The relationship between temperature, pulse and respirations in children is of great importance and should therefore always be reported together.

The Pulse

Owing to the small size of the structures involved, even simple procedures such as taking the pulse or the blood pressure and obtaining a sample of venous blood may present special difficulties in children; the younger the child, the more difficult it may be to feel and count the pulse beat over the radial artery at the wrist as he may resent being touched and may struggle or cry; also, overlying fat may make it hard to feel the pulse and may alter the volume and make assessment difficult. It is often a good plan to try to take the pulse while the patient is sleeping and this is often best done over the temporal artery immediately in front of the ear or in the case of infants over the fontanelle. In some instances it may be more helpful to record the apex beat using a stethoscope. The pulse should be taken and counted for 1 min. Changes in the rate, volume or rhythm should be reported at once. In certain diseases, for instance in some types of congenital heart disease, the pulse can be plainly seen at the side of the neck, in others it is not palpable in the groin, as it is in normal children.

The pulse rate alters as the child grows older and during exercise, excitement or disease. An increased pulse rate (tachycardia) may be associated with pyrexia, the administration of certain drugs and following haemorrhage. An abnormally slow pulse (bradycardia) may be due to raised intercranial pressure. Infection and febrile conditions in infancy are not, however, necessarily accompanied by a rapid pulse as with adults, a fact which must be borne in mind when assessing a child's condition.

Taking the Blood Pressure

In infants and young children it is difficult to estimate the blood pressure with accuracy. Special narrow cuffs may have to be used. The cuff should cover two-thirds of the upper arm between the head of the humerous and the œlecron process of the elbow. Variations may be considerable even in healthy children, but average systolic readings are likely to be 60-80 mmHg and the diastolic pressure 50−60 mmHg in the first year and 100−110/80 (systolic/diastolic) at 10 years of age, while at rest. Measurements made when the child is eating, sucking or crying will be unrepresentative and usually too high (de Swiet *et al.*, 1989).

Daily blood pressure readings may be required in certain heart diseases, diseases of the kidney, when increased intracranial pressure is suspected and in the case of patients on steroid therapy. All children should have their blood pressure taken before having an anaesthetic. Children are sometimes frightened by the apparatus, and it may be wise to 'reassure' them by taking the teddy-bear's blood pressure first and letting them handle the rubber bulb, making the mercury rise and fall themselves.

Cyanosis

Lack of oxygen in the circulation causes cyanosis more readily in young children than in adults. Central cyanosis is always a serious sign. It should be relieved without delay by the administration of oxygen. It may be particularly marked in respiratory abnormalities of the newborn, congenital heart lesions and in obstructed breathing. Occasionally young children have breath-holding attacks which cause cyanosis. These attacks are often due to behaviour disturbances.

TYPES OF HEART DISEASE IN CHILDHOOD

There are two main types of heart disease in childhood.

1. Congenital malformations of the heart or great blood vessels.
2. Inflammatory lesions in the heart, causing carditis.

Both these will interfere with the action of the heart and lead to heart failure, in an attempt by the heart muscle to compensate for the extra strain placed upon it, thereby becoming weakened and failing to push the necessary amount of blood to the body.

Heart failure in childhood is usually acute. Chronic heart failure develops gradually.

Heart Failure

Instant recognition and treatment of developing heart failure in the infant is necessary in order to preserve life. The young baby may collapse in a matter of hours or days, while the older child or adolescent may take weeks before his condition becomes serious.

The most common causes of heart failure are due to:

1. Congenital heart disease.
2. Pulmonary conditions.
3. The anaemias.
4. Carditis.

Principles of care

Nursing action	Explanation
Maintain an upright, supported position.	Prevent abdominal organs pressing on the diaphragm and allow lung expansion.
Administration of oxygen by tent. (Older children by mask.)	The sluggish circulation and reduced cardiac output result in cyanosis, restlessness and irritability.
Light, loose clothing changed frequently.	Prevent any restriction to breathing.
Regular, frequent recording of body temperature. Mittens and socks to wear on extremities.	Heat lost easily due to sweating and poor circulation. Maintain body heat to reduce metabolic demands.
Frequent observation of pulse and respiratory rate.	Marked tachycardia and abnormal rhythms reported.
Chest physiotherapy may be indicated.	To encourage expectoration of thick viscid secretions which may otherwise block the airway.
Daily bath and postural position changed every two hours.	Poor peripheral circulation makes these children prone to pressure sores.
Give ordinary milk feeds of 150–175 ml/kg body weight/ 24 h by nasogastric tube in small frequent amounts.	Low exercise tolerance and undue exertion should be avoided.

Nursing action	Explanation
Older children require to be tempted with diet. Nursing history will provide likes and dislikes.	To maintain nutrition for normal body requirements.
Frequent mouth care.	Mouth breathing causes drying of mucosa and mouth ulcers.
Mild aperient may be necessary to prevent constipation and prevent abdominal distension.	Difficult defaecation may cause further heart strain.
Record daily weight and fluid intake and output.	Weight gain caused by fluid retention (the development of oedema) will be detected and patient's general growth observed.
Support parents and teach them aspects of nursing care.	Participation in giving care will reduce anxiety of child and parent.

Human milk is relatively low in sodium and if the baby has difficulty in sucking because of low exercise tolerance, the mother should be encouraged to express her breasts. If breast milk is not available SMA may be used.

Drugs

Digoxin acts as a tonic to the heart muscle enabling it to work with greater effect without increasing oxygen consumption. The initial digitalizing dose is higher than the subsequent maintenance dose. The pulse or apex beat should be taken before this drug is administered as undue slowing of the heart beat may occur. Other early toxic symptoms to observe are vomiting, anorexia and irregular or coupling of the heart beat.

Frusemide (Lasix) is a quick-acting diuretic which is given to stimulate the kidney to excrete water from the body and thereby salts also. The side-effects of this drug include rapid fluid loss leading to dehydration. Potassium levels in the blood should be assessed frequently and extra potassium given.

Aldactone (spironolactone), a longer-acting diuretic, is occasionally given in divided doses combined with Lasix in patients with severe heart failure.

Morphine is commonly given in order to sedate the patient and reduce the metabolism. This drug also reduces the respiratory rate.

Antibiotics are often prescribed prophylactically as the risk of infection is high in these children.

Play and activity
Children in heart failure tend to be irritable and tire easily, feeling great frustration at not being able to do all the things their friends are able to do.

While doing everything for the child initially, the parents and nurse should encourage him to make small efforts to help himself, e.g. cleaning his teeth, but at the same time watch how each small effort affects the patient.

Suitable toys and play activities which do not require too much energy should be chosen. Whilst the child is receiving O_2 therapy no friction toys should be given. Parents and the 'play leader' can do much to help keep the child happily occupied and allay restlessness.

The welfare and well-being of the parents may have a great effect on the patient's general condition. The mother's anxiety is easily conveyed unconsciously to the child and will increase his restlessness. If possible the mother should be resident with her child. Parents need to be well-informed about their child's condition and the nurse should be available to listen and support the parents. A social worker should be available to help with particular problems as they arise. The family health visitor and school nurse should be informed before the child is discharged.

Congenital Heart Disease

Congenital heart disease can be divided as follows:

Acyanotic	*Cyanotic*
Patent ductus arteriosus	Fallot's tetralogy
Coarctation of the aorta	Transportation of the great vessels
Ventricular septal defect	
Atrial septal defect	
Aortic stenosis	
Mitral stenosis	

Patent ductus arteriosus

The ductus arteriosus is necessary to the fetal circulation and failure to close after birth causes oxgenated blood from the aorta (which is under pressure as it leaves the ventricle) to be pumped back into the pulmonary artery where the blood is under low pressure. The flow of blood from the aorta into the pulmonary artery may reach great volumes and the cardiac output is increased. It is not clear why the ductus arteriosus should fail to close in some children although research has shown it to be commonly associated with hypoxia during and after birth. Statistics show that more girls than boys are affected; ratio of $2:1$.

Growth is often stunted although otherwise there may be no other symptoms. Diagnosis may not be made until the child is 3 or 4 years old, when a heart murmur may be heard on routine medical examination by a doctor. Ligation of the ductus arteriosus is best carried out as soon as the diagnosis is made. The operation is carried out through a left thoracotomy; the heart is not entered. Following successful surgery the patient can expect to lead a normal life.

Coarctation of the aorta

Coarctation means narrowing; in this case narrowing occurs along the course of the aortic arch. The blood supply to the distal part of the aorta is thus reduced, whilst pressure is high in the proximal part—that part of the aorta and the arteries supplied by it which lies between the left ventricle of the heart and the narrowing. The systolic blood pressure in the arm is high, the myocardium hypertrophies in an attempt to increase cardiac output; subsidiary or collateral vessels develop. Pulsation in these vessels can be felt on the chest and back, but the femoral pulse is feeble or absent.

Operation consists of resecting the coarcted area with direct anastomosis. The age that this is performed depends a great deal upon the condition of the individual child and the surgeon, but the surgical correction is recommended before adult life.

In successful cases the prognosis is good. The circulation becomes normal, the blood pressure falls to ordinary levels and the patient is able to lead an active unrestricted life.

Ventricular septal defect

Septal defects between the right and left ventricle vary in size. Small defects (maladie de Roger) are characterized by loud systolic heart murmurs, but the child is often completely asymptomatic and the prognosis is good. No treatment is indicated. It has been reported that some defects close spontaneously.

With large septal defects the situation is different. Due to the higher pressure in the left ventricle, a shunting of blood occurs from the left to right ventricle during systole. This increases the work load of the right ventricle and hypertrophy occurs.

Symptoms may be severe, with marked feeding diffi-

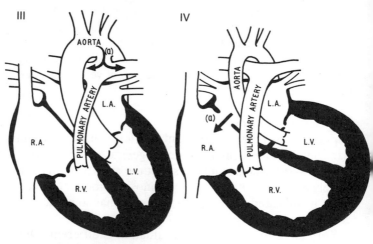

FIG. 20 Congenital malformations of the heart and great vessels. I. Fallot's tetralogy: (a) ventricular septal defect; (b) dextroposition of aorta; (c) pulmonary valvular stenosis; (d) thickened wall of right ventricle. II (a) indicates pulmonary valvular stenosis; III (a) indicates patent ductus arteriosus; IV (a) indicates atrial septal defect.

culty, frequent upper respiratory infections and dyspnoea. Growth is impaired. Urgent treatment is required. Operative repair is carried out with the aid of a heart–lung bypass machine. The defect may be repaired by direct closure or with a specially prepared patch, sutured in position. With surgery the prognosis is favourable but the outcome depends upon the amount of resistance which has developed in the pulmonary vascular bed.

Atrial septal defects

An atrial septal defect is an abnormal opening in the atrial septum resulting in shunting of blood from the left to right atrium. This produces an increase in the right ventricular output and resultant pulmonary engorgement. The diagnosis is suspected by the presence of a soft blowing systolic murmur in the area of the pulmonary artery that may be found at a routine medical examination.

The child usually appears slight, noticed to tire easily with poor exercise tolerance. Susceptibility to pneumonia and rheumatic fever is increased. Operative repair is possible both by closed and 'open-heart' surgery. Since the prognosis for most of these children is good, the risks of operative repair have to be carefully considered for each individual child.

Aortic stenosis

When a thickening of the aortic semilunar valves occurs it is spoken of as aortic stenosis. The narrowing restricts circulation and causes a lowering of blood pressure in the peripheral arteries; hypertrophy of the left ventricle develops as the heart attempts to overcome the obstruction. Valvotomy is carried out by opening the heart and operating under direct vision.

Fallot's tetralogy
The tetralogy of Fallot varies in severity but is characterized by the combination of four defects.

1. Pulmonary stenosis.
2. Ventricular septal defect.
3. Over-riding aortia.
4. Hypertrophy of the right ventricle.

As a result some of the right ventricular output goes to the aorta. Cyanosis in varying degrees occurs, which is most marked on exertion. It is the most common defect causing cyanosis in patients surviving beyond 2 years of age.

Attacks of paroxysmal dyspnoea may occur in children with Fallot's tetralogy, especially before the age of 2 years. The child becomes distressed with deep cyanosis and air hunger which may be followed by loss of consciousness and convulsions. The child should be placed in the knee-chest position to increase cardiac efficiency and oxygen should be given if available. Older children learn amazingly well to adapt their activities, so that during play they take frequent rest pauses and adopt the characteristic squatting position.

Correction of this anomaly is a major procedure in which the cardiac bypass machine is used. The best age for such surgery depends upon the individual patient.

Transposition of the great vessels
In this anomaly the aorta arises from the right ventricle instead of the left ventricle and the pulmonary artery from the left ventricle. Unless surgical treatment can be given, death usually takes place within a few weeks. A palliative procedure has been developed: *Rashkind balloon atrial septostomy* which creates an atrial septal defect sufficient

to maintain similar right and left atrial pressures. This procedure is carried out under a local anaesthetic at cardiac catheterization, before the age of 2 months whilst the septum is reasonably supple. A surgical septostomy through a thoractomy is performed in the older infant and child, i.e., Blalock–Hanlon operation (Aloan, 1987).

The Mustard Procedure has been devised to bring about an internal redirection of blood flow in order that deoxygenated blood will flow into the pulmonary artery. This major surgery is carried out very selectively with the use of the cardiac bypass machine usually after the age of 6 months. The colour change in the child is most dramatic. He often feels for the first time that he can play without having to sit down at the slightest exertion. The correction may not be adequate to maintain a reasonable level of activity when the child is older.

FIG. 21 Parents with a child receiving intensive therapy.

Cardiac Surgery

The recent advances in cardiac surgery are related to improved diagnostic scanning techniques allowing more accurate and detailed diagnosis. This enables the cardio-thoracic team to prepare the child and his parents for surgery to be performed, this frequently involves the use of intensive post-operative care and complex technology. In order to give comfort and support to their child parents should always be offered residential accommodation and be fully involved with each stage of the procedure.

Pre-operative nursing management

Nursing action	Explanation
1. The child is admitted 3–4 days before operation; introduce parents and child to other families in the ward.	To allow time for physical examination and assessment to take place and for the exploration of the new surroundings for the child and his parents.
2. The surgeon should interview the parents before they sign the operation consent form.	To explain the procedure and discuss operative risks involved.
3. Explanation, according to age, should be given to the child. Opportunities for equipment to be used post-operatively to be demonstrated and played with as part of the play experience in the ward.	To offset anxiety when recovering from anaesthetic.
4. Investigations will include blood taking for cross-matching, bleeding and clotting times, haemoglobin and electrolyte estimations.	To ensure that the child is fit for operation and to ensure the child's safety at operation and post-operatively.

Nursing action	Explanation
Chest X-ray and electro-cardiographs and electroencephalograms.	
5. Recordings of blood pressure, temperature, pulse and respirations.	If there is any evidence of infection the operation will be postponed.
6. Height and weight recorded.	For estimation of drug dosage and fluid replacement.
7. With the physiotherapist teach the child breathing exercises for lung expansion.	To enable the child to cooperate post-operatively.

Post-operative nursing management

1. For the first 24 hours nursed flat with a board beneath the mattress.	In case of need for emergency resuscitation purposes.
2. An individual nurse at the child's bedside.	To closely observe for detailed changes in the child's condition.
3. Quarter-hourly observation and recording of all vital signs. Any marked changes or trends are reported immediately.	Early warning indications of impending change, e.g. haemorrhage, shock, etc.
4. Intravenous fluid/blood transfusions should run according to instructions.	To replace blood loss and maintain hydration.
5. Urinary catheter released every hour and recorded on fluid balance chart.	Indication of return of renal functioning.
6. Chest drains are observed for patency and drainage which is measured and recorded.	Indicates returning lung expansions or haemorrhage.
7. Post-operative analgesia, e.g. pethidine or Omnopon.	Reduces shock and pain.

Nursing action	Explanation
8. Chest physiotherapy and passive limb exercises given. Child turned 2-hourly.	To encourage lung expansion, prevent chest infection and to prevent general circulatory complications.
9. Parents should see their child immediately post-operatively. Reinforce pre-operative explanations of care.	Best method of relieving anxiety of the child and his parents.
10. Nasogastric tube on free drainage and measurement. Nil by mouth.	Indication of return of normal intestinal peristalsis.
11. Frequent mouth care.	To avoid soreness of the mouth and promote comfort.

After 24 hours

1. Removal of urinary catheter.	If kidney function is satisfactory.
2. Gradually sit child up then slowly mobilize to sit in a chair.	To prevent vascular and chest complications.
3. Deep breathing exercises continued.	To fully expand lungs.
4. Intercostal chest drains are removed after a satisfactory chest X-ray.	Lungs are usually fully expanded 24–48 h post-operatively.
5. Small amounts of clear fluids offered orally and when these are tolerated the nasogastric tube is removed. Light diet gradually introduced.	Gastrointestinal function gradually returns to normal.
6. Increasing active play occupation provided.	Will encourage return to normal activities.

Nursing action	Explanation
7. Patients should be encouraged to participate in child's care.	Will aid child's recovery.
8. Glycerin suppository may be necessary to aid bowel action.	To prevent constipation and straining.
9. Sutures usually removed after a week.	

If the recovery period continues uneventfully the child is discharged home about the 10th day post-operatively. Parents should be advised as to the best routine to follow at home for the needs of their child. The child initially should be encouraged to rest in the afternoons, gradually doing more and more. After relief of a serious cardiac disability babies often find themselves enjoying their feeds for the first time. They are inclined to take them greedily, demanding more than is offered. The temptation to over-feed must be resisted to avoid overdistension and pressure on the diaphragm.

A follow-up appointment for all patients to visit out-patients is given usually 4–6 weeks after discharge. It is most rewarding for the nurse to see her patients when they come back looking very well, able to play more games with their friends and also to notice the relief of tension and anxiety in the family.

Assisted Ventilation

The aim of assisted ventilation is to maintain gas exchange in the lungs (see p. 56). The child is attached to the ventilator by a tracheal tube. It may be necessary for a child to have assisted ventilation immediately following major cardiac surgery.

Principles of care

Nursing action	Explanation
Aspiration of the tracheal tube at least 2-hourly or when secretions can be heard rattling in the tube.	To maintain a patient airway.
Carried out gently and swiftly.	The ventilator is temporarily disconnected to allow aspiration to be carried out.
Care of the tube. Secure tube with tapes.	To avoid dislodging the tube.
Support ventilator tubing weight.	To prevent weight pulling tube out.
Observation of patient. Record of the patient's pulse, respirations and temperature is kept. Colour observed.	Monitor change in condition.
Observation of ventilator. Rate of ventilator, inspiratory and expiratory flow, tidal volume and flow of gases are recorded.	To identify any change in patient or machine.
Humidification flow is observed and condensation in tubing removed.	All children require humidified gases to be administered.
Administration of respiratory depressant drugs.	To maintain syncronization with the ventilator.
Child should never be left unattended.	In case child becomes disconnected from machine.
Parents should be encouraged to talk to the child. Communicate by writing or drawing. Tell stories, play records, etc.	Although the child cannot respond by talking he will enjoy the stimulation which will help to allay anxiety.

Weaning the child from the machine
Either the child can be encouraged to breathe spontaneously during increasing lengths of time of disconnection from the ventilator, or the trigger mechanism is adjusted to encourage the child to greater effort in establishing the onset of inspiration.

Hypothermia

The ability of certain organs of the body to remain undamaged if deprived of oxygen at normal temperature is known to vary and it is known that the brain tissues are the first to suffer, the maximum period of deprivation for the brain being 3 min without causing irreparable damage. By cooling the body to temperatures as low as 12°–15°C (53°–60°F) the metabolism is slowed down and therefore the oxygen requirements reduced. Operations involving a temporary interruption of circulation can therefore be undertaken while the patient is in a state comparable to that of a hibernating animal.

Cooling of the body can be achieved by the use of ice packs, by immersion in cooled water or by allowing the blood to flow through a cannula and tubing from the superior vena cava to a refrigerating circuit and pumping it back into the circulation via the inferior vena cava.

Care of Intercostal Drainage

Following intrathoracic surgery one or two tubes are stitched into position to allow fluid and air to escape from the pleural space. The drainage tube connects to a drainage bottle either containing a measured amount of water or a 'Redivac' sealed bottle. This forms an air-tight seal.

Expansion of the chest on inspiration increases the intrapleural vacuum and as fluid and air drains out the lungs re-expand. Drainage must be carefully measured, and fluctuations in the tube noted. The tubes should be 'milked' at frequent intervals to prevent blockage of the tube lumen.

When the lungs are fully expanded drainage ceases; following X-ray confirmation of this, the tube is removed under aseptic conditions carefully sealing the tube entry point with sterile vaseline on a gauze dressing to prevent air entry.

The tube leading to the drainage bottle must be clipped off securely when changing the bottle and it must never be raised above the level of the patient, or air and fluid may be sucked back into the pleural space.

Special Diagnostic Procedures

Angiography
Radio-opaque dye is injected into the venous circulation. Serial radiographs or cine-recording follows the passage of the dye through the heart, outlining abnormal shunts or any obstruction. This procedure is commonly combined with cardiac catheterization.

Cardiac catheterization
Under deep sedation or a general anaesthetic an opaque catheter is inserted by way of a vein, commonly one of the femoral veins, into the superior vena cava, the right atrium, right ventricle and pulmonary artery. Pressures and oxygen saturations are measured repeatedly during the procedure revealing a great deal of information about the function of the heart. The use of serial radiographs and/or cine-recording enables the doctor to follow the progress of the catheter.

Catheterization of the left side of the heart in the absence of any shunt is much more difficult and must be performed either through the aorta or by perforation of the atrial septum within the heart as an Rashkind's procedure.

Cardiac catheterization is not without risk. This procedure should be carried out in specialist paediatric centres. After the procedure the child should be carefully observed for blood loss from the site of the venous incision, and resultant shock. Circulation to the limb of the affected side should be carefully observed and the pulses palpated. Nursing care is aimed at keeping the child quiet and rested. Oxygen and humidity are given if necessary. Providing all observations are satisfactory the child may be up and about in 24–48 h. The wound should be kept dry and the sutures removed about the seventh day.

Haematocrit
The haematocrit or packed cell volume becomes elevated with cyanosis and is accompanied by an increased viscosity of the blood. This increased viscosity heightens the patient's susceptibility to cerebral thrombosis.

Echocardiogram
This non-invasive technique demonstrates the outline and structures of the heart. When demonstrated upon a television screen the structures are in 3-dimensions, the single plate is flat. This technique is new and requires skilled interpreters of the pictures obtained (Rowlands *et al.*, 1984). The benefit of its use is that the child is not subjected to invasive diagnostic procedures. The child is required to remain still during the procedure and may require sedation to do this.

Inflammatory Heart Diseases

Although endocarditis, myocarditis and pericarditis are separate entities, any one of them is bound to affect all parts of the heart as the various structures are intimately connected.

Inflammation may be caused by toxins reaching the heart as in pneumonia, influenza, general septicaemia and especially diphtheria, and the result may be heart failure. Alternatively the heart may be affected by bacterial invasion, e.g. bacterial endocarditis. Inflammatory heart disease is one of the possible complications of rheumatic fever and chorea. Permanent cardiac damage may result.

Bacterial endocarditis

Bacterial endocarditis is an acute or more commonly a sub-acute infection of the endocardium and this condition often follows throat, dental or middle ear infections caused by *Streptococcus viridans*. Bacterial endocarditis usually arises as a complication of congenital or rheumatic heart disease. It is rare in childhood.

The symptoms are similar to those of rheumatic carditis but the child is extremely toxic. He looks seriously ill, the eyes are sunken and surrounded by deep shadows and though he seems weary he tosses about restlessly. Pulse and respiration rates are increased and the temperature may rise to 40°C (104°F) or more. The skin becomes dry, the urinary output is diminished, the tongue is furred, the lips dry and inclined to crack. Petechial spots may appear on the skin.

The child will be nursed in a similar manner as that described for a child with cardiac failure.

Drug therapy is directed towards overcoming the infections by giving large doses of the appropriate antibiotic, usually one of the penicillins given intravenously. Steroids are prescribed because of their anti-inflammatory effect and to minimize the production of scar tissue.

Recovery may be complete but the illness and period of convalescence may extend over many months. A careful follow-up by the paediatrician must be maintained over several years. Antibiotic prophylatic cover will be required if the child requires later any procedure which increases the risk of bacteria gaining access to the blood stream, e.g. dental extractions.

Complications

1. Embolism as a result of breakdown from the septic valves.

2. Permanent damage to the valves requiring operation at a later date.

REFERENCES

Aloan, C.A. (1987). *Respiratory Care of the Newborn*, p. 184. New York: J.B. Lippincott Co.

de Swiet, M., Dillon, M.J. and Littler, W. (1989). Measurement of blood pressure in children: recommendations of a working party of the British Hypertensive Society. *British Medical Journal* **299**, 497.

Rowlands, L. (ed.) (1984). *Recent Advances in Cardiology*, p. 32. London: Churchill Livingstone.

FURTHER READING

Graham, G. (1980). *Heart Disease in Infants and Children*. London: Edward Arnold.

Jordon, S.C. and Scott, O. (1989). *Heart Disease in Paediatrics*, 3rd edn. London: Butterworth.

Levin, D.L. (1984). *A Practical Guide to Paediatric Intensive Care*, 2nd edn. St. Louis, MO: C.V. Mosby.

Nursing Times (1980). *Intensive Care of the Newborn*. London: Macmillan Journals.

Talkington, S. and Raterink, G. (1987). *Every Nurse's Guide to Cardiovascular Care*. New York: Fleschner Publishing Co.

Thompson, D.R. (1982). *Cardiac Nursing*. London: Baillière Tindall.

7 The child with rheumatic and collagen problems

All the diseases described in this chapter are thought to be due to a hypersensitivity or an autoimmunity reaction. In persons affected by any of these conditions, the normal immune reaction is replaced by an abnormal sensitivity to infection or a definite destructive reaction within the body. In addition to the conditions described in this chapter, the following diseases are sometimes included in this broad group:

Anaphylactoid purpura (see p. 204).

Idiopathic and symptomatic thrombocytopenic purpuras (see p. 216).

Nephritis, nephrosis (see pp. 382 and 387).

Ulcerative colitis.

ACUTE RHEUMATIC FEVER AND RHEUMATIC CARDITIS

In acute rheumatic fever there is commonly a history of a sore throat or tonsillitis 2 or 3 weeks before the onset of symptoms.

Streptococcus pyogenes is usually the causative organism, but this is not always present on culture when a throat swab is taken. The infection may have been overcome although the streptococcal toxin has set up an autoimmune reaction in the body.

The child suffering from acute rheumatic fever often has a moderate pyrexia, a raised pulse rate and general toxic signs such as headache, vomiting, furred tongue, sweating and constipation. The child may complain of polyarthritis and the severe pain may affect one joint one day and others the next. Occasionally a faint, slightly pink rash appears on the trunk and this may recur intermittently (erythema marginatum). Rheumatic nodules are sometimes found over the elbows, shins, knuckles, knees, occiput and spine. These nodules are usually a sign that the illness is taking a serious course and they are rarely found unless the heart has become affected.

Principles of Care

The child requires exertion to be reduced to a minimum. Bed rest is enforced, the child doing as little for himself and being nursed in a recumbent position. The nurse will have to explain this if the child is old enough and capable of cooperation.

The child requires to be nursed in a warm, quiet corner or room where there is minimal danger of other children or passers-by knocking the bed. Even a slight vibration may cause the child to cry out in pain. A firm mattress should be used and the weight of the bedclothes relieved with a bedcradle. The painful joints may be relieved by support with a small pillow, and pads of warm cotton wool may give comfort.

The nurse can use her nursing skill and imagination in many ways to relieve pain and boredom and to make the irksome rest and the difficulties of taking food in a recumbent position as bearable as possible. The use of plastic straws eases the drinking problem. Appropriate play activities will need to be planned which enlist the help of the child's visitors. Radio and television help to allay boredom and keep activity to a minimum.

The temperature, pulse and respiration are observed every 4 hours. The pulse should be noted, particularly for quality and rhythm as well as rate. The sleeping pulse should be recorded every 3 hours to detect early signs of carditis. A fluid balance chart is kept and an imbalance in the intake and output may be an early sign of cardiac failure. Provided bed scales are available the child's weekly weight should be checked.

Progress is monitored by the erythrocyte sedimentation rate together with sleeping pulse recordings. A gradual increase in exercise is allowed as the clinical picture improves. If general symptoms persist and cardiac symptoms persist or occur, rheumatic carditis may have followed the attack of acute rheumatism.

Endocarditis, with some involvement of the myocardium, is the most common manifestation and the pathology is similar to that of endocarditis in the adult. The lesions resulting from the inflammatory process are scarring and growth of vegetation around the cardiac valves causing permanent damage such as heart failure, mitral stenosis, aortic valve incompetence and pericarditis. The child with rheumatic carditis will be in bed for a number of weeks.

Drug Therapy

Salicylates are the specific drugs for the treatment of acute rheumatic conditions to provide analgesia and minimize the inflammatory process. Relief from pain may be very rapid. Signs of intolerance should always be watched for and reported at once. These include nausea, tinnitus, vomiting, deafness, albuminuria, a discrete erythematous rash and purpura.

Steroids are used to prevent cardiac damage. They are used with caution and are found to be particularly valuable in severe cases of acute rheumatic fever with carditis.

Prophylactic antibiotics against recurrent streptococcal infections is sometimes prescribed and usually carried on for a period of five years or until the child leaves school, whichever is the longer.

Digoxin may be ordered if there is any cardiac incompetence due to carditis, together with frusemide (Lasix) if oedema presents.

CHOREA (SYNDENHAM'S CHOREA, 'ST VITUS' DANCE')

Chorea is characterized by involuntary, uncoordinated and purposeless movements. The onset is often insidious but emotional factors do appear to play a part in starting the disease. The child becomes fidgety, frequently dropping things and his handwriting deteriorates. Emotionally the child becomes labile. The movements cease during sleep.

Principles of Care

Cot sides should be used to prevent the child falling out of bed and in severe cases these may need to be padded to prevent injury. The child may be nursed with the aid of sheepskins and bedcradles to prevent friction sores. Sudden noises and lights should be avoided and all excitement kept from the patient. Drinking and feeding may present difficulties due to the continuous movements, and it may be necessary to resort to nasogastric tube feeding. The mouth should be given special attention as the child frequently bites his tongue, lips or cheeks and ulceration easily occurs. Axillary temperature must be taken to prevent accidents, and a sleeping pulse rate recorded.

Complete recovery may be expected after several weeks but there is a tendency for recurrence and the danger of cardiac involvement is considerable.

JUVENILE ARTHRITIS
(STILL'S DISEASE)

Still's disease or juvenile arthritis (Fig. 29) is an inflammatory condition of the joints, similar to the more common, crippling condition known as rheumatoid arthritis in adults. Although not common in childhood, Still's disease is of interest to the paediatric nurse because of the characteristic manifestations and the careful nursing called for in this disease.

Still's disease most commonly starts between the age of 18 months and 6 years and the earlier the onset the less favourable the prognosis. The cause remains unknown.

Clinical Presentation

The first manifestation of the disease may be a single swollen joint (often the knee). A carefully taken history may reveal recurrent complaints of a stiff neck or stiffness in other joints. Occasionally the onset is acute and may easily be mistaken for acute rheumatic fever. The child is feverish and complains of general malaise. Pain and swelling of the joints may be both acute and severe. More often, however, the disease develops gradually. The usually bright child becomes listless, miserable and pale. Loss of appetite soon causes him to lose weight and he fails to make general progress. He has a high, swinging temperature, the skin is moist and clammy and the blood sedimentation rate is raised (50–100 mm in one hour) and the Rose Waaler test may be positive. The haemoglobin level falls and there may be a mild degree of tachycardia. On examination, subcutaneous nodules may be found although more rarely than in rheumatic fever. As the illness progresses the joints become more painful and swollen and the overlying skin looks white and shiny, though at the same time it may be hot to the touch. Peri-articular swelling and wasting gradually cause the fingers to take on a spindle-shaped appearance.

As a rule the fingers, wrists, elbows and knees, feet and cervical spine are affected most and the swellings and deformity occur symmetrically. Despite marked swellings in the acute stages, the joints are not always permanently damaged, though fibrous ankylosis is very often the cause of extensive crippling and may necessitate corrective orthopaedic surgery. Osteoporosis may be considerable and may be the cause of pathological fractures. Occasionally a fine erythematous rash appears and may not fade for many weeks. Both the peripheral lymphatic glands and the spleen may be enlarged. Pericarditis is an occasional complication.

Treatment

In the acute stage this aims at resting both the child and the affected part, and splints are applied to avoid deformity. The child should be nursed in a well-ventilated room and the bed should be protected from any jarring movement. Whenever possible he should be carried onto a balcony or into the garden but draughts and colds should be avoided. The bedclothes should be light and bedcradles should be used. Sandbags, small pillows and foot rests, and light plaster of Paris splints help to make the patient more comfortable and may prevent deformities. Even in the acute stages, physiotherapy should ensure movement through the whole range at least once daily. Movement

may be made easier by heat therapy prior to physiotherapy and this can be achieved by the use of radiant
heat, wax baths or infra-red ray treatment, but it should
be remembered that the child must not be left even for a
short time during such treatment.

The diet should be attractive and nutritious and should
contain adequate amounts of vitamins. Fresh fruit is
wholesome and may help to prevent constipation. Poor
general health and immobility make careful attention to
all pressure areas important. Schooling and adequate
occupation should be provided to keep up the child's
morale and interest. At the same time occupational
therapy will help to keep the affected joints moving.

Drug Therapy

Salicylates which abolish pain and fever in acute rheumatism are also effective in Still's disease and continue to
be the drug of choice in this condition despite the association of aspirin within Reye's syndrome (Brewer, 1986;
British National Formulary, 1989). Iron is given to combat
anaemia and occasionally a small blood transfusion may
help to build up the child's health generally, as well as
raising the haemoglobin level. Steroids are used with
some success, but the side-effects which occur, and the
need to keep up the steroid therapy, limit their usefulness.
If only one or two joints are affected, intra-articular
hydrocortisone may be of value. However, if this treatment is used for weight-bearing joints, caution must be
observed lest the relief of symptoms leads to excessive use
of the joint thus causing further damage.

Prognosis

Inadequate or late treatment may lead to complications
which include general ill health, retarded growth, defor-

mities and blindness from iridocyclitis. About half the children suffering from Still's disease and treated within a year of onset may be expected to have no residual joint lesions 5 years later; the disease may, in others, burn itself out over a period of 1–2 years.

OTHER COLLAGEN DISEASES

Sometimes a hypersensitivity or autoimmune reaction affects the connective tissue, and in that case one of five rare diseases, grouped together as collagen diseases, may occur. These diseases are briefly described below. They may have a poor prognosis in spite of treatment with steroids and death is often caused by renal failure. The serum proteins are abnormal and the erythrocyte sedimentation rate is raised.

Henoch-Schönlein's Syndrome (Anaphylactoid Purpura)

Henoch-Schönlein's purpura, which is one of the collagen diseases, is seen fairly commonly in childhood, but rarely before the age of 3 years. The small purpuric haemorrhages seen on the skin are at first of a purple colour but later they turn a dusky red and still later, brown, until they gradually disappear. A faint urticarial rash is usually present. The areas most commonly involved are the legs, the back of the elbows and arms, the lumbar region and buttocks. Any pressure, such as sitting on a bedpan, may cause localized purpuric spots. If the haemorrhages involve the intestinal tract, there may be severe abdominal pain of a colicky nature which may last for several hours. This may be followed by the passage of bright blood or a melaena stool. The child may be shocked and occasionally an intussusception may complicate the picture. For that reason there is a certain danger in giving drugs such as pethidine to relieve pain, as this may mask symptoms which should urgently be recognized. The Henoch-Schönlein syndrome may also involve the large joints causing pain and swelling although there is no actual haemorrhage into the joint itself. As different joints become involved, pain flits from one site to another but it never leaves permanent damage or stiffness.

Often no specific treatment is considered necessary and with bed rest the child gradually improves and the rash fades after about 2 or 3 weeks. Steroids may, however, be given if the erythrocyte sedimentation rate is high or if there is albuminuria. There is a tendency for recurrence.

Complications
Complications include nephritis and intussusception, which are dealt with in the usual way.

Principles of care
Nursing care is symptomatic. Distraction and relaxation techniques can also be effective especially in the older child (Foster *et al.*, 1989) in promoting pain relief. Relief of pain for the affected joints may be given by applying pads of warmed cotton wool. Gentle massage may bring some comfort. A painful limb may be elevated on a small pillow and a bedcradle should be used to take the weight of the bedclothes. Pressure from the rim of a bedpan should be excluded by padding it with an air ring or by using a rubber pan.

Polyarteritis Nodosa (Periarteritis Nodosa)

Polyarteritis nodosa is an acute inflammation of the small arterioles, with aneurysm formation which can sometimes be quite easily felt as nodules under the skin. The damage to the arterioles may lead to thrombosis and to haemorrhage. The main signs and symptoms are fever, tachy-cardia, joint and muscle pains and proteinuria which may progress to renal failure. There is hypertension and a polymorphonuclear leucocytosis, and anaemia is common. Temporal arteritis may cause severe headaches and possibly cerebral haemorrhage. Renal and muscle biopsy will confirm the diagnosis.

Dermatomyositis

Dermatomyositis has an insidious onset. Muscle, skin and subcutaneous tissues become inflamed. The muscles are stiff, tender and swollen and become weak with atrophy, contractions and fibrosis. The heart muscle may be affected, causing myocarditis and tachycardia. There is a typical, violet-coloured rash on cheeks and eyelids, circumoral pallor, and an erythematous and sometimes urticarial rash on trunk, limbs and knuckles. The subcutaneous tissues become inelastic and there is a low grade pyrexia and progressive disability which may include muscles of respiration, speech and swallowing. The urinary creatinine levels are greatly elevated in the acute phase, and muscle biopsy and electromyogram confirm the diagnosis. The condition may become chronic with signs similar to scleroderma, but in spite of steroid therapy acute cases may die of cardiac or renal failure or inter-current infections.

Lupus Erythematosus

The disseminated form of lupus erythematosus is rare in childhood, and has an even worse prognosis than in later life. The most characteristic lesion is a purplish-red, raised and indurated 'butterfly' rash over the cheeks and nose. All the mesenchymal tissues are affected, leading to hypertension, anaemia, pyrexia, painful swelling of joints, enlargement of liver and spleen, pleurisy, endocarditis, proteinuria and renal lesions. The bone marrow is depressed, causing leucopenia, and the blood sedimentation rate is very high. Atypical antibodies from the auto-immune reaction—lupus erythematosus (LE) cells—can be seen in blood tests and are specially diagnostic. Treatment is with prednisone 1–2 mg/kg/day initially, but other immunosuppressive agents such as azathioprine 2–5 mg/kg/day may be given.

REFERENCES

Brewer, E.J. (1986). Collagen vascular disease. In *Current Paediatric Therapy*, pp. 353–357. Philadelphia: Saunders.

British National Formulary (1989). London: HMSO.

Foster, R., Hunsberger, M. and Anderson, J. (1989). *Family-Centered Nursing Care of Children*, p. 1551. Philadelphia: Saunders.

FURTHER READING

Ansell, B.M. (1980). *Rheumatic Disorders in Childhood*. London: Butterworth.

Brewer, E.J. (1982). *Juvenile Rheumatoid Arthritis*, 2nd edn. Philadelphia: Saunders.

Brunner, L.S. and Suddarth, D.S. (1990). *The Lippincott Manual of Paediatric Nursing*. London: Harper and Row.

Whaley, L.F. and Wong, D.L. (1987). *Nursing Care of Infants and Children*, 3rd edn. St. Louis, MO: C.V. Mosby.

Williams, G.F. (1981). *Children with Chronic Arthritis*. Massachusetts: P.S.G. Publishing.

8 The child with haematological problems

Anaemia, the most common disorder of the blood in childhood, is due to a reduction in the quality or the quantity of red blood cells (erythrocytes), and reduces the oxygen carrying power of the blood. Apart from a decrease in the number of red blood cells or the quantity of haemoglobin present, alterations in the shape and size of these cells may also occur.

Classification of Anaemias

Deficiency anaemias
Decreased blood formation due to:
   (a) Too few red blood cells.
   (b) Too little haemoglobin in red cells.

Haemolytic anaemias
Increased haemolysis (blood destruction) due to:
   (a) Production of abnormal red blood cells.
   (b) Abnormal destruction of red blood cells.

Haemorrhagic anaemias
Due to blood loss, acute or chronic.

Clinical Picture of Anaemia

When the onset is insidious the child is noticed to be listless, apathetic and tiring more easily than his playmates.

The young baby often refuses feeds or may not complete them. The older child sometimes complains of headaches, giddiness and blurred vision. In the younger child pica (dirt eating) may be observed, this usually stops once the cause of the anaemia has been treated.

The child is difficult over eating, refusing previously well-liked foods. Episodes of sepsis and upper respiratory tract infections are very common, often necessitating frequent absence from school. In severe cases, dyspnoea and some puffiness or oedema of the lower limbs may be present. On physical examination the doctor may hear a cardiac murmur.

Some children with anaemia appear pale, but this is deceptive as red cheeks or a dark skin may hide severe anaemia. The colour of the conjunctivae or of the mucous membrane are more important to observe as these will appear pale in the anaemic child.

When anaemia develops rapidly, e.g. after haemorrhage, the child will appear limp and breathless with a marked tachycardia within a very short time.

Whenever anaemia is suspected it is important that a specimen of blood is obtained before treatment is commenced in order that the primary cause of the anaemia be detected as quickly as possible.

DEFICIENCY ANAEMIAS

Hypoplastic and Aplastic Anaemia

Failure of the bone marrow to manufacture erythrocytes completely is called *aplastic anaemia* but fortunately this is rare. *Hypoplastic anaemia* or underproduction of erythrocytes may occur. These conditions may be caused by certain drugs, e.g. chloramphenicol, benzene, radiation and viruses, but often the cause is unknown. Diagnosis is established by bone marrow puncture. The white cells and platelets are usually also reduced, so that these children suffer from infections and bleeding as well as anaemia.

Treatment consists of giving whole blood or packed cell transfusions in order to provide the mature red cells. These transfusions need to be given repeatedly and one-day admissions to hospital will be necessary. Steroids may also be given.

If a compatible donor is available, bone marrow transplantation is the treatment of choice (Miller and O'Reilly, 1984) resulting in a 3-year survival rate of 50–70% of children treated this way.

NUTRITIONAL DEFICIENCY ANAEMIA

Iron Deficiency

Iron deficiency is the most common of the nutritional deficiency anaemias and indeed of all the childhood anaemias. Iron is essential for the production of haemoglobin and deficiency may be due to:

1. Insufficient iron in the diet.
2. Prematurity, multiple births or maternal anaemia before birth of the baby.
3. Failure to absorb iron in the gastrointestinal tract following neonatal surgery, or with malabsorption syndromes, e.g. coeliac disease.

Iron deficiency anaemia is most common in those infants fed on a milk-only diet after the age of 4–5 months, when all the reserves of iron stored in the liver have been used up. Infants born before term are particularly at risk for the development of this condition as the stores of iron in the liver are built up during the last months of pregnancy. The onset is gradual. Increased susceptibility to infection is often the first indication that anaemia may be present.

In later childhood this anaemia most frequently is caused by a snack food diet lacking in iron or follows infection, especially of the gastrointestinal tract. Intestinal parasites combined with infection and a poor diet will add to the iron deficiency.

Folic Acid and Vitamin B$_{12}$ Deficiency

Folic acid and vitamin B$_{12}$ are essential for the synthesis of nucleoproteins for the maturation of red blood cells. A deficiency of these constituents results in the red blood cells being immature and larger than normal (megaloblastic).

Management

Prophylactic administration of iron to all pre-term infants from the age of 1 month.

Mixed feeding to all babies is introduced from about the age of 4 months. Some paediatricians advocate iron supplements from the age of 12–16 weeks until mixed feeding is fully established. As with other medicines this should never be added to the milk feed but given separately.

Children often accept iron medicines more readily than they do pills. They can be given either through a straw or from a spoon. Older children should be encouraged to brush their teeth after taking the medicine, as they may produce some discoloration of the teeth. For all ages it is best to give the prescribed preparation before a meal.

As well as giving iron supplements the appetite should be stimulated with an attractive, well-balanced diet rich in iron-containing foods:

| Eggs | Liver | Chocolate | Dried fruits |
| Meat | Fish | Fruit | Wholemeal bread |

It is important that adequate amounts of vitamin C, copper, folic acid and vitamin B are also present in the diet as these are also essential for the development of mature red blood cells.

It should be remembered that anaemic children tire more easily than their friends, and will often need a rest during the day or a quiet play period instead of joining in more boisterous games.

In severe cases a blood transfusion may be necessary to replace the missing haemoglobin and stimulate the bone marrow. Intramuscular iron is seldom for children but intravenous iron may be given at the commencement of treatment for severe anaemia.

When anaemia is associated with malabsorption syndrome the underlying cause must be treated with the addition of vitamin and iron supplements to the diet.

HAEMOLYTIC ANAEMIAS

Haemolytic anaemias are due to excessive and rapid breakdown of red blood cells, and patients may become jaundiced as the haemoglobin released from the broken-down cells is converted into the bile pigment, bilirubin. Treatment consists of repeated blood transfusions. The most important haemolytic anaemia in childhood is haemolytic disease of the newborn which is considered on p. 61.

Acute Haemolytic Anaemia

Acute haemolytic anaemia is characterized by a rapid destruction of red blood cells, so that haemoglobin and red blood cells fall dramatically in a very short time. The spleen is enlarged, petechial haemorrhages may occur in the skin, mild pyrexia may be present and the child is listless, fractious and acutely ill. Vomiting and diarrhoea may aggravate the condition. The illness is usually cured by blood transfusion, but may continue as a chronic acquired haemolytic anaemia which needs to be controlled by the use of steroids.

This disease may be caused by drugs, sulphonamides and antimalarial agents in susceptible people who can be shown to have a deficiency of the enzyme G6PD (glucose-6-phosphate dehydrogenase) in their red blood cells. This deficiency is inherited as a sex-linked trait, and is most common in people of negro descent, Italians, Greeks, Oriental Jews and Arabs.

Acholuric Jaundice (Hereditary Spherocytosis)

The cause of this haemolytic anaemia is the unusual fragility of the red blood cells resulting in rapid haemolysis producting jaundice. The spleen is enlarged and firm. Latent periods and exacerbations occur. Crises are often caused by infections and at such times the jaundice deepens, the child may complain of severe abdominal pain, his general condition is poor and may even give rise to anxiety.

Blood transfusion may be needed during a crisis, otherwise a good diet with therapeutic amounts of iron as indicated by the haemoglobin level and prompt treatment of any infection is needed. Splenectomy may be necessary but should only be performed when the child is free from infection and able to tolerate operation. Removal of the spleen produces a clinical cure and prevents the risk of traumatic injury to the enlarged spleen. Children who undergo splenectomy are rendered susceptible to bacterial infection and long-term prophylactic oral penicillin is given (Foster *et al.*, 1989).

Thalassaemia

Thalassaemia (or Cooley's haemolytic anaemia) occurs in families of Mediterranean origin. The cause is the failure of change from fetal haemoglobin to the more mature adult form. Severity of the disease is determined by inheritance.

In the homozygous child (inherited from both parents) anaemia is very severe, marked by extreme fatigue and apathy; repeated infections occur. The child will be noticed to be 'pot-bellied' due to the enlarged liver and spleen and growth is stunted.

Treatment consists of frequent fresh blood transfusions with long-term desferrioxamine therapy to minimize the accumulation of iron in the tissues (haemosiderosis). Folic acid 5 mg daily should also be given. The long-term prognosis is poor.

Sickle Cell Anaemia

Sickle cell anaemia is common amongst black races. An abnormal form of haemoglobin is present in this disease, with the beta chain amino acid sequence being altered. During low oxygen concentration these abnormal red cells distort and become 'sickle' shaped. This haemoglobinopathy results in excess haemolysis and may occur in two forms. Inheritance of the recessive gene from both parents (homozygous) results in severe anaemia and jaundice, with repeated attacks of pain and fever. The pain is caused by the effect of sickled cells becoming impacted in capillaries where oxygen tension is low, such as intestine, joints and kidneys. Symptoms can be brought on by a child having an anaesthetic. Anaemia results from the rate of destruction of red cells exceeding the rate of production. Treatment is aimed at allowing the child to lead as normal a life as possible and protect against possible infection. Repeated transfusions of packed blood cells will be necessary in order to maintain the level of haemoglobin.

The minor form of sickle cell disease (heterozygous) may go undetected, but it should be remembered that the disease may be passed on to the next generation.

N.B. Susceptible individuals should ideally be screened for this disease during childhood and before a general anaesthetic is given. Genetic counselling should be offered to all parents of children with the disease, and to adolescents and young adults with the minor form of the disease before becoming parents.

HAEMORRHAGIC ANAEMIAS

Anaemia can result from the loss of red blood cells from the circulating blood through haemorrhage. The condition may result from a large sudden haemorrhage or from prolonged chronic bleeding from one or numerous small sites.

Purpura

Purpura may be the sign of an underlying disease rather than a disease in itself. Characteristic, spontaneous haemorrhages appear in the skin and mucous membrane of the body, causing bruising, petechiae and frank bleeding of the gums, kidneys, intestinal tract, conjunctivae and the brain. The causes of purpura in childhood may be classified under the following headings.

1. Purpura due to primary or secondary platelet deficiency.

2. Purpura due to vascular defects. This may be congenital or acquired.

3. Purpura due to congenital defects of blood plasma, such as prothrombin.

4. Raised capillary pressure.

Purpura due to platelet deficiency

Idiopathic thrombocytopenic purpura occurs without a known cause. Repeated blood transfusions will be given in an attempt to treat the anaemia and control the bleeding which may be most severe and difficult to control. Steroid therapy, prophylactic antibiotics and intravenous gamma globulin may be given. Some of the more chronic cases may respond well to splenectomy. The majority of patients (80–90%) recover spontaneously in 6–12 months; most of these in fact do so within 8 weeks of diagnosis (Bussel and Hilgartner, 1987).

Symptomatic thrombocytopenic purpura occurs in such illnesses as leukaemia, aplastic anaemia, rubella syndrome, severe infections and some malignant diseases.

Familial thrombocytopenic purpura is one of the causes of haemorrhage in the newborn. Apart from giving platelet transfusions from time to time there is no curative treatment. Splenectomy may be performed when the child is older and this gives good results (see also Haemolytic Disease of the Newborn, p. 61).

Purpura due to vascular defects
May be either primary or secondary. In primary cases it is thought that a hypersensitivity response may be present which causes temporary permeability of the capillary walls. Henoch-Schönlein's purpura is the most common of this type.

Among secondary types the causes include scurvy, meningococcal meningitis and intolerance to drugs.

Purpura due to lack of essential constituents in the blood plasma

This occurs in haemorrhagic disease of the newborn and obstructive types of jaundice.

Disturbance of Clotting Mechanism

Haemophilia

Haemophilia is a bleeding disease which occurs almost exclusively in males; the sex-linked genes are transmitted by unaffected females who are carriers. The clotting time is prolonged by a deficiency of factor VIII, the anti-haemophilic globulin.

Freeze-dried human factor VIII or factor IX is available and when patients and their families have adjusted and accepted the treatment for haemophilia the appropriate freeze-dried factors can be self-administered or given by parents within the home. The dose is adjusted according to the size of haemorrhage, and hospital management of haemophilia is undertaken in haemophilia centres with the support and advice of the community nursing service.

Haemophilia and Human Immunodeficiency Virus (HIV).
Some haemophiliac children have developed antibodies to the Human Immunodeficiency Virus (HIV) due to transfusion in recent years with infected blood or blood products and are therefore at risk of developing Acquired Immunodeficiency Syndrome (AIDS) or AIDS Related Complex (ARC). However with improved donor screening, methods of HIV detection and heat-treatment of blood products this source of the infection has been substantially decreased, but not totally eliminated (Pratt, 1988).

The haemophiliac child should carry suitable identification at all times to alert first-aiders, medical and nursing staff should accidental trauma occur away from home.

The family health visitor and the school nurse should be kept fully informed of the changes in treatment and care. Genetic counselling should be offered to the parents when the disease is first diagnosed.

Christmas disease

Christmas disease is very similar to haemophilia. The condition is inherited in the same way but is not confined to male sufferers. Heterozygous females may rarely be affected in the same way as males.

The treatment and management is similar to haemophilia.

LEUKAEMIA

Leukaemia is a disease affecting the white blood cells. It is characterized by the presence in the circulating blood of immature leucocytes. The cause is unknown. The disease may occur at any age but is most common between 3 and 5 years (Steinherz, 1987).

Very often the child appears pale, lethargic and un-interested in normal activities. Bruising or bleeding from the nose and gums may occur as a result of a low platelet count. Sometimes the child complains of bone pain which may be accompanied by limping due to leukaemic infiltration of the cortex of the bone. The lymph glands may also be swollen.

Acute Leukaemia

Acute leukaemia is the most common malignant disease in childhood. It is classified according to the cell type involved.

Acute lymphocytic leukaemia (ALL)—85% of diagnosed cases.

Acute myeloblastic leukaemia (AML)—15% of diagnosed cases.

Principles of Care

Nursing action	Explanation
Careful handling to prevent bruising.	Low platelet count creates a tendency to bleed and bruise easily.
Test all urine, stools and vomit for blood.	To detect any hidden bleeding.
Brush teeth with small, soft brush. For mouth toilet use a cotton bud or gauze wrapped around a finger; forceps should not be used (Evans, 1990).	To avoid tissue damage and bleeding.
To relieve nausea and vomiting as a result of treatment, give anti-emetics as prescribed.	To alleviate distressing symptoms and promote comfort.
Mouth washes and toilet as necessary.	To clear debris from the mouth.
Reassure child and parents.	To relieve anxiety.
Monitor and record observations of temperature, pulse and respiration. Note condition of skin and of intravenous site.	For the early detection of infection.
Note child's appetite. Record body weight on a regular basis. Encourage eating of favourite foods and drinks.	Chemotherapy may suppress appetite and lead to weight loss.

Nursing action

Warmth of understanding and recognition of parents anxieties. Siblings too will need recognition and support.

Involve the support of the primary health care team and social services.

Encourage normal family life despite the possible long-term nature of the illness—education play activities, hobbies, etc.

Explanation

Difficult time for parents adjusting to their child's illness. Siblings may feel left out and suffer as in later years as a result (Doyle, 1987).

The child and family will require help and support in the home.

The continuity of normality will give reassurance to the child and family and alleviate boredom.

FIG. 22 Cytotoxic drugs administered by clockwork pump allows for normal activities to continue.

Drug Therapy

Combination therapy with cytotoxic drugs to induce remission in the treatment of leukaemia now ensures that the survival rate is 60–70% (Evans, 1990).

Cytotoxic drugs fall into five main groups:

1. Alkylating agents—Cyclophosphamide, Busulphan and Chlorambucil.

2. Anti-metabolites—Methotrexate, Cytosine-Arabinoside and Thioquanine.

3. Vinca Alkaloids—Vincristine, Vinblastine.

4. Antimiotic Antibiotics—Actinomycin D, Adriamycin and Bleomycin.

5. Miscellany, drugs that are not in the above groups—Nitrosoureas, *cis*-platinum and L-asparaginase.

Other groups of drugs in conjunction with chemotherapy, e.g. prophylactic antibiotics, steroids and analgesics, may also be given.

Routes of administration

Many cytotoxic drugs are given by the intravenous route to maximize their therapeutic effect. The use of central venous lines avoids the need for repeated venepuncture especially important for those children who are to receive repeated courses of treatment. All other routes of administration including the intrathecal one may be used either singly or in combination.

Side-effects of chemotherapy

Alopecia is an unavoidable side-effect of drug therapy and radiotherapy. This can be distressing to all members of the family. A wig may be provided, or caps or scarves worn.

The child and parents can be reassured that the hair will grow back again.

Gastrointestinal disturbances are common and need to be considered on an individual care basis. Anti-emetics with a sedative action are useful in the treatment of nausea and vomiting. Good dental and oral hygiene needs to be maintained to prevent the development of ulcers and oral discomfort.

The risk of infection is considerable as a result of immuno-suppression and neutropenia. Prophylactic antibiotics are usually prescribed. Measles and chicken-pox pose a particular threat to immunosuppressed children. It is therefore important to give human immunoglobulin and zoster immunoglobulin if the child has not had either of these diseases but has been in direct contact (Evans, 1990). The Department of Health (1990) recommends that all siblings and close contacts of immunosuppressed children should be immunized against measles, mumps and rubella.

N.B. Children who are immunosuppressed should not receive live virus vaccines until at least six months after chemotherapy has finished (Department of Health, 1990).

Needle phobia may be a cause of considerable distress to these children receiving repeated venepunctures. EMLA cream, a topical anaesthetic, applied to the skin site before venepuncture or injection can be helpful in relieving the pain. Relaxation, distraction and other non-pharmacological therapies (Foster, 1989) can also be beneficial.

Potential hazards of cytotoxic drugs
Cytotoxic drugs have been found to be carcinogenic, mutagenic and potentially teratogenic. Evans (1990)

states that 'the three guiding principles behind cytotoxic drug preparation and administration are to protect the handler, the environment and the patient'. The administration of these drugs must be according to the local health authority policy.

Radiotherapy

Cranial irradiation may also be given during the treatment of acute lymphoblastic leukaemia to prevent secondary leukaemic deposits in the central nervous system.

Bone Marrow Transplantation

Bone marrow transplantation has become an accepted treatment for childhood leukaemia. There are three types of bone marrow transplant available:

1. From an identical sibling.
2. From a matched or related or unrelated donor (allogenic).
3. Autologous transplant, where the child's own bone marrow is taken during remission and preserved until needed.

Following bone marrow transplantation the child is nursed in isolation with reverse barrier nursing in a special unit. The potential nursing problems will include:

The risk of infection due to a low white blood count as a result of chemotherapy and total body irradiation prior to bone marrow transplantation.

The early recognition of graft versus host disease, a serious complication that occurs when T-lymphocytes in the donated marrow react against tissues in the host. Graft versus host disease may be in acute form occurring in 70%

of transplanted children (Evans, 1990) or in a chronic form which may develop up to a year or more after the transplant. Skin involvement in the form of lesions and gastrointestinal problems occur.

Discharge home depends upon the child's physical and haematological condition. Long-term follow-up is needed to monitor condition and for maintainance therapy to be continued. Usually admission to hospital takes place to confirm the diagnosis and for treatment. Thereafter admission is kept to a minimum, the continuing care and treatment being carried out as an outpatient with close liaison with the primary health care team.

HODGKIN'S DISEASE

Hodgkin's disease affects the lymphoid tissues of the body, causing enlargement of lymph glands. Any group (or groups) of glands may be affected but it is usually the cervical or axillary glands that are involved. The disease is rare, and is most unusual under the age of 5 years. It is almost twice as common in boys as in girls (Leventhal, 1987).

The child is listless, anaemic and progressively becomes more ill. Waves of recurrent low grade pyrexia or 'Pel-Ebstein' fever is usually present. Remissions may occur. Treatment includes radiation therapy and chemotherapy. A cure rate of 90% is reported (Sullivan, 1987).

REFERENCES

Bussel, J.B. and Hilgartner, M.W. (1987). Intra-venous immunoglobulin therapy of idiopathic thrombocytopenia in childhood and adolescence. *Haematology/Oncology Clinics of North America* **1**(3), 465–482.

Department of Health (1990). *Immunisation against Infectious Disease*, pp. 4–5. London: HMSO.

Doyle, B. (1987). I wish you were dead. *Nursing Times* **83**(45) 44–46.

Evans, M. (1990). *The Child with Cancer: Nursing Care* (J. Thompson, ed.), Ch. 5. London: Scutari.

Foster, R.L., Hunsberger, M.M. and Anderson, J. (1989). *Family-Centered Nursing Care of Children*, Chs 29, 48. Philadelphia: Saunders.

Leventhal, B.G. (1987). Neoplasms and neoplasm like structures. In *Nelson Textbook of Paediatrics* (R.E. Behrman and V.C. Vaughan, eds), pp. 1079–1109. Philadelphia: Saunders.

Miller, D.R. and O'Reilly, R.J. (1984). Aplastic anaemia. In *Smith's Blood Diseases of Infancy and Childhood*, 5th edn (D.R. Miller *et al.*, eds), pp. 523–542. St Louis, MO: C.V. Mosby.

Pratt, R.J. (1988). *A.I.D.S: A Strategy for Nursing Care*, p. 38. London: Edward Arnold.

Steinherz, P.G. (1987). Acute lymphoblastic leukaemia of childhood. *Haematology/Oncology Clinics of North America* **1**(4), 549–566.

Sullivan, M.P. (1987). Hodgkin disease in children. *Haematology/Oncology Clinics of North America* **1**(4), 603–620.

FURTHER READING

Fleming, A.E. (1982). *Sickle-Cell Disease*. London: Churchill Livingstone.

Jones, P. (ed.) (1980). *Haemophilia Home Therapy*. London: Pitman Medical.

Jones, P. (1984). *Living with Haemophilia*, 2nd edn. Lancaster: Medical & Technical Publishers.

Miller, D.R. (1978). *Smith's Blood Diseases in Infancy*, 4th edn. St. Louis, MO: C.V. Mosby.

Thompson, J. (ed.) (1990). *The Child with Cancer: Nursing Care*. London: Scutari.

Willoughby, M.L.N. (1977). *Paediatric Haematology*. London: Churchill Livingstone.

9 The child with gastrointestinal problems

Daily oral toilet is as important in young children as in the older ones and in adults. The popular belief that the first teeth are unimportant as they will soon be replaced by the permanent ones is erroneous, and the child should be taught good habits with regard to dental care.

Cleaning the teeth with an attractive toothbrush and pleasant tasting toothpaste can be a pleasant part of the morning and evening toilet. Very young children are often reluctant to open their mouth, and so make effective cleaning difficult. It is therefore often best to let the child chew a piece of raw apple at least once a day as soon as the first teeth have come through—a most effective way of keeping the teeth healthy and clean.

THE MOUTH

Observations on the condition of a patient's mouth will often assist in diagnosis and treatment. Of special importance are the following points:

1. *Dry lips and tongue* which will be present in mouth-breathers and in those with high fevers and dehydration. At the same time the tongue will often be thickly coated.

2. *Herpes* which is often seen in patients with colds, high fevers and pneumonia. These small vesicles, grouped on a patch of inflammation around the mouth, are sometimes also called fever blisters.

3. *Pallor of the lips* which is caused by anaemia and may be a sign of loss of blood.

Important odours which a nurse should recognize include:

A sweet smell, where acetone is present.
The smell of stale blood in cases of bleeding from the tonsil bed or from the stomach.
Offensive smells which may be due to the presence of pus, as in retropharyngeal abscess and bronchiectasis.
A faecal odour in intestinal obstruction.
A urinary smell in uraemia.
A foul smell from the mouth occurs in the late stages of leukaemia.
Specific smells when poisons have been swallowed.

Treatment of any of these symptoms depends on their cause, but in all cases of sickness careful mouth toilet is an essential of good nursing.

Herpes Simplex

Herpes simplex is a virus infection which causes eruptions of vesicles. A common site is the lips in febrile illnesses causing swelling and blisters. The latter dry off and leave thick, uncomfortable crusts. The lesions are best treated by drying them up with dusting powder or applying Neocortef ointment. Dabbing the blisters with methylated spirit is painful and for that reason particularly unsuitable for children.

Catarrhal, Aphthous and Ulcerative Stomatitis

Catarrhal, aphthous and ulcerative stomatitis are varying degrees of generalized inflammation of the mouth. There is swelling and inflammation of the gums, coupled with ulcers on the mucous lining of the mouth. The tongue is coated and there is a foul smell. The patient seems ill, the temperature is often raised, he refuses his food and shows intense misery. Frequently these children are debilitated.

A swab is taken to determine the causative organism. In many cases of aphthous stomatitis, the cause is the ultra-microscopic virus of herpes simplex.

Principles of care

As these children dribble saliva because swallowing is so painful, the chin should be protected by applying Vaseline. A dish or a piece of absorbent material can often be arranged to catch the saliva. The application of Vaseline will give some relief from this painful condition by pro-tecting the ulcer from rubbing on the gums or teeth. Benzocaine lozenges to suck will also help. For persistent ulcers, Bonjela ointment may shorten the course of the ulcer. For Vincent's angina oral penicillin is usually effective, alternatively oral metronidazole (Flagyl) may be given. Very young children may have to have their arms restrained to prevent them from putting their fingers in their mouths. Isolation nursing (see p. 34) may be required to prevent cross-infection.

Bland, cool fluids containing plenty of glucose should be given at first and later the diet should contain extra milk and nourishment. Vitamins are important, but concentrated orange juice should be avoided as it stings on the open lesions. Semi-fluid foods which can be forti-fied by additional agents are often enjoyed. Teeth and tonsils should be inspected and, if necessary, treatment or tonsillectomy carried out to eliminate septic foci.

Gingivitis

Swollen, bleeding gums, may be present in general oral infections. They occur in ulcerative stomatitis, scurvy and in leukaemia, but sometimes may merely be due to poor oral hygiene. Careful mouth toilet and a well-balanced diet are essential. Certain drugs taken over a long period may cause gingivitis.

Teething

Gentle mouth toilet should be carried out. A mild analgesic may be ordered for relief of pain. Teething rings, which the infant can bite on, relieve the discomfort and there is nothing against them, provided they are kept clean and safely tied to the cot to prevent them from falling onto the floor.

Thrush

Thrush is caused by the fungus *Candida (Monilia) albicans*. It is mostly seen in bottle-fed babies and is a highly contagious condition. White or grey patches appear on the inside of the cheeks and lips, on the roof of the mouth and on the tongue and cannot be removed without damaging the mucous membrane. The baby will be reluctant to take his feed.

Thrush can be prevented by scrupulous cleanliness, especially with regard to feeding utensils, and by keeping the mucous membrane moist in case of high fever or dehydration. Babies on broad spectrum antibiotics are particularly prone to thrush because the drug kills the organisms which are normally present in the mouth and which can control the antibiotic resistant *Candida albicans*.

Principles of care
Because the condition is highly contagious, barrier nursing is essential. Feed bottles must not be returned to the common feed kitchen until sterilized.

The infection is treated by giving an oral antibiotic called Nystatin or Miconazole. The solution is usually dropped directly onto the tongue.

Complications

Infection may spread throughout the gastrointestinal tract and cause thrush septicaemia, a very serious condition. Severe cases are treated by giving hydroxystilbamidine in a solution of glucose and saline by intravenous infusion. Buttock lesions should be treated with local applications and the baby nursed with exposed buttocks.

Nurses can assist in the prevention of thrush by teaching mothers adequate, easy methods of hygiene in infant feeding.

Tongue Tie

Occasionally a child cannot stretch his tongue sufficiently to make it protrude beyond the teeth. This may cause feeding and speech difficulty so that the fraenum has to be cut in a minor operation. Mild degrees of tongue tie usually right themselves as the child grows older.

THE OESOPHAGUS AND STOMACH

Vomiting

Vomiting in the neonatal period should never be treated lightly. If it is persistent, recurrent, forceful or copious, admission to hospital should be arranged at once. Immediate operation for an obstruction may be necessary, and expert observations may prove life saving. In childhood the causes of vomiting are very varied (see Table 6) and some children seem to vomit at the slightest provocation and show little or no concern about it. Nonetheless,

TABLE 6 The causes of vomiting in childhood

Causes	Age	Content of the vomit	Remarks
Underfeeding	0–3 months	Recently taken feed	The hungry infant cries, swallows air and gulps the feed when offered
Indiscretion of diet	All ages	Undigested food	Milky curd in infancy
Congenital abnormalities	Infancy	Milk, mucus	Effortless or projectile
Pyloric stenosis	2 weeks to 4 months	Curd, mucus, occasionally blood	Projectile
Gastritis	All ages	Food, mucus, blood	Colicky pain often presents
At the onset of fevers	Young children	No characteristic	Accompanied by rise in temperature
Acute appendicitis	All ages	Food at first, bile later	Associated with abdominal pain
Toxic illness	All ages	Food, gastric fluid	Quickly causes dehydration
Whooping cough	All ages	Food and mucus	During or just after meals. After attack of coughing
Diabetes mellitus	All ages	Food	Heralds impending coma
Renal diseases	All ages	Fluid gastric contents	Mostly in late stages of the illness

TABLE 6 *continued*

Causes	Age	Content of the vomit	Remarks
Poisoning	All ages	Gastric contents	Must be saved with special care
Intolerance to drugs	All ages	Gastric contents	e.g. Salicylates. The drugs may have to be discontinued
Nervous conditions	All ages	Watery	Excitement, anxiety, habit
Cyclincal vomiting	After age of 2 years	Food at first, later gastric fluid only	Severe, general disturbance, Ketosis, may last several days
Mechanical	All ages	Gastric contents	May result from finger sucking, enlarged tonsils, mucopus in nasopharynx, air swallowing
Oesophageal reflux	Infancy	Feed, mucus, sometimes blood	e.g. Hiatus hernia
Intracranial pressure	All ages	Not related to taking food	Gastric contents, projectile, without warning
If associated with meningitis, constipation is often an accompanying feature

the nurse should remember that vomiting in most cases entails considerable effort and the child may feel dizzy, faint, cold and miserable. The nurse should always remain with the child, protecting the bedclothes and placing the patient in a comfortable position, and if necessary, drawing the curtains around the bed. The patient may find it comforting if the nurse holds a hand on his forehead and supports any recent abdominal wound. When the attack is over, the patient should be given a mouthwash, or have his teeth cleaned, and be left comfortable. Persistent vomiting may cause considerable loss of fluid and replacement by a parenteral route is sometimes necessary.

The vomit should always be inspected before it is discarded and an entry should be made on the patient's chart. The amount should be measured, the reaction tested with litmus paper, and the time and relation to mealtimes recorded. The nurse should notice whether the vomit is effortless, or forcible and projectile in nature. The presence of curds, blood, excess mucus, bile or foreign bodies should be reported at once.

Gastritis

The causes of acute irritation or inflammation of the gastric mucosa range from unsuitable diet; swallowing infected material; e.g. pus from sinusitis, or dental caries causing incomplete mastication; intolerance of drugs; swallowing an irritant such as a poison; gastroenteritis or chronic dilatation, as in pyloric stenosis.

Principles of care

As gastritis is, as a rule, a symptom of some other disturbance, the underlying cause must be found and appropriately treated.

If old enough, the child may complain of discomfort, nausea and vomiting. The vomit may contain mucus, or specks of fresh blood. Vomiting frequently relieves the distension and discomfort. Ordinary food is omitted from the diet for a few days to reduce irritation to the gastric mucosa. Clear fluids, mildly flavoured, are encouraged to prevent and correct any dehydration. The child generally has a poor appetite. The return to a full diet should be gradual. Lightly boiled eggs, soups, toast and ice cream are suitable as soon as the child is ready for more soild food.

When the illness is severe or long-standing, gastric lavage may be beneficial. Oral hygiene should be given frequently to the dry mouth and furred tongue.

Congenital Hypertrophic Pyloric Stenosis

Congenital hypertrophic pyloric stenosis is due to the thickening of the pyloric sphincter, causing a narrowing of the lumen. Signs of obstruction, gastritis and malnutrition develop.

Pyloric stenosis develops soon after birth and symptoms are first noticed at the age of 2–6 weeks. Mild cases or those which show late symptoms may improve spontaneously at the age of about 4 months, but early and severe cases require medical or surgical treatment.

Diagnosis
Diagnosis is often delayed as varying feeds are tried in an attempt to stop the baby from vomiting. At each change a temporary improvement may take place but vomiting and loss of weight soon recur and eventually the presence of pyloric stenosis is suspected.

Pre-operative nursing management

Nursing action	Explanation
Observation of vomiting. The amount, content and frequency should be recorded.	Large projectile vomits containing curds from previous feeds and flecks of blood from gastritis.
Intake and output fluid balance chart maintained.	The vomiting causes dehydration and the urine is dark and scanty. The skin is dry and fontanelle is sunken.
Assist doctor by administering a feed whilst the abdomen is examined for pyloric nodule.	Peristaltic action during feeding causes the pyloric muscle to contract.
Care of the intravenous infusion, and blood specimen taken for analysis of blood chemistry.	Replacement of fluids to correct dehydration and blood chemistry. The loss of chlorides in the vomit has a serious effect in altering the blood chemistry. Plasma bicarbonates are high and there is an increase in the non-protein nitrogen in the blood and urine. The toxic state (alkalosis) requires rectifying without delay and before operation.
Gastric lavage once or twice daily.	Clears the stomach of stale milk, curds and mucus. The tube is left *in situ* immediately before operation.
Normal preparation for theatre.	Surgery under general anaesthetic is the usual method of treatment.

Post-operative nursing management

Details of feeding vary from one hospital to another but the fundamental principles remain the same. If the baby is breast-fed every effort should be made to help the mother keep the milk supply going. The first feed offered to the baby may be 5 ml of boiled water. The baby may then, 4 hours post-operatively, be offered the breast for 1–2 min. The baby will then be given a breast feed 3-hourly, gradually increasing the time allowed for feeding, and thus increasing the amount of feed taken.

Alternatively the baby may follow a typical post-operative pyloric regimen as follows:

Hours post-operation

4–8	5 ml dextrose hourly
8–10	10 ml dextrose hourly
10–12	10 ml half-strength milk feeds hourly
12–18	15 ml half-strength milk feeds 2-hourly
18–24	30 ml half-strength milk feeds 2-hourly
24–30	30 ml full-strength milk feeds 2-hourly
30–36	45 ml full-strength milk feeds 2-hourly
36–42	60 ml full-strength milk feeds 3-hourly
42–48	75 ml full-strength milk feeds 3-hourly

After 48 hours, the baby may be expected to take normal feeds according to expected weight. One or two vomits during the early post-operative periods are not uncommon, and there may be a little delay in establishing normal gastric peristalsis. The problem is usually resolved or relieved with a further gastric washout; the baby is usually well and gaining weight by 72 hours, and may be discharged home once he is taking full feeds for 24 hours.

Gastric Lavage

The equipment required for gastric lavage in young children differs from that used for adults only in some minor detail. On account of the small amounts of fluid involved and the danger of causing distension and colic if too much fluid is allowed to run into the stomach or to accumulate there careful calculation of the amount of fluid flowing in and out should be made.

Babies and young children should be securely wrapped in a blanket to avoid any struggle, as little co-operation can be expected. The tube should be measured from the bridge of the nose to the lower end of the sternum to give an idea how far the tube needs to be passed in order to enter the stomach. The point is reached when the mark made on the tube, after measuring, reaches the level of the dental arch.

Children cannot be expected to assist with the passing of the tube by swallowing or deep breathing and it is best to feed the tube gently, but firmly along the floor of the mouth after lubricating it with a little sterile water. The assisting nurse, or a parent if present, may steady the child's head or support the chin as this helps to reduce the tickling sensation and excessive retching. After seeing gastric residue rise in the funnel, or after testing some resting juice which has been obtained by siphon action for reaction on litmus paper, fluid [e.g. normal saline at a temperature of 37.2°–37.8°C (99°–100°F)] is run into the stomach. The amount will vary according to the age and size of the patient. Gastric lavage in children should always be supervised by a qualified nurse who will be able to give advice from her own experience as to the correct quantity of fluid which should be used. By raising or lowering the funnel, fluid can be siphoned back. At the end of the procedure the nurse should make sure that no fluid is left in the stomach.

Nasogastric Tube Feed

When giving a feed by nasogastric tube, the technique and equipment are essentially the same as for a gastric lavage.

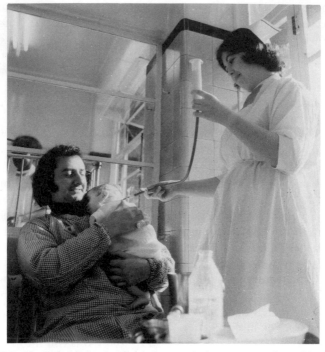

FIG. 23   Proud father holding infant son during naso-oesophageal feed.

The size of tube used is usually a smaller bore and usually passed through the mouth.

At the end of the feed the funnel should be allowed to empty down to the juncture of the funnel and tube, before adding a small amount of water. This ensures that the baby gets all the feed. If the tube is withdrawn before it has emptied completely, as much as 14 g of feed may be lost, a considerable proportion of the total if the small amounts sometimes involved in infant feeding are considered. Furthermore, as long as there is any fluid in the tube, there is always a danger that some may be aspirated into the trachea as the tube passes the larynx on with-drawal. As an additional safety measure, and in order to prevent this from happening, it is considered wise to pinch the tube whilst withdrawing it. The tube should always be withdrawn fairly quickly, and in one steady pull.

On completion of the feed, sometimes the tube is left *in situ* unspigotted to allow free drainage and prevent dis-tension of the stomach.

Hiatus Hernia

Hiatus hernia is a type of diaphragmatic hernia. The abnormality is caused by a defect in the muscles forming the diaphragm so that these do not fit closely around the distal end of the oesophagus, and part of the stomach is pulled through the opening into the thoracic cavity. Sphincter control is impaired and there is a constant reflux of gastric secretions and food into the oesophagus.

Principles of care

As time goes on the baby vomits mucus, food and even blood soon after feeds, and later at any time. He fails to gain weight as much food is lost in this way, and if the condition is not corrected, ulceration of the lining of the oesophagus results. The milky vomit may become streaked with blood. Treatment consists of keeping the baby sitting in an upright position and this position should be main-tained day and night, even when the baby is bathed or nursed. In this way the stomach is kept below the dia-phragm and vomiting made more difficult by force of gravity. It may help to thicken feeds with thickening agent.

Feeds should be given slowly. This allows the oeso-phagitis to resolve by preventing regurgitation ıng in some gain in weight. The diagnosis is confirmed by barium swallow and radiographs. In most instances the hernia is repaired by surgery.

The stomach is returned to the abdominal cavity and the defect in the diaphragm repaired. The surgical approach is usually through the abdomen but may be through the chest. As soon as condition permits post-operatively the child is nursed in a sitting position, particularly after feeds.

Abnormalities of the Oesophagus

There are a number of variants of the abnormalities of the oesophagus, and these may or may not involve the trachea.

1. Tracheo-oesophageal fistula without associated atresia of the oesophagus.

2. Oesophageal atresia, i.e. the oesophagus is not continuous but neither end communicates with the trachea.

3. Oesophageal atresia with associated tracheo-oesophageal fistula.

These abnormalities occur most commonly in low birth-weight babies. There is often a history of hydramnios during pregnancy. Symptoms vary according to the abnormality.

1. In the case of tracheo-oesophageal fistula not associated with atresia of the oesophagus, gastric reflux will cause inhalation of secretions and of hydrochloric acid from the stomach into the trachea causing ulceration of the mucous membrane.

2. As neither the saliva nor oral fluids can pass into the stomach the oesophagus soon fills up as much of the proximal end of the oesophagus fills and spills over, causing coughing

and choking as fluid enters the lungs. Inhalation pneumonia results.

3. When atresia associated with a communication between oesophagus and trachea is present, there is again obvious danger of reflux and inhalation of secretions and any feed that might be given.

Pre-operative management

Nursing action	Explanation
Gentle aspiration of the nasopharynx and mouth at regular intervals and when required.	Because the infant is unable to swallow secretions, coughing and choking occur.
Continuous or intermittent suction to a tube residing in the blind oesophageal pouch.	It is unwise to lower the head end of the cot as this would encourage reflux of stomach secretions into the lungs.
No oral feeds.	Because of oesophageal obstruction.
Care of the intravenous infusion.	To maintain hydration.
Normal preparation for operation.	Obstruction will be repaired under general anaesthetic.

Post-operative management

When the oesophageal blind ends are in close proximity to each other, a simple anastomosis may be carried out through a thoracotomy. This one-stage repair leaves a transanastomotic tube in situ for a week and tube feeding commences after 24 hours. The first oral feed will be a few drops of sterile water, given after seven days, th̶ ̶̶̶̶̶ncy of the anastomosis being tested. Post-operat baby should be handled as little as possible an venient to use an incubator.

If the proximal and distal ends of the oesophagus are too far apart to be brought together, a graft to bridge the gap is necessary. The graft may consist of some inert material or may be taken from the patient's own intestinal tract. It is usually necessary to do the repair in two stages. In that event the proximal end of the oesophagus is brought to the surface at the base of the neck, and through it secretions are discharged. A 'sham feed' of clear fluid is given at the same time as gastrostomy feed, so that the infant associates sucking and swallowing with the pleasure of a full stomach. This makes it easier to establish normal feeding when reconstruction of the oesophagus is completed. A gastrostomy is established through which the child can be fed (Whaley and Wong, 1987).

Feeds given through a gastrostomy tube are given slowly to avoid distension. The funnel is not raised above the height of the baby so that the feed flows gently and gas can escape when necessary. Special care is given to the skin surrounding the gastrostomy opening, and to the mouth.

Hydration and electrolyte balance are maintained by an intravenous infusion before and after surgery. Gentle physiotherapy is carried out to prevent chest complications.

THE INTESTINE

Constipation

Infrequent bowel actions are unlikely to be harmful, provided the stools are soft and passed without causing pain or distress. Few paediatricians are in favour of giving enemas or aperients and regular dosing should be discouraged unless specifically prescribed by the doctor.

Constipation is a symptom rather than a disease in

itself; the underlying cause should be found and treatment given accordingly. True constipation can, however, be responsible for a number of symptoms such as furred tongue, anorexia and vomiting, poor general circulation and sluggishness, restless sleep and bedwetting.

True constipation, that is to say dry, hard faeces passed with difficulty, may be due to a long list of causes including those mentioned below:

In young babies: underfeeding due to inadequate fluid or calorie intake or a failure of lactation (Jolly and Levene, 1985).

Congenital abnormalities: these may hold up the food or faeces or inhibit peristalsis. Among such conditions are congenital pyloric stenosis, intestinal atresia, stricture of the anus, Hirschsprung's disease, hypothyroidism, mental deficiency and atonia due to muscular dystrophy or debility.

Painful defecation: this may be due to local causes, e.g. anal fissure, which makes the child hold back the stool to avoid pain.

Parenteral causes: illnesses which result in a reduction in the circulating fluid volume such as febrile illness and conditions which cause oedema.

Psychological factors: these, or faulty habit training, may lead to infrequent bowel actions and so cause hard stools and painful defecation. Such psychological factors include maternal anxiety.

Principles of care
Dietary adjustments may be all that is necessary. Drinks of boiled water in between ordinary feeds, as well as extra orange juice, may prove sufficient. In older children a diet rich in roughage and adequate exercise; regular habit training should be encouraged. The child old enough to

co-operate should have an unhurried time on the toilet planned into his morning routine. Allbran, wholemeal bread, fresh fruit, green vegetables and prune juice are palatable and suitable high roughage additions to the daily diet.

Occasionally it is found that constipation has developed because the lavatory in the child's home is situated in a cold, dark or isolated part of a tenement building or house, so that the child is frightened of going there on his own. Alternatively, the toilet seat may be too high and, as the child's feet cannot touch the ground, he is frightened of falling in. Lack of time before leaving for school may be another, easily remedied cause of chronic constipation. Lack of exercise leading to poor circulation and muscle tone should be corrected. Television viewing has contributed to physical inactivity in recent years and all types of sport should be encouraged as a healthy counterbalance.

Severe cases of long-standing may need initial treatment by colonic lavage or enemas.

Anal fissure
The severe pain experienced on defaecation should be minimized by keeping the faeces soft with the aid of a correct diet and mild laxatives. Local anaesthetizing ointment such as amethocaine may be used.

Constipation with overflow
This is a term used for leakage of decomposed faeces around a mass of impacted faecal matter. The condition is mainly seen in children with psychiatric disturbances or children who are mentally handicapped. Treatment includes patient toilet training, aperients and, occasionally, manual removal under anaesthetic. For treatment to be successful it is important to find out the underlying cause. In the meantime the patient's mother, exasperated by the

constant soiling of clothes will need support and sympathy in order to gain her co-operation in treating the condition.

Observation of Faeces

The observation of faeces is an important duty of every nurse, it is of particular value in paediatric nursing. Children are often unable to describe symptoms accurately, and the abnormal stool preserved for inspection by an experienced ward sister or medical officer may frequently lead to the establishment of a previously doubtful diagnosis. The nurse should note such points as the colour, consistency, odour, shape and frequency of the stools. Any abnormal constituents such as blood, mucus or foreign bodies should be noted and any complaints of pain on passing the stool, treated as being significant (see Table 7).

Collection of specimens

The collection of faecal matter for investigation does not differ from that in adult nursing but, in the case of 24-hour specimens for very young children, a specially constructed chair may have to be used or the napkin lined with thin plastic.

The handling of bedpans and pots should at all times be reduced to a minimum. Soiled napkins should be saved with the corners tucked underneath the part on which the stool lies when first taken from the baby, placed in a receiver and covered. It is now ready for easy inspection. Any doubtful stool should always be saved and kept available for inspection by the paediatrician.

Intestinal Obstruction

Intestinal obstruction in childhood may be due to congenital abnormalities, strangulated hernia, intussusception,

TABLE 7 Types of stools in infancy and childhood

Description	Usual occurrence	Colour	Odour	Consistency	Frequently	Composition	Reaction
Meconium	First 2–3 days after birth	Tarry, changing to greenish-black	None	Semi-solid	3–6 daily	Normal	Neutral
Changing stools	Approx. 3rd–6th day of life	Dark green changing to yellow	None	Soft	5–8 daily	Normal	Acid
Breast-milk stools	In breast-fed babies	Mustard colour	Character-istic	Soft homo-geneous	5–6 daily	Normal	Acid
Cow's-milk stools	In artificially fed babies	A pale yellow-grey	Musty	Semi-formed, bulky	4–5 daily	Normal	Alkaline
Mixed feeding	In toddlers	Brown	Slight	Formed	1–2 daily	Normal	Varies
High protein content	In infancy	Grey	Sour and offensive	Dry and crumbling	1–2 daily	Excess protein	Alkaline
High fat content	e.g. Coeliac disease	Grey, clay coloured	Offensive	Bulky, greasy	Several daily	Excess fat de-ficient in bile	Acid

Condition	Cause	Colour	Odour	Consistency	Frequency	Contents	Reaction
High carbohydrate content	In infancy	Green	Slightly offensive	Relaxed, frothy	Frequent	Fermented faeces	Very acid
Soapy stools	Digestive disturbances	White	Offensive	Pasty	Several daily	Excess fat or deficient in bile	Neutral
Melaena	Swallowed blood, intestinal bleeding	Tarry-black	Characteristic sweet	Soft	Varies	Blood	Alkaline
Intestinal hurry	Gastro-intestinal infections	Green-brown	Characteristic offensive	Fluid, relaxed	Many times daily	Unconverted bile	Neutral
Crohn's disease Dissaccharide intolerance		Green-brown		Fluid	Many times	Reducing substances	Acid
Hunger stools.	Infancy	Dark green	None or sour	Small, dry	Frequent	Large proportion of mucus-bile	Acid
Over-feeding	Infancy	Bright green	Offensive	Frothy, fermenting	Frequent	Excess fat and carbohydrate	Very acid

TABLE 7 *continued*

Description	Usual occurrence	Colour	Odour	Consistency	Frequently	Composition	Reaction
Intestinal infections	Gastro-enteritis	Pale green	Characteristic offensive	Soft or liquid	Very frequent	Partially digested food, mucus	Varies
Fresh blood	1 Anal fissure 2 Ulcerative colitis 3 Dysentery 4 Rectal polyp	Bright red	1 None 2 } Offensive 3 } 4 None	1 Hard 2 } Liquid 3 } 4 Normal	1 Infrequent 2 } Frequent 3 } 4 Normal	1 Normal 2 } Mucus, 3 } bile, blood 4 Normal and streaks of blood	Alkaline
Red currant jelly stool	Intussus-ception	Bright red	None	Jelly-like	1 or 2 isolated stools	Mucus, blood	Neutral
Pea-soup stool	Typhoid	Green	Offensive	Liquid	Very frequent	Mucus, pus, blood	—
Pus, mucus	Pelvic abscess	Normal or green, streaked with pus	Offensive	Relaxed	Once after rupture of abscess into bowel	Pus, mucus	—

volvulus, a swallowed foreign body or pressure from a tumour. The classical symptoms are the same as in adults, namely vomiting, pain, absolute constipation and abdominal distension. Urgent operation to relieve the obstruction is necessary otherwise there is a danger that the constriction of the blood supply may lead to gangrene of the strangulated portion of the gut, and the continued vomiting may result in dehydration and loss of electrolytes. A nasogastric tube is passed and the stomach contents aspirated before giving an anaesthetic. An intravenous infusion will be necessary.

Duodenal atresia
Duodenal obstruction in the neonate is due to narrowing or absence of the duodenum lumen. There is often a history of hydramnios in pregnancy and other abnormalities may be present.

Vomiting starts within 4 hours of birth and the vomit may contain bile.

Principles of care. The infant pre- and post-operatively requires the usual care after major surgery for intestinal obstruction. To avoid strain on the anastomosis, the transanastomotic tube may be in situ via the nasogastric route or alternatively through a gastrostomy. Feeding, either orally or through the transanastomotic tube, is commenced when bowel sounds are heard. Feeds given into the jejunum are given in very small amounts, at approximately 1 ml/min.

Volvulus
A different kind of obstruction occurs in volvulus, when a loop of bowel gets twisted round itself causing complete obstruction, but symptoms and treatment are similar to the ones described above. After opening the abdomen,

the site of volvulus is sought and the gut untwisted and anchored to the peritoneum. Resection and anastomosis are rarely necessary.

Intussusception

Intussusception, a partial or total obstruction of the bowel, is caused by invagination of a piece of bowel into the bowel beyond it.

Intussusception is one of the most urgent emergencies of early childhood, though on occasions repeated attacks occur, which rectify themselves. Acute intussusception is seen usually at the time the infant starts a weaning diet and it is possible that irritation of the bowel causes a small area of inflammation and oedema in the ileocaecal or ileocolic region. A high proportion of children show signs of a recent virus infection causing oedema of the lymphoid tissue of the bowel. This swelling is then the starting point of the telescoping. A portion of the bowel becomes invaginated and is dragged onwards towards the rectum by peristaltic movement.

Principles of care. The infant is, as a rule, a well-nourished healthy baby of 4 months to 2 years. The mother will explain that he suddenly seemed to have severe abdominal colic which made him draw up his legs and that these pains had been recurring at intervals, between which the baby seemed normal and contented. At first the pain may recur every hour or ½ hour but it soon becomes more frequent and its severity causes shock, with pallor, sweating and a cold clammy skin. The baby soon becomes exhausted. At first a normal stool may be passed but this is followed by complete constipation due to the obstruction, except for the passage of blood-stained mucus—the typical 'red currant jelly stool'. Vomiting may occur but is not a constant symptom.

Following admission to hospital nothing is offered orally because the infant may require surgery. A barium enema may be performed to assist diagnosis and may result in reducing the intussusception, preventing surgical intervention. More usually an operation is performed and the infant is prepared for theatre, passing a nasogastric tube to aspirate the stomach contents to avoid inhalation of vomited food. The abdominal skin, the umbilicus and the groins are washed with soap and water, or the child is bathed if the condition permits.

Post-operative care is usually straightforward. Oral fluids are given in small amounts when bowel sounds are heard—some hospitals start on a 'pyloric schedule'—but in most cases the child can return to a light, normal diet within 3 or 4 days. The intravenous fluids are discontinued when oral fluids are established. Any vomiting, the passage of flatus and the first stool are reported as they are an important guide to treatment. The wound is often left exposed, or covered with a small dressing, and the stitches are usually removed on the eighth and tenth day respectively.

Resection of bowel
Whenever extensive resection of bowel has been carried out, the child's diet will have to be carefully regulated as abnormalities of digestion and absorption result. Disturbances of growth, electrolyte balance, blood formation and vitamin absorption must all be prevented.

Crohn's Disease

The cause of Crohn's disease is not known and potential causative factors are being investigated including environmental, heredity, immunological and other agents (Harries *et al.*, 1982). The disease is primarily one of young people although children of a younger age are increasingly being seen with this condition. About 20% of affected children will have a family relative with this condition (Foster *et al.*, 1989).

Presentation
Abdominal pain is the most common initial complaint with diarrhoea, pyrexia, loss of weight and anorexia. Failure to thrive is the reason for seeking medical help in 20–30% of children (Gryboski and Hillemier, 1980).

Treatment
A combination of therapies which involves both medication (including suphasalazine and steroids) and surgery with colectomy and ileostomy.

Nursing interventions
The major problems identified for the patient will include:

Controlling diarrhoea. A record should be kept of the number of stools passed daily and their association with types of food, stress and activity. This will assist the child, by helping him to learn the association with particular foods that he should avoid such as spices, onions, etc. Anti-diarrhoeal preparations, e.g. Lomotil, are often helpful and they also help to relieve any cramping pain.

Diet. Dietary counselling will be required for the child and parents in order to identify those foods which aggravate symptoms. The child may also require a great deal of encouragement to eat as he will often associate feelings of discomfort, nausea and pain with eating. If the child is severely underweight total parenteral nutrition may be required.

Comfort. Excoriation of the anal region is often severe and scrupulous skin care will be needed. If the child is on bed rest nursing measures will be necessary to prevent skin breakdown. Pain relief will be important, which includes not only the giving of the appropriate medication but also quiet diversional activities and counselling for the child and the family.

Acute Appendicitis

There are few conditions in childhood that present a more confusing picture than acute appendicitis. Among the conditions which may lead to this diagnosis erroneously are tonsillitis, mesenteric adenitis, urinary tract infections, pneumonia, diaphragmatic pleurisy, meningitis, anaphylactoid purpura, dysentery, gastroenteritis, and premenstrual pain. Assessment of all symptoms and sometimes a period of careful observation will, however, establish the correct diagnosis. Because of the extensive examination necessary to establish the correct diagnosis, the nurse may have to be prepared for an ear, nose and throat swab a neurological examination, a rectal swab, a clean specimen of urine, blood picture and chest X-ray.

Acute appendicitis is rare before the age of 2 years and most common at 5–12 years. The onset may be insidious with anorexia, listlessness, nausea or one or two attacks of vomiting and constipation. Alternatively the child may become acutely ill with little warning. The temperature may rise to between 37.2° and 38.4°C (99°–101°F), the pulse may become rapid and the expression, anxious. The tongue is furred and there is halitosis. The child is irritable and resents being touched or examined. If the appendix lies deep in the pelvis—pelvic appendix—the symptoms may include frequency of micturition and diarrhoea due to irritation. If the appendix is retrocaecal the abdominal signs will be masked and diagnosis made very difficult.

Pain may be vague and intermittent to begin with but it

gradually moves to the para-umbilical region and within 12 hours settles in the right iliac fossa.

On examination there is guarding and tenderness, and rectal examination causes the patient to flinch or cry out in pain as the finger points towards the right side. Abdominal rigidity may be caused by cold or general protest and for that reason it is particularly important in children that the doctor's hands should be warm and that a moment or two should be spent in gaining the child's confidence. Occasionally a sedative has to be given before a satisfactory examination can be carried out. If a white cell count is done, it is found to be raised to as much as 30 000 white cells/mm^3 (mainly polymorphonuclear cells).

Once diagnosis has been made, operation should not be delayed. Peritonitis occurs readily as the poorly developed peritoneum is less resistant to infection in a child than in later life, and infection does not localize well in childhood. The appendix walls is thin and the appendix perforates more often than in adults and with more serious results. Operation and after-care are the same for children as for adults and in an uneventful case the child can be expected to be up for bedmaking on the first day after operation and playing happily in the wards on the second day.

Complications: perforated appendix

Acute appendicitis which cannot be diagnosed or treated in time may lead to perforation and set up peritonitis or form a pelvic abscess. When perforation has occurred, there may, for a time, appear to be some improvement in the child's condition. The pain subsides, he seems more relaxed and may fall asleep. However the temperature and pulse rate will rise and the rigidity will spread and, after a few hours, it becomes evident that he is seriously ill and in spite of operation, complications have now become unavoidable.

Peritonitis

The course of peritonitis is now usually controlled by chemotherapy, but severe cases do occur and merit description, as good nursing care has considerable bearing on a satisfactory outcome. Peritonitis may be caused by surgical emergencies such as ruptured appendix, perforation of the bowel due to ulcerative colitis, ascending infection from the vagina and infection in the blood stream. In newborn babies the infection may enter via the umbilicus. The causative organisms include the staphylococcus, *Escherichia coli* (bacterium), the tubercle bacillus; gonococcus and pneumococcus.

In the case of a perforated appendix, the causative organism is usually *Escherichia coli* and the fluid in the peritoneal cavity soon becomes infected. The onset is mostly very acute.

Pre-operative nursing management

Nursing action	Explanation
2- to 4-hourly recording of temperature.	Infection causes temperature to rise to 39.4°–40.6°C.
Observation of pain. Warmth to relieve abdominal pain.	In young children pain may not be localized in abdomen. Rapid shallow respirations prevent movement of diaphragm and abdomen. Legs may be drawn up to chest.
General observations including measurement of fluid balance.	The child will show symptoms of severe toxaemia with grey skin colour with a malar flush. Eyes are bright but sunken.
Oral hygiene.	Oral feeding discontinued due to vomiting and impending surgery.

Nursing action	Explanation
Intravenous therapy.	To maintain hydration.
Nursed sitting up.	To localize peritoneal fluid in pelvis and prevent pain.

At times the free fluid in the abdomen may fail to absorb and become infected. A generalized septicaemia may develop or, in more favourable cases, the pus will localize and form a pelvic abscess. Adhesions may form between the convolutions of the bowel and later give rise to colic and obstruction.

Subphrenic abscess
Rarely, the pus localizes below the diaphragm causing an abscess which is difficult to palphate and diagnose. Treatment is by surgical drainage.

Pelvic abscess
Pelvic abscess rarely requires surgical interference. The pus localizes and, in the majority of cases, the abscess eventually ruptures into the rectum. Pus and mucus are passed when the child has his bowels opened. This complication delays recovery by a week or two but is rarely very serious, although the child may have considerable pain.

Paralytic ileus
When the serious complication of paralytic ileus arises, peristalsis ceases and there is complete constipation; no flatus is passed and the abdomen is distended and resonant when tapped. Vomiting may be severe and continues even when the normal stomach contents have been vomited; the vomit consists only of gastric and intestinal secretions mixed with bile.

Treatment consists of resting the bowel completely until

peristalsis is re-established. Continuous gastric suction, or frequent aspirations by syringe through a nasogastric tube are carried out until there is no more aspirate and bowel sounds can be heard through a stethoscope.

Fluids are given only by the intravenous route until peristalsis is once more present. The child will need a good deal of nursing attention. He is usually restless and needs comforting. Hands and face should be sponged from time to time; the mouth treated regularly; the position of the limb into which the infusion is running, adjusted and supported by small pillows and the hands restrained to prevent him from pulling out the aspiration tube. Thirst may be troublesome and occasionally it may be permissible to give very small, infrequent cubes of ice to suck. Once peristalsis has started again, recovery is rapid and the child is, as a rule, eager to have his meals; he gains strength rapidly. Initially, the introduction of oral fluids should be slow and as the condition improves the process may be speeded up by introduction of easily digested foods.

Appropriate antibiotics are prescribed according to the seriousness of the causative organism, determined by blood culture and from a swab of the discharging wound.

Mesenteric Adenitis

Children often complain of abdominal pain for which there is no obvious explanation. The pain is not usually severe and neither guarding nor tenderness on examination are marked. There may occasionally be vomiting. The condition resolves itself without treatment and recurs from time to time. Although the symptoms are unconvincing, laparotomy is sometimes performed in order to exclude acute or subacute appendicitis. It will then be seen that the mesenteric lymph nodes are enlarged. It is thought that the enlargement is due to a generalized reaction of lymph tissue to infection. The condition is not a serious one but because of the possibility of appendicitis or renal tract disease, it should never be taken lightly.

Hernia

A hernia is a protrusion of an organ from the cavity in which it is normally contained. The following describe two types of hernia commonly encountered in children.

Umbilical hernia

Umbilical hernia is a very common condition of childhood. It is entirely harmless, although it is unsightly, but may cause parents much worry and may be thought by them to be the cause of such disturbances as wind and colic. The defect consists of a small, oval-shaped weakness in the linea alba, through which a loop of gut protrudes, and in the majority of cases it disappears spontaneously during the first 3 or 4 years of life. Small umbilical hernias rarely call for treatment but larger ones resolve more rapidly if surgical treatment is given. This is a simple repair of the hernia and can be done as a minor operation as an outpatient or as a day case. Trusses, adhesive strapping and elastic bandages are useless.

Inguinal hernia

Inguinal hernias occur due to a developmental weakness in the abdominal wall and are usually first seen when the child cries, strains at stool, or coughs (particularly during the paroxysms of whooping cough). A small lump appears just lateral to and above the crest of the pubic bone. Occasionally this lump spreads down into the scrotum. It usually disappears when the child is at rest, or if he is held with shoulder and head lower than the rest of the body. In the majority of cases, operation is the treatment of choice. The operation is a minor one, consisting of locating and excising the hernial sac; it can be carried out in an out-patients' theatre, or the child can be admitted as a day case. Post-operatively the child is allowed the freedom of the cot as soon as he feels like it, and he can be allowed up on the day after the operation.

Inguinal hernias occur more frequently in boys than in girls because in development before birth, or in some cases during infancy and early childhood, the testes migrate through the inguinal canals into the scrotum. There is therefore a certain weakness in the abdominal wall in boys due to the fact that the inguinal canal is patent and the track through which the testes descend has not become obliterated. If either of the testes remains undescended it has to be brought down into the scrotum by a surgical operation (orchidopexy). Often at operation for undescended testicles, a hernial sac is also found and herniotomy performed.

If an inguinal hernia is sufficiently large or the neck of the hernial sac very narrow, the hernia can become ir-reducible and there is a danger of intestinal obstruction. As the child draws up his legs in pain and cries, the abdominal pressure increases and so aggravates the state of affairs. A sedative should be given and the buttocks and foot end of the cot raised. Occasionally the child is put into a warm bath or is nursed in a gallows-type of exten-sion. Alternatively an ice-bag is suspended over the area to reduce the engorgement caused by the constriction of vessels in the inguinal canal. As the child relaxes, gravity causes the intestinal loop to slip back into the abdominal cavity, and the hernia reduces itself. Once this kind of situation has arisen, operation and repair should be carried out at an early date. If the hernia cannot be reduced by any of these methods, an operation should be carried out before a strangulated hernia occurs, as if this happens the blood supply to the loop of the gut is cut off, and this leads to gangrene of the loop.

Jaundice

Jaundice is the yellow staining of the skin and conjunctiva of the eyes by pigments absorbed from the blood instead of being excreted in the bile, as in a healthy person. It is therefore a symptom and not a disease in itself and there are several causes, some of which are dealt with in the appropriate chapters in greater detail. Jaundice arises if the breakdown of red cells is so rapid that the liver cannot cope with it. The unconjugated bilirubin in the circulation then rises. If, in the case of babies, it exceeds the normal level of 340 μmol/litre (20 mg/100 ml) of blood, bilirubin will be deposited in the ganglia of the nervous system, resulting in spasticity and mental handicap. Low birth-weight babies and those with haemolytic disease are at particular risk, and frequent estimations of the serum bilirubin levels have to be performed and appropriate treatment given when danger point is reached. The main causes of jaundice in childhood can be grouped under the following headings.

The haemolytic types

These are due to excess destruction of red cells, i.e. at a greater rate than the liver can deal with. As these bile pigments are not excreted by the kidneys but are eliminated by the liver, stools and urine retain their normal colour. Examples are:

1. Haemolytic disease of the newborn (see p. 61).
2. Acholuric jaundice (see p. 213).
3. Transfusion jaundice.

Obstructive jaundice

This is caused by an obstruction in the bile ducts so that bile pigment cannot reach the duodenum. Stools are pale or even colourless but the urine is heavily coloured, and the skin is tinged yellow to olive colour. Examples are:

1. Biliary atresia.
2. Obstruction from pressure of a tumour or a cho-ledochus cyst.
3. Very rarely obstruction by gall-stones or roundworms.

Jaundice due to sepsis

The principal examples are infection spreading from the umbilicus of the newborn, or general infection spreading via the blood stream and causing liver damage. In these instances the jaundice is rarely very deep.

Infective or acute virus hepatitis

This type of jaundice frequently appears in epidemic form. Serum hepatitis comes under this heading and this is caused by contamination with virus-infected blood or needles used for injections and blood tests. The urine is dark while the faeces are pale or colourless. There is a similar neonatal 'giant cell' hepatitis.

Other conditions accompanied by jaundice are congenital syphilis, galactosaemia, cystic fibrosis of the pancreas, physiological jaundice and Weil's disease.

Congenital atresia of the bile duct

In spite of the fact that atresia of a bile duct is congenital, symptoms may be at first either missed or mistaken for physiological jaundice. Contrary to the jaundice in the physiological variety, the jaundice in the case of obliteration of the bile duct fails to improve and the baby becomes more deeply jaundiced until he is almost an olive colour

(Mowat, 1979). The urine and saliva are stained with bile, the stools are grey, clay coloured or white and the liver is enlarged and firm. The obstruction to the normal flow of bile is due to a complete block, or absence of a segment of the common bile duct, so that bile cannot pass through it.

Diagnostic laparotomy is performed to pinpoint the site of the atresia and to take a liver biopsy. If a gall bladder is present, a radio-opaque substance is injected and this will outline the anatomy of the biliary tract under X-ray (cholecystography).

If a bile duct of adequate size is present, surgery, which aims at anastomosing it to a loop of bowel, is performed. Complications commonly occurring are: breakdown of the anastomosis; leakage of bile and attendant excoriation of skin; and post-operative bleeding due to delayed clotting time, despite pre-operative cover with vitamin K.

If surgical relief is not possible, the jaundice gradually deepens, liver and spleen enlarge and cirrhosis of the liver develops. The child is then a candidate for liver transplantation.

THE COLON, RECTUM AND ANUS

Megacolon

Megacolon means enlarged colon. It may be:

1. The result of chronic constipation.
2. Due to a narrowing of the rectum.
3. Caused by an absence of the parasympathetic ganglia of the rectum, e.g. as in Hirschsprung's disease.

The treatment of the first two causes may require initial manual evacuation of the rectum under general anaesthesia, and frequent rectal washouts using normal saline and aperients. These measures must be combined with toilet training to redevelop normal bowel habits. In cases where the megacolon is secondary to chronic constipation, the nurse should appreciate that there may also be present quite a severe degree of psychological disturbance, and the help of the psychiatrist may be needed.

Hirschsprung's Disease

Hirschsprung's disease (Fig. 24) is due to the absence of the parasympathetic ganglia in the rectum and occasionally farther along the intestine, perhaps even beyond the sigmoid colon. As peristaltic action is initiated and maintained by these nerve cells, normal bowel movements do not take place and the intestine above the affected part becomes grossly dilated, while the rectum is, as a rule, empty, smaller than usual and frequently in spasm.

The disease is present at birth, but delay in diagnosis may occur, depending on the length of the aganglionic segment. Constipation is the presenting symptom, and there is often a delay of passage of the first meconium stool (Tripp and Candy, 1984), which in the majority of normal babies is passed in the first 24 hours of birth.

Principles of care

Children with Hirschsprung's disease look miserable and unhappy, with thin wasted limbs in contrast to the big distended abdomen. The baby is often reluctant with his feeds and he will be inclined to vomit. As the condition progresses, visible peristalsis may be observed across the drum-like abdomen. Occasionally foul-smelling flatus and thin 'ribbon-like' stools are passed. Characteristic rumbling noises can be heard; these are known as borborygmi. At intervals the mucous lining of the bowel becomes inflamed and the stagnated, putrefied, offensive bowel content is passed. This enterocolitis can at first be

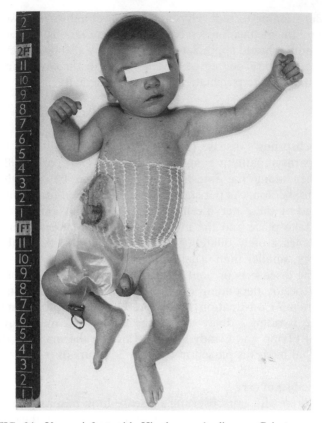

FIG. 24 Young infant with Hirschsprung's disease. Colostomy performed. Major surgery involving a radical pull through delayed until after the age of 6 months.

mistaken for gastroenteritis and may rapidly lead to a dangerous loss of body fluids, requiring intravenous replacement. Characteristically, the distension and constipation may be relieved by digital examination of the rectum or by irrigation, and the child's condition will improve for a short period. Chest complications are common, as the distension of the abdomen impedes respiration by pressure on the diaphragm.

Babies suffering from Hirschsprung's disease cannot thrive unless treated, surgery being the only hope of survival. Commonly, if the affected segment is a relatively short one, the child will present at a later age as a failure to thrive, appearing puny and stunted in growth. It is good nursing observations and reporting that lead to Hirschsprung's disease being diagnosed. Accurate recording of the number of bowel actions, and the nature of any stools passed, will bring abnormalities to the notice of medical staff at an early date. The putrefied smell often associated with bouts of diarrhoea, and the abdominal distension which causes the umbilicus to evert and the abdominal veins to be unusually prominent, are often first observed through daily handling and nursing care of the patient.

Barium enema
Diagnosis may be confirmed with the aid of a barium enema. When Hirschsprung's disease is suspected the normal pre-examination bowel preparation is omitted.

Rectal biopsy
A submucous biopsy is taken to demonstrate the absence of ganglion cells. This can now be obtained with a special instrument using suction, which avoids the need for general anaesthesia.

Anorectal manometry
This demonstrates the absence of the normal reflex inhibition of the internal anal sphincter on rectal distension, and is useful as a screening test.

Surgical management
Most commonly, Hirschsprung's disease is diagnosed as an emergency, the child presenting with acute symptoms and requiring immediate surgical intervention. A colostomy will be performed and surgery delayed until the child is 6–12 months old, or the symptoms have subsided.

The immediate pre-operative preparation is the same as for any other major abdominal operation. An intravenous infusion is set up, and a nasogastric tube passed.

Colostomy
General management of a colostomy in children differs little from that in an adult. In the immediate post-operative period there is danger of bleeding from the bowel and this is best stopped by the application of a firm bandage and a gauze pad soaked in a solution of adrenaline 1 : 1000. Occasionally the protruding bowel becomes strangulated and the opening in the abdominal wall has to be enlarged. A loop of bowel may prolapse through the incision and if this happens a pack of warm, sterile saline is applied until the patient can be taken back to the theatre. The delicate skin of children needs particularly careful attention. The surrounding area and buttocks should be washed frequently and no soiled pads left on longer than necessary. A barrier cream should be applied. If washouts are ordered they are done with a very soft catheter for fear of perforating the bowel.

With care the bowel can be regulated so as to produce a semi-formed stool which is easily passed but not too messy, and bowel actions can be reduced to twice daily. Extra nourishment and vitamins should be given, keeping in mind the fact that absorption can take place only in part of the length of the digestive tract.

It is important to remember the effect such an operation may have on the parents. As a rule they can be reassured that the colostomy is merely a temporary measure. Permanent colostomy, performed for a congenital abnormality of the lower bowel, will of course cause great distress to the parents and they will need a long period of adjustment and sympathetic support. Parents should be taught how to change the colostomy appliance and encouraged to participate in the child's care. Older children should change the appliance for themselves with the support of parents or nurse (Elcoat, 1986). Children with a permanent colostomy can be fitted with a colostomy belt and a normal life should be possible.

Surgical correction

The two most common operative procedures for Hirschsprung's disease are Swenson's (Fig. 25) and Duhamel's (Fig. 26) operations. Each involves laparotomy, mobilization of bowel, resection and reconstitution of the lower alimentary tract and often a temporary colostomy for the post-operative period.

Prior to operation a course of phthalysulphathiazole is given to sterilize the bowel. Any anaemia is treated and

FIG. 25 Swenson's operation. *Left*: The colon is mobilized, the rectum prolapsed through the anus allows an anastomosis. *Right*: Completion of the operation with the bowel returned to the pelvis, the ganglionic bowel (A) is anatomosed to the rectal stump.

FIG. 26 Duhamel operation. Aganglionic bowel (B) is pulled down behind the closed rectum through the internal sphincter until the normally innervated bowel (A) is pulled through and fixed to the distal rectum. The aganglionic section that is pulled through is excised and the spur (C) is crushed with a clamp applied at the end of the operation.

blood is taken for grouping. The immediate pre-operative preparation is the same as for any other major operation. An intravenous infusion is set up, and a nasogastric tube passed.

Post-operative management
Intravenous therapy will be needed for the first 24 hours or so, as the child will be allowed nothing by mouth. During this time careful mouth toilet will be required to keep the mouth moist. Frequent observations must be recorded including a quarter-hourly pulse rate. If the pulse rate is rising a doctor should be informed, as in Hirschsprung's disease this is often a sign of fluid loss from an inflamed bowel. A nasogastric tube will be in position and should be aspirated 1- to 2-hourly. Providing the amount of aspirate is low and bowel sounds are heard, feeding with clear fluids can be commenced 24–48 hours after operation. The intravenous infusion can then be discontinued. Gradually, over the next few days, a normal diet is introduced.

The perianal skin may become sore, and should be washed frequently and a barrier cream applied. As the child's condition improves ambulation can be encouraged. Sutures are removed at about the eighth post-operative day if the wound is well healed. The colostomy is cared for and is closed about 2 weeks later.

Prognosis is excellent for these children. Regular bowel training is necessary at first. The mother is taught to give her child an adequate intake of roughage and fluids to avoid constipation. Occasional laxative may be required.

Rectal Prolapse

When a section of mucous membrane comes down and presents at the anal orifice, the condition is known as rectal prolapse. Only rarely do all the coats of the rectum come down in this way and if this happens the condition is called *rectal procidentia*.

Rectal prolapse is a common occurrence in children of about 9 months to 3 years. There are several underlying causes and each will have to be treated before improvement can be expected from either medical or surgical therapy. The following are the usual causes: poor muscle tone, as in diseases of the nervous system; malnutrition and wasting disease, in which the supporting fatty tissue is absent; stress from coughing, as in whooping cough; longstanding diarrhoea causing irritation of the lower bowel; general mismanagement; behaviour problems; poor toilet training, long periods spent sitting on the pot; and finally, mental handicap.

Principles of care

When a rectal prolapse occurs it should be dealt with calmly and the prolapse gently reduced. In most cases it can easily be pushed back by steady pressure with a piece of damp cotton wool while the patient is lying on his back. Alternatively, very young children can be held up by their legs when gravity may cause the prolapse to reduce itself. It may help if, after reducing the prolapse, the nurse holds the child's buttocks together for a few minutes, while she distracts his attention by telling a story or playing with him.

Good, consistent toilet training is a very important part of the treatment, but young children should not be allowed to sit on their pots for long, nor should undue importance be attached to a daily bowel action.

Surgical intervention is rare and occurs in intractable or long-standing cases. There is no pre-operative treatment although some surgeons may order a rectal washout before the patient is sent to the theatre. Post-operatively, the buttocks may be strapped together for 4 or 5 days. Extra fluids, a roughage free diet and liquid paraffin are given, to ensure soft stools and easy bowel action without straining.

Anal Stenosis

Some babies are born with anal stenosis. This abnormality is not recognized on first examination but the baby will pass toothpaste-like stools and will be seen to strain at defaecation. Treatment consists in performing dilatations and giving laxative drugs.

According to the abnormality, signs and symptoms will vary. If the condition is missed, the three typical signs of obstruction, vomiting, abdominal distension, and complete constipation, will develop in the case of severe stenosis or absence of an anal opening. If the anal opening is displaced, meconium will appear in an abnormal position.

Diagnosis
Diagnosis is made by thorough inspection, by digital examination and by radiographs. The baby is held upside down under the X-ray screen and this causes intestinal gases to rise to the apex of the blind pouch. A marker is placed over the anal dimple and the distance between this and the apex is measured. In this way a concise diagnosis can be made and the distance between the blind end of bowel and the perineum can be determined.

Treatment
Treatment depends on the type of abnormality. Very briefly, anal stenosis is treated by dilatation and laxatives; hidden anus with normal rectum, by incision of the covering membrane and dilatation; anal opening on the perineum but in a forward displaced position, by incision of the perineum and stitching of rectal mucosa round the new opening, followed by dilatation over a period of months. Rectourethral and rectovaginal fistulae require major surgery and the creation of temporary or permanent colostomy.

Imperforate Anus

During the first examination of the newborn baby, careful inspection of the perineum must always be included. Failure of the baby to pass meconium must always arouse suspicion that an abnormality of the anus is present. The deformity may be superficial or deep. The anus may merely be hidden by skin which covers a normal rectum and sphincter, or the opening of the anal canal may be displaced forward on the perineum. In more severe deformities the rectum forms a fistula, which in the male communicates with the urethra and in the female with the vagina, there being a gap between the anal dimple seen on the perineum and the blind end of the bowel. Surgical repair is usually attempted.

REFERENCES

Elcoat, C. (1986). *Stoma Care Nursing*, pp. 123–127. London: Baillière Tindall.

Foster, R., Hunsberger, M. and Anderson, J. (1989). *Family-Centered Nursing Care of Children*. Philadelphia: Saunders.

Gryboski, J. and Hillmeier, C. (1980). Inflammatory bowel disease in children. *Medical Clinics of North America* **64**, 1185–1202.

Harries, A.D., Baird, A. and Rhodes, J. (1982). Has the rising incidence of Crohn's disease reached a plateau? *British Medical Journal* **284**, 235.

Jolly, H. and Levene, M.L. (1985). *Diseases of Children*, 5th edn. Oxford: Blackwell Scientific.

Mowat, A.P. (1979). *Liver Disorders in Childhood*, pp. 79–93. London: Butterworths.

Tripp, J.H. and Candy, D.C.A. (1985). *Manual of Paediatric Enterology*, pp. 12–13. London: Churchill Livingstone.

Whaley, L.F. and Wong, D.L. (1987). *Nursing Care of Infants and Children*, pp. 464–467. Washington, DC: C.V. Mosby.

FURTHER READING

Harries, J.T. (1977). *Essentials of Paediatric Gastroenterology*. London: Churchill Livingstone.

Jolly, H. and Levene, M.L. (1985). *Diseases of Children*, 5th edn. Oxford: Blackwell Scientific.

McLaren, D.S. and Burman, D. (1982). *Textbook of Paediatric Nutrition*, 2nd edn. London: Churchill Livingstone.

Mowat, A.P. (1979). *Liver Disorders in Childhood*, pp. 79–93. London: Butterworths.

Walker-Smith, J. (1979). *Diseases of the Small Intestine in Childhood*, 2nd edn. London: Pitman Medical.

Walker-Smith, J.A. (1986). *Diarrhoea and Malnutrition in Childhood*. London: Butterworths.

Young, D.G. and Martin, E.J. (1979). *Young and Weller's Baby Surgery*, 2nd edn. London: Harvey, Miller and Metcalf.

10 The child with metabolic problems

Metabolic disorders should be suspected when there is mental handicap, abnormal hair or skin texture or colour, abnormal urine output or colour, excessive thirst, abnormal appetite and failure to grow. With such conditions, the urine and the blood should be examined. Special biochemical tests can be carried out. A number of these diseases originate from an absence or abnormality of an enzyme which is essential for a particular metabolic process.

RICKETS

Rickets occur as a result of lack of fat-soluble vitamin D in the diet and from lack of sunshine. Calcium and phosphorus metabolism fail, and serious, typical signs and symptoms occur.

Improved standards of living and nutrition, and a well-developed welfare service have caused rickets—once known as the English disease—to become rare amongst the indigenous population in the British population. The disease is seen amongst immigrant families, particularly Asian families, where the vitamin content of the traditional diet is often low, and may even be negligible if strict vegetarianism is adhered to.

Prevention

1. A well-balanced diet with vitamin supplements up to the age of 5 years.

2. As much time as possible spent in the sunlight. Exposure of the baby's cheeks to sunlight for even a few hours is said to be sufficient for a day's requirement of vitamin D.

3. Co-operation between doctors, midwives, health visitors, teachers and nurses to identify children at risk and those showing early signs of tiredness, pain and weakness in the lower limbs and often with a poor posture. Emphasis on the value of sunlight and vitamin supplements should be made to Asian families, with the help of the local community leaders and link workers to overcome any language problem.

Active Rickets

The groups at risk are infants, toddlers and young adolescents. It is caused by lack of vitamin D, which is essential for the utilization of calcium and phosphorus for good bone growth. Neither human nor cow's milk provide sufficient vitamin D for the baby's needs after the first weeks of life. The deficiency may also be produced by prematurity, lack of exposure to sunshine, faulty diet and inability to absorb the fat-soluble vitamin D in diseases such as coeliac disease. The risk period for vitamin D deficiency is during the winter, especially in northern cities where the daylight hours are shorter than in the south.

Signs and symptoms
In severe cases, the entire bony system of the body can be involved. The sutures and fontanelles of the skull are late

FIG. 27 A child with well-developed rickets. Urine bag in position for collection of specimen.

in closing and together with bossing of the forehead give the skull the so-called 'hot cross bun' effect. Thinning of the cranial bones causes a resilience known as *craniotabes*. Dentition is delayed and the teeth are defective. The affected infant sits up and walks late, the bones are soft, arms and legs are bent and the epiphyses are enlarged. Respiration causes sucking in of the softened ribs, which results in a horizontal groove, known as *Harrison's sulcus*, running round the anterior aspect of the chest. At the same time, beading at the juncture of the ribs and sternal cartilages forms the *rickety rosary*. The pelvic bones may become flattened and the angle of the neck of the femur on its shaft alters and eventually leads to limping, and in girls to obstetric complications in later life.

The abdomen in children with rickets is protuberant and there is a tendency to respiratory tract infections, sweating, diarrhoea and vomiting. The child is often miserable and sleeps little. Tetany, carpopedal spasm and laryngismus stridulus are all now rare complications.

Treatment
This consists of giving adequate amounts of vitamin D and minerals in the diet, which should be rich in milk, butter, fortified margarine, fresh eggs, green vegetables, meat and oily fish. This will require adjusting according to religious dietary laws.

The diet should be supplemented by vitamin D concentrates. Daily doses of 5000–50 000 iu (international units) of vitamin D or of calciferol by intramuscular injection or by mouth may be ordered in the active, acute stage.

The wearing of thick napkins should be avoided as they may cause bowing of the femora by holding the legs apart. Deformities are prevented by restricting walking and crawling in the acute stages and by nursing the infant on a firm, flat mattress.

Advice and education should be given to the parents to prevent recurrence of the disease and to protect the remaining members of the family. The health visitor and general practitioner will be able to provide local support.

PHENYLKETONURIA

Phenylketonuria is an inherited metabolic disorder, in which there is a failure to metabolize the amino acid, phenylalanine (Holton, 1985). This is due to the absence of the liver enzyme, phenylalaninase.

According to Nyhan (1980), the majority of children with phenylketonuria are fair, with blue eyes, a marked tendency to eczema, a small head, large alveolar arches and widely spaced teeth. Their growth is stunted and they are late in sitting up. There is a peculiar musty odour to the urine of these children and they often suffer from epileptic fits.

The basis of treatment lies in the dietary limitation of phenylalanine (Nyhan, 1980). Some of this essential amino acid must be given for normal tissue growth and repair, but not enough for an abnormal accumulation to develop in the blood. For treatment to be effective it must commence between the age of 2–6 weeks. Therefore, the early detection of phenylketonuria is of utmost importance if mental handicap is to be prevented.

The Guthrie test

A drop of blood is taken from a heel prick direct onto a filter paper and sent to the laboratory for specific culture tests, which will show whether there is an increased level of phenylalanine in the blood. The normal phenylalanine level is $0.06–0.12$ mmol/litre ($1–2$ mg/100 ml).

The test is reliable after the first week of life.

The diet

The basis of treatment lies in the dietary limitation of phenylalanine (Nyhan, 1980). Some of this essential amino acid must be given for normal tissue growth and repair, but not enough for an abnormal accumulation to develop in the blood.

Infants. Human milk is lower in protein and phenyl-alanine per unit of nitrogen than cow's milk. A 15% solution of Minafen (Cow & Gate) before each breast-fed lowers the intake of protein and phenylalanine by reducing the amount of breast milk taken.

Small amounts of cereal can be started at 3–4 months. Reduced protein foods are not introduced until breast-feeding is discontinued.

Older children. Aminogran (Allen & Hanbury's). The changeover from Minafen/breast milk to Aminogran should be made slowly. Ketovite vitamin supplements are essential to maintain health.

Successful treatment is monitored by maintaining dietary treatment according to serum phenylalanine levels, below 0.03 mmol/litre.

GALACTOSAEMIA

Galactosaemia is a familial disease caused by an inability to metabolize galactose and so leading to intoxication of the body and brain cells. The result is mental deficiency, cataract and cirrhosis of the liver. The baby fails to thrive, is drowsy, refuses his feed and vomits. Jaundice may be present from the first day of life. Oedema may give a false impression of a satisfactory gain in weight. The stools are loose and the liver becomes enlarged.

Treatment

Treatment must be started at once if it is to be effective. It entails substituting all feeds containing galactose or lactose by special preparations such as Nutramigen or Galactomin. Where these are not available, soya bean 'milk' to which Casilan, cane sugar, coconut oil, minerals and vitamins can be added, may be given.

Diagnosis
Whenever there is a familial history of the disease a simple test can be carried out on the cord blood, or alternatively a urine test will show the presence of galactosuria. Any finding of sugar in the urine must always be reported at once so that more specialized laboratory tests can be carried out.

DISORDERS OF LIPOID AND GLYCOGEN STORAGE

This group of diseases includes such rare conditions as xanthomatosis, Schüller-Christian syndrome, Gaucher's disease, Niemann-Pick disease and lipoidosis. In the last, abnormal amounts of various lipoids are stored in the reticulo-endothelial system. The chief damage is in the brain cells, but in spite of this, diagnosis can be confirmed by a simple rectal biopsy involving approximately 1 cm of full thickness bowel wall.

HYPOGAMMAGLOBULINAEMIA (IMMUNODEFICIENCY DISEASE)

Hypogammaglobulinaemia is a rare condition mostly seen in boys and the principal manifestation is a marked tendency to infections, as the lack of gamma globulin prevents antibody formation.

Treatment
Gamma globulin is given by weekly injections and in some cases prophylactic antibiotic treatment is ordered. Where a suitable donor can be found, bone marrow transfusion is given. This, combined with reverse barrier nursing in the initial phase of the disease, offers the best hope of a normal life.

STEATORRHOEA

Steatorrhoea is a symptom rather than a disease in itself and is the passage of fluid or excessively soft stools containing an unusual amount of fat.

Steatorrhoea may be caused by some disturbance in the function of the small intestine and the amount of fat present in the stools may vary from amounts so small that they are only found in the process of careful analysis, to visible, oily globules on the surface of the stools.

Signs and symptoms

The stools have a characteristic, highly offensive smell. Their appearance is putty-coloured, unformed and bulky and their frothy quality suggests the presence of fermentation. Occasionally fatty globules can be seen on the surface. The frequent loose evacuations may alternate with periods of constipation. Abdominal distension, redness around the anus, excoriated buttocks and rectal prolapse often accompany the steatorrhoea.

The affected child fails to thrive.

The abnormal fat losses and frequent stools may cause secondary symptoms such as a voracious appetite and tetany due to loss of calcium, which in turn results in a low blood calcium level, dehydration, stunted growth and lassitude.

Investigations

Investigations depend on the suspected, underlying cause and may include:

Heaf test and X-ray of abdomen (tuberculosis).

Barium meal and X-ray (congenital abnormalities affecting the gut).

Glucose tolerance curve (this is flat in coeliac disease).

Analysis of duodenal secretions and stools for tryptic activity (fibrocystic disease of the pancreas).

Sweat tests.

Examination of stools for ova, cysts, starch granules and excess of fat.

A fat balance may be done as one of the investigations.

Three-day stool collection for fat content estimation.

Stool collection for fat estimation. The simplest form of faecal fat estimation is carried out on stools collected over three consecutive days. The normal excretion being 5 g of fat in a 24-hour period, the excess is estimated. If a more accurate estimation is required an estimation of the amount ingested against that excreted is calculated.

All faeces must be collected and it is useful to line nappies or bedpans with cellophane or plastic material during the test period. The faeces can then be easily lifted into the collecting receptacle.

COELIAC DISEASE

Coeliac disease is a chronic condition which is commonly diagnosed during childhood, but is now less common (Stevens *et al.*, 1987). Peak frequency is between 9 and 18 months (Foster *et al.*, 1989).

The disease is caused by malabsorption of food from the intestines. There is abnormal sensitivity to gluten, found in wheat, rye and possibly also barley and oats (Brunner and Suddarth, 1986).

Signs and symptoms

Children with coeliac syndrome are stunted in growth and underweight and X-ray examination reveals osteoporosis (rarefaction) and immature development of bone due to poor vitamin absorption and calcium deficiency. Excess gas formation caused by fermentation of malabsorbed food causes abdominal pain and vomiting. The patient has a large, protuberant abdomen. The buttocks are wasted and the skin hangs in loose folds. The stools are bulky, putty coloured, unformed and greasy and have a characteristic, putrefied smell. The child may have his bowels opened several times a day (Jolly and Levene, 1985).

The child himself looks frail, stunted, pale and wizened, and usually utterly miserable, though the face may at first look round and well. The hair is sparse and dry, the limbs thin as drumsticks and cold to the touch. Poor muscle tone reflects itself in bad posture and rectal prolapse is common. Anaemia is a usual feature. The appetite is very poor and capricious. These children often have the strangest whims and their feeding may tax the ingenuity and patience of the nurse and his parents to the utmost.

Investigations
Analysis of stools, i.e. fat content, a complete blood count, a glucose tolerance test, a xylose excretion test and jejunal biopsy may all be performed. The jejunal biopsy is done with the aid of a Crosby capsule and may reveal characteristic flatness of the mucosa of duodenum and jejunum. A gluten challenge may be offered.

Jejunal biopsy. The child is starved for 4–6 hours before the procedure commences. Sedation may be prescribed. The doctor usually passes the capsule into the stomach. Gastric movement and peristaltic movement passes the capsule into the duodenum. With the aid of radiographs to ensure the capsule is in the jejunum, the capsule is 'fired'. The capsule is withdrawn containing the biopsy specimen of intestinal mucosa.

Following completion of the biopsy, the child is allowed to rest 12–24 hours. The child is observed for signs of

haemorrhage or perforation. Diet is gradually reintro-
duced over a 24-hour period, providing complications of
perforation and haemorrhage do not occur.

Principles of care
Admission to hospital cannot always be avoided, but the
stay should be cut to a minimum while investigations are
carried out, diagnosis confirmed and treatment established. Occasionally these children are acutely ill and
during that time require more intensive nursing care.

Because of weight loss and emaciation, skin and mouth
require special attention. Mouth toilet is carried out frequently and pressure areas treated.

As soon as possible, these children should be allowed to
get up and lead a normal life. Play activities are important
in stimulating interest and speeding recovery. Having a
parent resident will not only help the young patient but
will also teach the mother much about the handling of her
child and about the special diet (Whaley and Wong,
1987).

Diet
The main treatment is the introduction of a diet which is
free of gluten, which is contained in wheat and rye.
Gluten-free bread, cakes and rusks can be obtained and
gluten-free flour is available to make into cakes, bread,
biscuits and puddings. Lists of proprietary foods that are
gluten free is available from a dietician. At first, the fat
content of the diet may be restricted and extra protein
added. However, if all foods containing wheat and rye are
omitted, a normal amount of fat can soon be taken.

A satisfactory diet can be given, without much extra
work, if foods made of maize (corn), rice, sago, and
tapioca (not semolina) are substituted for those made of

wheat, rye, barley or oats. Extra vitamin A and D, folic acid and iron should be given.

The diet is continued for life, although small amounts of gluten may be tolerated as the child grows and becomes an adult. Gluten should be avoided during at least the first 2–5 years after diagnosis. The mother should be told that even minor deviations from the prescribed diet in the early stages of the disease may cause serious relapse.

Prognosis
The improvement is rapid following introduction of the diet. The stools soon become less bulky and offensive, the appetite improves and the child gains weight and is happier. Provided care is taken with the diet, this improvement should be maintained.

Complications
Complications include intercurrent infections; oedema due to low serum protein; rickets and terany due to impaired absorption of the fat-soluble vitamins.

As excess amounts of potassium and fluids are lost in the large stools, 'coeliac crises' due to electrolyte depletion occasionally call for urgent action. The child suddenly becomes severely dehydrated, lethargic and collapses. The temperature may rise by several degrees. Intravenous therapy may be necessary to correct both the blood chemistry and the dehydration.

CYSTIC FIBROSIS (MUCOVISCIDOSIS)

A multisystem disorder cystic fibrosis is characterized by a disturbance of exocrine gland function, resulting in raised levels of sodium chloride in the sweat and thick mucous secretions from the secretory glands. In the United Kingdom it is the most common of the inborn errors of metabolism, with an incidence of 1 in 2000 births. Most children with cystic fibrosis present in early life but the diagnosis can be made at any time, depending upon the severity of the symptoms (Byers, 1989). It is the most common life-threatening genetic disease in white-skinned people and is less common in those with a black skin (Foster *et al.*, 1989). More than one child in the family may be affected as the disease is transmitted as a recessive gene carried by each parent.

The production of the abnormal mucus results in chronic lung infections, pancreatic insufficiency and intestinal obstruction in the newborn (meconium ileus).

Signs and symptoms
Unlike the child suffering from coeliac disease, children with cystic fibrosis are friendly and good tempered. The appetite remains good in the absence of general infection but in spite of this there is failure to gain weight, growth is stunted, the abdomen is distended giving the child a 'barrel-like' appearance. The stools are pale and bulky, bowel actions are frequent and the smell is characteristically offensive (Whaley and Wong, 1987). Repeated chest infections are often a presenting symptom, the gastro-intestinal symptoms being revealed in the history.

When the disease is well-established at birth, intestinal obstruction results due to the failure to pass meconium. This is because the enzyme which would normally liquefy the meconium is absent. Urgent treatment either by surgery or treatment by Gastrografin enema under X-ray control is required.

Specific investigations

Boehringer meconium strip is smeared evenly with meconium and placed in water. Cystic fibrosis is diagnosed by the appearance of a bright blue colour at the end of the strip.

Sweat test is carried out by placing the child's washed fingers on an agar plate containing silver nitrate and potassium chromate. In cystic fibrosis the excess of chlorides in the sweat show up by the fingerprint impression being grey. For a more accurate test a sample of sweat may be collected on a weighted piece of filter paper (free from sodium chloride) after inducing local sweating with pilocarpine iontophoresis. The filter paper is handled with forceps and taken to the laboratory in a sealed container for chemical analysis. A child with cystic fibrosis usually excretes more than 60 mmol of sodium chloride per litre.

Duodenal intubation allows specimens of duodenal juice (including pancreatic enzymes) to be aspirated and analysed. The child is starved for 4 hours prior to the procedure and a Ryle's tube is passed. The child lies in a right lateral position and gastric motility and peristaltic action conveys the tube into the pyloric sphincter and into the duodenum. The location of the tube in the duodenum can be made by noting the change from an acid to an alkaline reaction.

Tryptic activity is examined in specimens of faeces. Trypsin is a proteolytic enzyme which is one of the pancreatic enzymes which may be absent or diminished in cystic fibrosis.

Principles of care and treatment

Nursing action	Explanation
Prescribed pancreatic enzyme preparations are to be taken with all meals.	To replace the enzymes blocked in the pancreas.

Nursing action	Explanation
Care to prevent irritation of the skin around the mouth.	The enzymes are strongly alkaline.
Diet. An intake of 150% of the recommended daily calorie allowance is advised to include high calorie drinks and snacks. A normal fat content may be allowed although medium chain triglyceride fats may be recommended if steatorrhoea is present.	Due to malabsorption problems loss of weight, poor growth and diminished energy may occur. A relationship between improved nutritional status and increased pulmonary muscle strength has been demonstrated (Mansell, 1984).
Vitamin supplements.	In particular, fat-soluble vitamin deficiencies are likely to occur.
Supplementary salt, particularly in hot climates.	Excessive sweating with high salt content is characteristic of the disease.
Chest physiotherapy with postural drainage and percussion. Parents are taught how to carry this out. The regimen is prescribed on an individual basis.	To clear the lungs of the thick tenacious mucus. Will be required for the rest of child's life.
Humidification of air breathed.	Helps to ease expectoration.
Prevention of cross-infection. Nurse away from children with other infections.	Poor lung drainage makes child susceptible to infection.
Frequent baths and changes of clothes.	Because of excessive sweating will promote patient's comfort and coolness.
Careful explanation to parents. Genetic counselling.	The disease is inherited by recessive genes.

Nursing action	**Explanation**
Suggest the help and services of the medical socialworker. Alert parents to Cystic Fibrosis Society.	Social and emotional problems may arise. Contact with other families in the society will provide on-going support.
The health visitor, school nurse and the community paediatric nursing service are informed of discharge.	To continue management and support at home.
Intravenous antibiotics may be prescribed which the parents and/or child can be taught to give at home.	

During recent years, the prognosis of children with the chronic and disabling condition of cystic fibrosis has much improved as a result of vigorous treatment and the prevention of respiratory infections and other complications. Adolescents require considerable counselling and support as they may become resentful about the long-term nature of the illness, its physical limitations, diet and therapy which may adversely affect compliance with regimens. The parents should be encouraged to treat their child in as normal a way as possible. Muller *et al.* (1988) suggest that other members of the family should be involved at an early stage in the exercises and treatment regime prescribed to minimize feelings of alienation. Some health authorities now have adolescent units which provide an environment that recognizes the special needs of these young people.

As more young people are surviving into adulthood sensitive arrangements should be made for their transfer to an adult physician at a time that suits the family and the adolescent. Time and discussion should be allowed for this to take place, especially as the teenager and family may have known the paediatric team over very many years. The time at which this occurs should depend upon on all the family circumstances to ensure the least disruption to lifestyle rather than solely on chronological age.

Since 1984 a number of children with severe respiratory disability have been successfully treated with heart/lung transplantation, but this treatment remains in its early stages.

REFERENCES

Brunner, L. and Suddarth, D. (1986). *Manual of Nursing Practice*, 4th edn, Ch. 37. Philadelphia: Lippincott.

Byers, C. (1989). Managing cystic fibrosis. *Paediatric Nursing* **1**(6), 14–18.

Foster, R., Hunsberger, M. and Anderson, J. (1989). *Family-Centered Nursing Care of Children*, Ch. 41. Philadelphia: Saunders.

Holton, J.B. (1985). *Inherited Metabolic Disorders*. London: Chapman and Hall.

Holton, J.B. and Tyfield, L. (1980). *The Child with Phenyl-ketonuria*, 2nd edn. West Yorkshire: NSPKU.

Jolly, H. and Levene, M.L. (1985). *Diseases of Children*, 5th edn, pp. 283–286. London: Blackwell Scientific.

Mansell, A.L. (1984). Short term pulmonary effects of total parenteral nutrition in children with cystic fibrosis. *Journal of Paediatrics* **104**, 700–705.

Muller, D.J., Harris, P.J. and Wattley, L. (1988). *Nursing Children: Psychology, Research and Practice*. London: Harper Row.

Nyhan, W.L. (1980). Understanding inherited metabolic disease. *Clinical Symposium* **22**(5), 13, 31.

Stevens, F.M., Egan-Mitchell, B., Cryan, E. *et al.* (1987). Decreasing incidence of coeliac disease. *Archives of Disease in Childhood* **62**, 465–468.

Whaley, L.F. and Wong, D.L. (1987). *Nursing Care of Infants and Children*, 3rd edn. St. Louis, MO: C.V. Mosby.

FURTHER READING

Anderson, C.M. and Goodchild, M.C. (1976). *Cystic Fibrosis*. London: Blackwell Scientific.

Ellis, R. *et al.* (1980). *Inborn Errors of Metabolism*. London: Croom Helm.

Francis, D.E.M. (1987). *Diets for Sick Children*, 4th edn. London: Blackwell Scientific.

Holton, J.B. (1985). *An Introduction to Inherited Metabolic Disorders*, 2nd edn. London: Chapman and Hall.

Holton, J.B. and Tyfield, L. (1980). *The Child With Phenylketonuria*, 2nd edn. West Yorkshire: NSPKU.

Sinclair, L. (1979). *Metabolic Disease in Childhood*. London: Blackwell Scientific.

11 The child with endocrine problems

Diseases of the endocrine system are comparatively rare in childhood but when they occur they may have a serious effect on mental and physical growth and maturation.

THE THYROID GLAND

Thyrotoxicosis

Over-secretion, causing thyrotoxicosis, is very uncommon in childhood. If it occurs, methyl thiouracil, carbimazole or potassium perchlorate and very occasionally surgery are employed in its treatment, in much the same way as for adults.

Hypothyroidism

Under-secretion of the thyroid gland causes cretinism in children. The condition, though congenital, is sometimes missed at birth as the infant carries a small amount of thyroid secretion from the maternal circulation. As the amount decreases, general metabolism is slowed down and symptoms appear.

Signs and symptoms
Children with congenital hypothyroidism have certain, typical characteristics. Their skin is cold, coarse and dry

with a yellow appearance. The hair is brittle, sparse and lacks lustre and the hair line grows low down on to the constantly puckered brow. A broad, flat nose with a depressed bridge lies between the small widely spaced eyes. The lips are thick and as the tongue is apparently too large for the mouth—it protrudes. The abdomen is large, and constipation and umbilical hernia are common features. Pads of fat over the clavicles make the neck appear short. As bony development is retarded, the fontanelles are late in closing, the head seems disproportionately large and the first teeth are late in coming through. The entire appearance is heavy, coarse and dull. As general metabolism is suppressed, the temperature is subnormal and the pulse rate slow. Anaemia is common. Speech develops late and some achieve only an elementary vocabulary. The voice is croaky and unmelodious. All milestones are late and, if left untreated, the child will be severely mentally handicapped.

Although not all these characteristics are noticeable at birth, the nurse may first notice the umbilical hernia and the constipation and, if she is alert and well-informed, may link these symptoms with the low temperature and sluggish pulse. Most are poor feeders, at least partly due to the abnormally large tongue which makes sucking difficult and also causes attacks of suffocation. An observant nurse or midwife can contribute greatly to a good prognosis as early treatment is the key to success.

Investigations

The ones likely to be carried out are: blood cholesterol and serum lipid levels, both of which tend to be raised; creatinine and protein-bound iodine levels, which are abnormally low; X-ray of bones to estimate the bone age; electrocardiogram and blood picture. A radioactive iodine-123 (^{123}I) uptake and scan are performed to identify the location, size and function of the thyroid tissue.

Treatment
Treatment should be started without delay and will have to be continued throughout life in order to replace the thyroxine which the abnormal gland cannot produce. Treatment may be so successful that the child develops normally. However, a great deal depends on the age at which treatment is begun. The treatment consists of giving thyroxine in dosages just below the point at which signs of intolerance appear. The initial dose for infants is 25 µg daily and this is increased until tachycardia, diarrhoea and wakefulness suggest that the dosage has passed the tolerance level. Tolerance may be higher during the cold season than in the summer months. The maintenance dose is fixed slightly below the maximum reached during the stabilizing period.

Nursing care and observations
During the initial stage, nursing care is symptomatic. The infant should be kept warm and the nurse feeding the baby will have to be both experienced and very patient. Suppositories or Milk of Magnesia will have to be given for the constipation and the skin should be kept supple with baby creams or lotions. Care must be taken when the baby is placed in his cot and it is safest to lie him on his side to guard against the danger of respiratory obstruction caused by the large tongue.

Once thyroid therapy has been started, the nursing observations will be the principal guide in determining the maintenance dosage. Signs of response, such as an increased pulse rate and a rise in the body temperature, are all due to an increase in the metabolic rate. There is an improvement in the infant's colour and activity and a drop in weight due to the disappearance of the excess fat. The bowels will start to act regularly. The infant will be more alert and interested in his feeds.

The nurse should keep full and accurate observation charts. The feeds may have to be large for a time to satisfy the newly found appetite and to supply adequate nourishment for the sudden progress. It is well worth while to arrange for a little extra attention by the mother or nurse to encourage every attempt at play and to help the infant develop his activities and mental achievements.

THE PITUITARY GLAND

The chief importance of the pituitary gland is probably its influence on the other ductless glands. Abnormalities of the anterior lobe cause gigantism if there is over-secretion, dwarfism if there is under-secretion. Abnormalities of the posterior lobe cause diabetes insipidus.

The abnormalities may be congenital or may be caused by pressure from intracranial tumours or by inflammatory conditions such as encephalitis. None of these conditions are sufficiently common to warrant description in a small handbook and the reader is referred to larger text books for greater detail.

The hormone activity of the gland, however, is of great interest. The pituitary gland produces adrenocortico-trophic hormone (ACTH) which makes the adrenal cortex produce hormones with three effects:

1. On carbohydrate metabolism.
2. On mineral metabolism affecting blood electrolytes.
3. On growth and maturity, including masculinization if there is excess in the female.

Growth Hormone Deficiency

Some children fail to grow normally, even though they were of normal weight and length at birth and the parents are known to be of average height and build. This type of growth failure is commonly due to deficient secretion of growth hormone from the anterior lobe of the pituitary. Replacement therapy can be given by regular intra-muscular injections of synthetic growth hormone, usually over a period of 2–3 years at a specialized referral growth clinic.

THE ADRENAL GLANDS

Diseases of the adrenal and suprarenal glands are extremely rare in childhood and are usually due to tumours, injury at birth resulting in haemorrhage, or infections such as tuberculosis. Both the diagnosis and treatment are difficult, though the discovery of cortisone has contributed much to the understanding of the diseases caused by over- or under-secretion of the glands.

Tumours of the medulla are often malignant and cause metastases in the liver, lungs and bone tissue. Surgery in the less malignant type of tumours, however, carries a hopeful prognosis. The adrenal medulla produces adrenaline and noradrenaline which, like cortisone, have a place in the treatment of asthma and shock.

Over-activity of the adrenal cortex leads to sexual precocity in both sexes and to virilism in the female. The over-activity may be present before birth and in this case causes pseudohermaphroditism (see below). In the young child over-activity causes sexual precocity and virilism and if the anterior pituitary gland is secondarily affected, Cushing's syndrome will result. True Cushing's syndrome is rare in childhood but is often simulated when a child is having too large a dose of steroids. The child characteristically becomes 'moon-faced', looking flushed and bloated. Obesity develops, with pads of fat accumulating on the upper part of the back, producing a 'buffalo hump' together with a fat abdomen and hips. In contrast the limbs remain thin. Growth of hair occurs on the face and body, together with purple striae on the trunk. Acne is common. Hypertension is usually present, and the child may complain of headaches. Glycosuria may also be found on routine testing.

Adrenogenital Syndrome

Very occasionally in some children there is difficulty in determining the sex of the child, owing to the malformation of the external genitalia in the male or masculinization of the genitalia in the female. This occurs as a rare genetic disorder. For a correct sex determination to be made it is necessary for chromosome studies to be carried out. To avoid distress to the parents and to the child in subsequent development it is important, in all these cases, that necessary examination of the blood, urine and smears from the buccal membrane are undertaken before the birth is registered. Nurses should see to it that these children are not subjected to unnecessary examinations, as even very young children are sensitive to handling of the genital area.

Great understanding and counselling are needed in helping the parents to understand and adjust to the condition of their child. Cortisone therapy and plastic surgery may be beneficial to some of these children. Surgery is usually performed in the first year of life to avoid psychological trauma at an older age (Foster *et al.*, 1989). Long-term follow-up to assess progress and appropriate adjustment of therapy will be required.

Steroid therapy
The adrenal cortex produces hormones with three effects:

1. On carbohydrate metabolism.
2. On mineral metabolism affecting blood electrolytes.
3. On growth and maturity, including masculinization if there is excess in the female.

In addition, excessive amounts can damp down inflammatory reactions by interfering with antigen–antibody reactions and can cause the production of ACTH by the pituitary to be lowered.

Cortisone or similar preparations such as prednisone, prednisolone or triamcinolone can be given by mouth and hydrocortisone by injection for the following purposes:

1. To make up for deficiency of the adrenal activity as in shock or in Addison's disease.
2. To suppress the production of ACTH in cases of precocious sexual development of a masculine type.
3. To suppress antigen–antibody reaction, as in rheumatic fever, rheumatoid arthritis, some types of nephritis, asthma and haemolytic anaemia.

The use and choice of steroid depends upon the child's disease and condition, balanced against the known adverse effects of steroid therapy (see Table 8).

Long-term treatment
When long-term corticosteroid therapy is given, the maintainance dose should be kept as low as possible to minimize the side-effects. When treatment is to be discontinued, the dose should be reduced gradually over a period of several weeks.

The parents should be given a 'steroid card' giving details of dosage, together with the drug name and

TABLE 8 Adverse effects of steroid therapy and its management in children

Main adverse effects of steroid therapy in children	Due to	Principles of care
Weight gain Oedema Hypertension Disturbed electrolytes Tiredness Lethargy	The mineralocorticoid effect upon sodium and potassium metabolism	Daily weighing. Regular measurement of blood pressure. Maintain fluid record charts. Low salt diet
Suppression of growth	Excessive loss of calcium and phosphorus	Adequate calcium and protein in diet. Stunted growth may be mitigated by giving steroids only on alternate days
Glycosuria, which may lead to diabetes mellitus	Glucocorticoid effect on carbohydrate metabolism and insulin utilization	Daily urinalysis for glucose
May allow potentially very damaging infection to pass unrecognized, e.g. tuberculosis	Modification of tissue reaction resulting from suppression of antigen–antibody reaction	Keep child away from known infection. Be aware of risk and record child's temperature appropriately
Altered behaviour pattern		Note and report any change from usual behaviour

possible complications to be alert to. They should also know that if for any reason they need to seek other medical or dental care for their child the card should be presented to the practitioner before treatment is commenced. Anaesthetists also need to know if a child is taking or has been taking corticosteroids, as adrenal suppression may cause a precipitous fall in blood pressure during anaesthesia.

DIABETES MELLITUS

Diabetes mellitus is the most common endocrine disease of childhood. Children with diabetes suffer from deficient insulin action caused either by a diminished insulin excretion by the islets of Langerhans in the pancreas, or due to the presence of insulin antagonists which render any insulin produced ineffective for carbohydrate metabolism, resulting in glycosuria, ketosis and eventually coma.

It is now recognized that diabetes mellitus is not a single disease but rather a complex of clinical signs and symptoms or a syndrome. There is an agreed international classification system (National Diabetes Data Group) and the various types of diabetes are divided as follows:

Type 1: Diabetes mellitus—insulin dependent and non-insulin dependent.
Type 2: Gestational diabetes.
Type 3: Altered states of carbohydrate metabolism.

Because most children fall into Type 1 this text will concentrate on this group.

In children, the onset of diabetes is usually very sudden and, although never actually responsible for the disease, infections such as tonsillitis or measles, and emotional stress seem to act as the trigger starting off the symptoms.

Signs and symptoms

Most obvious, and therefore often first noticed, is the sudden excessive thirst, coupled with frequency of micturition or the onset of enuresis in a previously clean child. The output of urine is large but in spite of this it is of high specific gravity. The child grows listless and fractious. As dehydration occurs, the skin becomes dry and he is constipated. The breath may smell of acetone. The tongue is dry but, as a rule, it remains clean but abnormally red. Loss of weight may be rapid and considerable and a proportion of children develop an unusual appetite.

The penis or vulva is often red and irritating due to the high sugar content of the urine, and the child may complain of abdominal pain. As ketosis increases, vomiting sets in and may hasten the occurrence of diabetic coma. The urine contains glucose and ketones.

Investigations

These include testing of urine, blood sugar estimation and glucose tolerance tests. Serum bicarbonate, blood pH and plasma carbon dioxide will need estimating if ketoacidosis is present.

If possible, tests involving needle punctures and fasting should be spaced and not all done the first day after admission, as it is important to preserve the young patient's confidence since he will probably be starting on a lifetime of daily insulin injections.

Treatment

Some specialists like to treat these children as outpatients as they feel that the child should be assessed and stabilized under his usual living conditions. The majority feel, however, that the child should be admitted to hospital so that the investigations and the initial stabilizing can take place under controlled and known conditions. The fact that in hospital the child's activities are, of necessity, restricted should always be borne in mind. The mother should be asked about the child's normal routine, and exercise should be given so that the child's usual energy output is maintained.

Children with diabetes should never be kept in bed unnecessarily. From the start, a healthy attitude and interest should be fostered and any special diet should be accepted as a natural part of the young diabetic's routine.

It is essential that children with diabetes wear an identification bracelet or badge at all times.

Nursing goals

Foster *et al.* (1989) has defined the goals for the care of a child with Type 1 diabetes as:

1. Metabolic control of the child's diabetes
2. Self-care by the child or the family through education about illness management and
3. Normal growth and development of the child and family.

The diet

With the present-day insulins, which are very stable and long-acting (e.g. the Lente group), the child, once stabilized, can be kept free from reactions by allowing his appetite to regulate his blood sugar levels. It will be found that if he has been unusually energetic he will also be very hungry, and if he has sat quietly for a time his appetite will decrease. Periodic tests to estimate the serum cholesterol levels are done. If the level rises, foods containing cholesterol are omitted from the diet (e.g. eggs) as a persistently raised serum cholesterol level predisposes to vascular changes in later life. Children receiving an unrestricted diet are much less likely to have the psychological problems which children who are placed on a restricted diet tend to develop. However, some paediatricians continue to advocate a strictly controlled diet on the grounds that it lessens the chances of future vascular complications.

For children who are learning about the importance of the diabetic condition, there are playing cards, charts and games, e.g. Diaguest (Beckton-Dickenson), a children's diabetes quiz game, which help them to memorize the new knowledge. 'Rupert and his Friends' (Ames, Slough) is a useful booklet that can also be used as a teaching aid.

Insulin Therapy

The dose of insulin will have to be readjusted until the condition is stabilized. This may not happen until some weeks after discharge home. Adjustment will usually become necessary when the child has an infection or any severe emotional upset; as he grows and increases in weight; and especially at the time of puberty. The aim is to find the dose which will enable the child to live a normal life on a diet adequate for growth, energy and enjoyment of life. It is here assumed that the reader has already a sound understanding of the types of insulin available and of the various syringes and their markings, as well as of the principles involved in insulin therapy (see Table 9). In these aspects there is no difference when dealing with young diabetics as compared with adults, but the approach to the problem of diabetes in childhood is important and specialized.

Both the parents and the child should be taught how to give injections, monitor blood glucose and test urine as needed, and, to understand the principles involved. By the age of 8 years it should be possible to teach most children to inject themselves with insulin and to draw up the dose, even if it is still checked by the parents (Fig. 28).

FIG. 28 Diabetic child injecting herself with insulin using automatic injector.

The site of the injections should be as varied as possible in order to prevent thickening of the tissues and local fat atrophy which, though harmless, causes unsightly depressions and irregularities in the contours of the limb. The injection should be given fairly deeply with the needle almost at right angles to the skin.

General points
Both the child and parents should be helped to come to grips with the disability and the latter should not be allowed to make the child into an invalid by misplaced

TABLE 9   Some recommended insulin regimens

Insulin	Regimen
Short-acting insulin mixed with Intermediate-acting insulin	Twice daily (before meals)
Short-acting insulin mixed with Intermediate-acting insulin	Before breakfast
Short-acting insulin	Before evening meal
Intermediate-acting insulin	Bedtime
Short-acting insulin	Three times daily (before breakfast, mid-day and evening meal)
Long-acting insulin (e.g. Ultratard)	Bedtime
Short-acting insulin mixed with Intermediate-acting insulin	Before breakfast (sufficient in some cases)

solicitude. Both the parents and the child, once old enough, should be taught the fundamentals of the illness and should be allowed to practise blood glucose, urine testing and the giving of injections well before discharge, so as to gain confidence and dexterity in so doing.

It is a good plan to allow children to experience one or more insulin reactions while still under supervision in hospital, so that after discharge, they will be able to guard, in good time, against any serious hypoglycaemic reaction.

Insulin is now standardized on a single strength insulin of 100 units/ml (U 100). This has the advantage of simplifying the measurement of dosages because it will be possible to read off the units of insulin directly on the U 100 syringe.

Education

Most diabetic children can attend normal schools provided the teachers know of their condition. Hypoglycaemic reaction is often heralded by naughty or unusual behaviour, and glucose or a lump of sugar may correct the hypoglycaemia without much disturbances. Teachers should have sugar or glucose available, but, when old enough, the young diabetic should be made responsible for recognizing and dealing with a hypoglycaemic reaction by taking sugar from an own emergency supply which should always be carried by the child. It is usually possible to allow diabetic children to have the usual school meals, as the high carbohydrate content of school puddings supplies the extra amount needed during the exertion of the afternoon games period.

Holidays

Under controlled conditions and supervision, the Diabetic Association runs holiday camps which have the added value that the children meet other diabetics, often learn much from each other and come to realize that they are not alone with their diabetes.

Hyperglycaemic or Diabetic Coma

The signs of oncoming coma are essentially the same in children as in adults, but a child's behaviour may differ according to age. Thus a very young child may demand to be put to bed or may curl up in a corner and fall asleep. Shock and dehydration often come on very rapidly and both may be severe.

Hypoglycaemic or Insulin Coma

Insulin coma comes on even more suddenly than diabetic coma. It often happens that the child is hard to wake in the morning and, when roused, looks pale and apprehensive and shows a peculiar emotional behaviour.

Points of importance
If there is any doubt about the nature of the reaction, the child should be given some glucose, as little harm can be done by hyperglycaemia, while insulin coma may require urgent relief. It is useful to remember that 2 slightly heaped teaspoonfuls of sugar in water equal approximately 10 g of carbohydrate.

Administering Insulin—Education of Child and Parents

Aim
The child with diabetes and at least one parent should be fully competent in the preparing, drawing up and the giving of insulin.

Checklist

1. Do they all understand the need for insulin injections? Ask the parents, and the child where possible, for an explanation in their own words. Correct any misunderstandings. Provide with the literature that is available.

2. Provide syringe and needles and opportunities to take these apart. Note their different pieces, structure and the measurements on the side of the barrel. Answer any questions fully.

3. Emphasize the need for cleanliness of hands, skin of injection site, and equipment for the prevention of any infection.

4. Discuss the need to rotate injection sites. Suggest it might be helpful for the child, initially, to keep a chart showing this rotation. The child may like to design one of his own; a decorated body outline is often a good idea.

5. Insulin. How this is obtained and the need to maintain supplies, and where to store vials, which should be in a cool place. Instruct carefully in the calculation of insulin dosage.

6. Finally, drawing up of the insulin and administering an injection. 'Try-outs' with sterile water on 'teddy' or oranges, or thick foam pads should be supervised. The giving of insulin under supervision is the final goal.

The assimilation of this new knowledge may take several days or weeks depending on many variable factors, e.g. age of the child, intelligence of the child and the parents, the impact of anxiety and stress impeding uptake of new knowledge. The nurse needs to be prepared to repeat each stage frequently and to reassure the child and the parents as to the progress being made. Set realistic goals for the family to achieve in realizing the aims set.

REFERENCE

Foster, R.L., Hunsberger, M.M. and Anderson, J. (1989). *Family-Centered Nursing Care of Children*. Philadelphia: Saunders.

FURTHER READING

Baum, J.D. and Kinmouth, A.L. (1985). *Care of a Child with Diabetes*. Edinburgh: Churchill Livingstone.

Brooke, C.G.D. (ed.) (1989). *Clinical Paediatric Endocrinology*. Oxford: Blackwell Scientific.

Drury, M.I. (1986). *Diabetes Mellitus*. Oxford: Blackwell Scientific.

Farquhar, J.W. (1981). *The Diabetic Child*, 3rd edn. London: Churchill Livingstone.

Hughes, I.A. (1986). *Handbook of Endocrine Tests in Children*. Bristol: John Wright.

McLean, T. (1985). *Sam Metal. The Story of a Diabetic*. London: Hodder and Stoughton.

12 The child with neurological problems and learning difficulties

Basically, examination of a child's nervous system is the same as for an adult. A child, however, is unable to describe his symptoms accurately and he will often be irritable and uncooperative. It will always help if the child's mother or a nurse whom the child knows and trusts can be present to assist the paediatrician. It is important to allow plenty of time for the child to settle in the unfamiliar surroundings.

Most of the history of the child will be obtained from the mother and it is traced back to include information about pregnancy and delivery. It is important to know whether there were any signs of cyanosis or asphyxia at birth and whether the baby was pre-term or born at term. The paediatrician will also want to know if there is any family history of epilepsy, mental handicap or any other illness.

EXAMINATION OF THE NERVOUS SYSTEM

The paediatrician will note any abnormality of the skull such as bossing, asymmetry, head circumference and the size of the fontanelles. In certain cases, such as suspected cerebral lesions or intercranial tumours, it may be important to notice the way in which the child holds his head.

The child may be unable to accurately reach objects held out and may have a tremor of the hand. In certain diseases the way in which the child rises from the floor to a standing position is in itself diagnostic. Sometimes the absence or presence of normal skills gives the best guide towards assessment and diagnosis.

An assessment of the child's behaviour will be made in order to establish:

Motor development.
Activity patterns.
Speech development.
Cognitive development.
Sensory evaluation.

To test the reflexes is important. Reflexes in the very young infant are unusually brisk and the plantar reflex is still extensor and only becomes flexor, as in the adult, when the child starts to walk.

Assessment of Consciousness

A comatosed state has been defined by Whaley and Wong (1987) as:

... diminished alertness as a result of pathological conditions occurs as a continuum and is designated as the comatosed state, which extends from somm- nolence on one end to deep coma at the other.

Levels of consciousness are determined by observing the child's response to his environment. Several scales of coma assessment for adults have been introduced in order to standardize practitioner interpretation and description of consciousness levels. The most universally used scale is the Glasgow coma scale. This scale, devised for adult evaluation, consists of a three-part assessment, eye

TABLE 10   Adult Glasgow coma scale with scores

Behaviour	Response	Score
Eye opening	Spontaneous	4
	To speech	3
	To pain	2
	None	1
Verbal response	Orientated	5
	Confused	4
	Inappropriate words	3
	Incomprehensible sounds	2
	None	1
Motor response	Obeys commands	5
	Localizes	4
	Flexion	3
	Extension	2
	None	1

TABLE 11   Paediatric coma scale (Adelaide scale)

Behaviour	Age	Response
Eye opening		Spontaneous
		To speech
		To pain
		None
Best verbal response	5 yrs	Orientated to place
	12 mths	Words
		Vocal sounds
	6 mths	Cries
		None
Best motor response	6 mths–5 yrs	Obeys commands
		Localizes pain
	6 mths	Flexion pain
		Extension pain
		None

opening, verbal response and motor response and then arranged in order of increasing dysfunction. Whilst the Glasgow coma scale (Table 10) can be used for the older child and adolescent it requires modification for use with the younger child. An example of such a coma scale modification is the Adelaide scale (Table 11) (Simpson and Reilly, 1982). The modifications in the Adelaide scale primarily affect the verbal and motor responses in recognition of the individual child's developmental stage and neurological maturity.

When assessing levels of consciousness it is helpful to have a parent or familiar adult present to help elicit a desired response. An infant or child may not respond in an unfamiliar environment or to unfamiliar voices (Whaley and Wong, 1987).

SOME NEUROLOGICAL PROCEDURES

Lumbar Puncture

Lumbar puncture is the same for children as for adults and is done for the same reasons. Using a language which the child understands, explain simply why lying in an uncomfortable position for this procedure is required. An explanation should also be given to the parents. This will help to reassure the child and gain co-operation. The mother may wish to be present to hold the child or to sit by the child's head to comfort. It is, however, important to have complete control when holding the child. Very young children are often best lifted onto a table or a well-padded locker. Really adequate control is, as a rule, best achieved by the following means. The child is made comfortable on the pillow or mattress and the back flexed as much as possible in order to separate the spinous processes of the vertebrae. The person holding the child

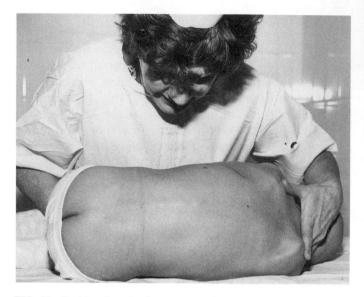

FIG. 29   Position for a lumbar puncture (a face mask may be worn by the nurse).

then hooks one arm round the neck, the other round the crook of the flexed knees and allows the hands to meet in front of the patient, so forming a complete circle with hands and arms and the child's body (Fig. 29). Although safely restrained the child can breathe adequately and the holder does not tire easily as the pull on their own hands gives them strength and support. The child should be adequately still, neither struggling nor crying while the pressure is being read, lest false readings be obtained.

Whenever it is thought that lumbar puncture may have to be done repeatedly, a sedative or light anaesthetic should be given so as to minimize possible fear and psychological trauma.

In children, headaches rarely follow lumbar puncture

and the routine of keeping the patient flat and the foot of the bed raised is not necessary unless air has been injected as for the purpose of an air encephalogram.

Ventriculography

For ventriculography the head has to be shaved, as the blunt cannula is introduced through the scalp, directly into the ventricles. In young infants this can be done through the still-open fontanelle or the still-ununited sutures. In older patients it is necessary to make burr holes in the skull. Approximately 40 ml of filtered air or pure oxygen is then injected after withdrawing a similar quantity of cerebrospinal fluid.

In either case, radiographs are taken immediately after the air has been injected. By placing the patient in different positions the movement of the air through the ventricular system and the shape, size and position of the ventricles can be clearly seen. This procedure may be carried out following a brain scan to demonstrate more detail in brain structures.

Aftercare

1. Record temperature, pulse, respiration and blood pressure at frequent and regular intervals until stabilized.

2. Observe for signs of raised intracranial pressure.

3. Keep the child quiet and comfortable. Give analgesics as prescribed for any headache.

Radio-opaque Methods

Angiography is used when it is desirable to outline blood vessels of the brain. An injection of a radio-opaque dye is made into the main carotid artery in the neck. As the dye circulates through the arteries their outline can be seen on the X-ray screen or film. Pictures are taken in rapid succession. In this way abnormalities such as angiomata of the brain can be clearly seen and accurately located.

In cases of suspected non-communicating hydro-cephalus, contrast or radio-opaque media may be injected into the ventricle through the anterior fontanelle or through burr holes, and the site of a hold-up may be seen in the radiograph. Radio-opaque substances may also be injected into the spinal cord to discover the site of a spinal tumour.

Possible complications

These may include: bleeding from injection site, hemi-paresis, disturbances of blood pressure, convulsions, and infection.

Aftercare

1. Frequent observations of the injection site for any oozing or haematoma formation.

2. Pulse, temperature, respiration and blood pressure recordings at regular intervals.

3. Report any indication of speech disturbance, altera-tion in responsiveness or muscle weakness.

Electroencephalogram

It is known that rhythmical electric charges of a certain pattern and frequency are exhibited in the human brain and that both pattern and frequency change in disease. Recordings can be made by means of electrical leads placed on the patient's scalp. The graphs obtained are typical of certain diseases and are a valuable aid to diag-nosis. It is desirable to have a fully co-operative patient, capable of obeying instructions (e.g. to open or close his eyes) and this is often achieved by arranging for the mother or for the child's own nurse to be present. Frequently, however, a sedative has to be given.

Brain Scan

This is a non-invasive technique which demonstrates any tumour or other pathology in the brain.

A radioactive substance is first given to the child either orally or intravenously. This radioactivity diffuses into any

FIG. 30 Child in a scanner.

abnormal cerebral tissue and is picked up by the scanner which prints out the uptake as a picture.

The child should lie quietly and still during the scan and this should be explained before the procedure.

EPILEPSY AND CONVULSIONS

Epilepsy and convulsion should, like cough be regarded as symptoms rather than diagnostic entities.
Brett, *Children in Health and Disease*

Febrile Convulsions

These occur in about 5% of children under the age of 5 years, especially in those with a similar history in siblings or in a parent. The convulsion is associated with the rapid rise in temperature which may herald the onset of an infection. Immediate treatment is to control the convulsion with intravenous or rectal diazepam or clonazepam. The parents should also be given advice on how to prevent the convulsions from recurring: by giving paracetamol orally and to keep the child cool whenever he becomes feverish. Some of these children may develop epilepsy later in life.

Infantile Spasms

These usually begin between the age of 3–18 months. A typical attack involves repeated flexion of the head and trunk forward whilst the arms are raised up. Numerous attacks occur daily. The prognosis is poor. Commonly associated with mental handicap, the spasms may lead to major convulsions from about the age of 4 years.

Treatment is aimed at controlling the spasms with one

of the anticonvulsants. Corticosteroids and ACTH have been used successfully in improving the associated EEG abnormality and also in reducing the number of attacks.

Petit Mal

This rarely occurs before the age of 3 years.

Attacks of minor epilepsy may be so mild that they are only noticed by those who are in constant contact with the patient. The loss of consciousness is so fleeting that, after a momentary pause, the patient immediately resumes his activities as if nothing had happened. The eyes may take on a momentary dazed look or there may be a feeling of giddiness or a loss of postural control.

Major Epilepsy

The stages of a major epileptic attack are the same in children as in adults, but children frequently become irritable or cling to their mothers as if seeking comfort during the period of aura. Occasionally there is no loss of consciousness nor are there true convulsive movements but the child shows considerable behaviour disturbances or temporary loss of memory and, in some cases, un-explained headaches or abdominal pain are thought to be of epileptic origin.

A variety of drugs are used to control convulsions. These include carbamazepine, phenobarbitone, Mysolin, Epanutin or various combinations of anticonvulsant drugs. Some of these drugs have serious side-effects and the nurse should be well-informed about them, and make careful observations.

In dealing with a child in a convulsion, the principal concern is to keep the child from harm. If up and about, the nurse should lay the child on a bed or on the floor away from any harmful object. The child's head should be turned to the side to allow saliva to drain freely and to prevent inhalation. Tight clothing should be loosened. If the attack occurs in bed, pillows are best removed. Avoid restraint.

As consciousness is regained, the patient is likely to be bewildered, and reassurance and comfort should be given. A warm drink may help restful sleep.

In hospital, an airway and swabs are usually kept near the beds of known epileptic children but these should be covered and out of sight of both child and visitors. While looking after the patient the nurse should make careful observations. Parents may well be very used to managing the child during a fit and able to participate in observing for changes.

Observations
How did the fit start? Was there an aura, noise in the ears, or flash or light? Were there any movements? Where did they begin? Where did they spread to? Were the movements tonic or clonic? Was there a tremor and eye movements?

Did the patient lose consciousness? Were the eyes open or closed? If closed, could they be opened? Towards which side were they turned? If lightly touched, did the eyes blink? Was there incontinence, cyanosis, and/or breath holding? Did the patient bite his tongue? What was the duration of the fit? Was the patient drowsy or confused after the fit? Did the patient show abnormal or unusual behaviour after the fit? What could the patient remember about the fit?

General principles of care
The aim should always be that the child with epilepsy is encouraged to lead as normal a life as possible. Both the

parents and the child should be given every opportunity to ask questions and to discuss freely the nature of the illness and of the fits.

Some of these children may have an associated degree of mental handicap although many are of normal or of high intelligence. Schooling provision should be considered on an individual basis in full consultation with the parents and the education authorities.

Behavioural disturbances, e.g. temper tantrums or overactivity, are common and psychiatric help may be indicated. Every encouragement and support should be given to the child to promote independence, e.g. in accepting responsibility for medication. The only limitations on physical activities should be that children should not be allowed to swim or to climb on their own.

MENINGITIS (INFLAMMATION OF THE MENINGES)

Meningitis is more common in children than in adults. The main types are classified according to the causative organism:

1. Pyogenic, e.g. meningococci, pneumococci, staphylococci.
2. Viral or aseptic meningitis.
3. Tuberculous meningitis.

Presentation
Initial presentation depends upon the age of onset, but includes:

Headaches and pain in back of neck.
Vomiting and nausea.
Fever.

FIG. 31 Extreme opisthotonos due to cerebral irritation in a young baby.

Irritability, restlessness with a high-pitched meningeal cry.

Photophobia.

Later signs:

Increasing drowsiness.
Resentful at being touched.
Opisthotonos (see Fig. 31).
Convulsions.

Diagnosis

Established by lumbar puncture and laboratory examination of the cerebrospinal fluid. Blood culture and throat swabs should be taken, together with blood for a full blood count and electrolyte estimation.

Treatment

Appropriate antibiotics intravenously or intrathecally.

Principles of care

1. Provide minimal nursing intervention in a quiet room or space that is compatible with the child's condition. Barrier nursing may be required to prevent the spread of infection (see p. 427).

2. Frequent observations to monitor child's response to treatment:

Temperature, pulse and respiration.

Blood pressure.

Head circumference in the young infant should be measured.

Neurological status and behaviour.

Intake and output, to assess renal function.

3. Basic comfort care, particularly of pressure areas and mouth. Position semi-conscious or unconscious child on side and turn at regular intervals. Frequent suction to nasopharynx to prevent aspiration of secretions.

4. Assess nutritional status:

Oral feeding if child is conscious and able to tolerate adequate amounts.

Nasogastric feeding if child is semi-comatosed or unconscious.

Intravenous infusion.

Whatever route is chosen, the aim should be to provide at least sufficient kilojoules (Calories) to meet energy requirements and enough fluids to maintain hydration.

5. Provide stimulation as the child progresses with suitable play activities according to age and interests.

6. Support for parents. Encourage their participation in care. Provide opportunities for questions to be asked about their child's progress and future.

N.B. Prophylaxis for close contacts of children with

meningococcal or *Haemophilus influenzae* meningitis may be indicated.

Prognosis
In most instances complete recovery may be expected, but much depends on early diagnosis and prompt, effective treatment. The outlook is most serious in very young infants and the prognosis should always be somewhat guarded.

Complications
Complications include neurological disturbances, hydro-cephalus, mental deficiency, paralysis, deafness and con-vulsions. A special point worth remembering is that, in young infants, meningitis may occur in a *sub-acute form.* There may be little or no fever; diarrhoea and vomiting may lead to dehydration and sunken eyes and fontanelle. Together with these misleading symptoms neurological examination is difficult and often atypical in babies, and only lumbar puncture can confirm the diagnosis of meningitis.

ACUTE ENCEPHALITIS

Acute encephalitis may be caused by viral infections, specific fevers and, rarely, by vaccination.

Signs and symptoms
The onset of the disease is very acute with high fever, severe headache, vomiting, visual disturbances and some-times convulsions and loss of consciousness. Patients may be so confused as to become irrational and violent to an extent which necessitates restraint.

Treatment
Antibiotics may be given to treat any secondary infection.

Steroids are often prescribed although their value in the treatment of encephalitis is not clear.

Principles of care
Generally supportive and along the same lines as the care of a child with meningitis (see p. 319).

Tracheostomy and/or mechanical ventilation may be required for the comatosed child.

The prognosis is variable, emotional and behavioural problems are common in the convalescent phase of the illness which may be prolonged.

INTRACRANIAL TUMOUR

Intracranial, space-occupying lesions are fairly common, particularly in children of 5–10 years old. Treatment is surgical combined with chemotherapy and radiotherapy. According to their situation the lesions cause complications by pressure, e.g. pressure on the pituitary gland, causing diabetes insipidus. Some of these tumours are malignant and inoperable but in many cases there is reasonable hope of successful treatment. The commonest site is the cerebellum and the pressure here causes the patient to suffer from vomiting which is difficult to control. Papilloedema is usually present and the child is grossly ataxic.

Principles of care
Care will need to be related to the individual child's treatment and general condition. The aims will include the alleviation of pain and other distressing symptoms, and the provision of emotional support to the parents and child. Surgical treatment will involve shaving the child's head which may cause added distress to child and parents. Reassurance with the possibility of a wig post-operatively helps to allay anxiety.

CEREBRAL PALSY

Cerebral palsy is caused by defect or disease of the brain affecting the upper motor neurones and is liable to occur any time before, during or after birth. The disease is not progressive.

Children suffering from cerebral palsy have difficulty in carrying out co-ordinated movements. The adductor muscles of the thigh in particular go into spasm (the scissor attitude). The gait is unsteady or clumsy, and is often reminiscent of a drunken man, charging forward, dragging a foot and stumbling about, or the movements may be slow and writhing. The incoordination of the respiratory muscles leads to frequent chest infections. Speech is difficult if the lip, tongue and laryngeal muscles are affected and the child may grimace in an attempt at forming words. What speech is possible is often explosive and the abnormal functioning of the respiratory muscles causes the child to make uncontrolled, animal-like noises. This may intensify the impression that the child is mentally abnormal. In addition he has difficulty in swallowing and he may have a constant dribble of saliva down his chin. Poor mastication causes dental decay, anaemia and malnutrition.

Many spastic children have a squint caused by muscle spasm, and visual disturbances such as double vision are common. Hearing defects are often associated with cerebral palsy, and these and the visual defects are often partly responsible for the delay in acquiring speech and learning to read.

Principles of care and treatment
The aim is to make a full assessment and then set to work on those muscle groups and abilities which give hope of response and seem capable of development.

Teamwork is the essence in the treatment of cerebral palsy.

This 'teamwork' concept will need to include the parents and other members of the child's family as participants in order to be fully effective.

The education of the child with cerebral palsy must depend to some extent on the degree of handicap. The new technology of electronics and silicon chips has made enormous advances in developing aids to help these children, even for those with severe motor problems.

SPINA BIFIDA

Spina bifida is a congenital abnormality due to a defect in the formation of the skeletal arch enclosing the spinal cord. It occurs most frequently in the lumbar region but may be present anywhere along the spinal column or even on the skull.

There are various degrees of this abnormality. In the mildest there is nothing beyond the bony defect. At other times a patch of hair or naevus over the spinal defect should lead the nurse to suspect the presence of spina bifida. Next in severity is the meningocele, in which case the spinal meninges herniate and the sac contains cerebrospinal fluid. If the sac contains nerve tissue as well as fluid the lesion is called meningomyelocele (Fig. 3.2).

When a baby with a meningocele is born, immediate steps should be taken to assess the problem and prepare for possible surgery, the lesion must be kept moist with saline soaks or with a bland non-adherent, non-greasy dressing, as any damage at this stage may aggravate the neurological damage, already present. Paediatric surgeons generally feel that early surgery should be restricted to those with mild or moderate neurological involvement.

The operation aims to give the lesion a good cover of skin. The skin is undermined, often right round to the umbilicus, and drawn together over the meningocele. Direct suture is usually possible after the underlying sac of meninges has been excised. The skin cover gives good protection, prevents infection (e.g. meningitis), helps to reduce paralysis and makes the care of the baby easier for all concerned.

Post-operative management and care

1. Maintenance of a clear airway together with careful positioning of the infant to protect the operative site and to relieve wound tension. The infant may be nursed prone or, alternatively, in slings suspended from the roof of the incubator.

2. Nutrition. Oral feeding can usually be commenced 4–6 hours post-operatively depending upon the infant's condition. A nasogastric tube may be kept in position for a few hours after operation for aspiration of stomach contents at frequent intervals.

FIG. 32 A newborn infant with meningomyelocele.

3. Prevention of infection:
   Dressings only when indicated by the surgeon.
   Application of urine bag or tube to prevent soiling of the dressing.
   Monitor body temperature.

4. Measure and chart head circumference daily to detect developing hydrocephalus. Early signs of developing hydrocephalus include a tense fontanelle.

5. Wound care. Suction drains usually removed about 48 hours after operation, sutures about 8–10 days later.

6. Family support. Encourage parents to visit their baby and participate in care. Talk over their baby's progress with them and answer all questions. Be prepared for a repetition of questions which is a result of natural anxiety.

7. Physiotherapy. Passive exercises will need to be provided initially by physiotherapists and later the parents should be instructed in how to continue with the programme at home.

8. Prepare parents for discharge. Liaise with the paediatric liaison health visitor to ensure continuity of care.

Conservative care
When surgery is delayed or even impossible, parents and nurses should then use their ingenuity in the way they protect the protruding lesion. Polyurethane rings are most satisfactory.

Special care should be taken to prevent trophic ulceration and to keep these babies warm, bearing in mind the fact that many are paralysed and lack sensory appreciation.

Feeds often need to be small and frequent, taking account of fluid and calorie requirements.

Long-term care
The degree of handicap varies from one child to another, and each poses a different set of problems. Whilst each must be considered individually, the main areas of concern can be considered under the following headings.

Urinary problems may range from stress incontinence to complete loss of sphincter control. Some children develop over-distending bladders with the consequent risk of infection which will require intensive treatment with antibiotics. Where the bladder becomes over-distended, a method of manual expression of urine can be taught to the mother and later the child. Girls, particularly, present problems: if incontinence pads and protective plastic pants do not provide the answer intermittent catheterization may be required. Boys can use a penile clamp or a fitted penile urinal. It is important to ensure that these childen can take plenty of fluids by mouth.

Bowel control. Most of these children can achieve bowel continence with good management. This involves giving a low residue diet together with an enema once or twice a week.

Voluntary defecation can also be achieved in some children, by straining at stool after a meal or hot drink. Care muse be taken that the rectum does not become impacted with faeces, thus causing overflow incontinence.

Orthopaedic handicaps. Intensive physiotherapy, training and splinting will all help in the management of any limb deformities. Most of these children can be taught to walk using calipers, and walking aids, although great care must be taken in view of the skin anaesthesia which makes them very vulnerable to trophic sores and ulceration. Some children will need to use a wheelchair and a surprising agility can often be achieved, sometimes to the envy of their friends!

Hydrocephalus. Although hydrocephalus will usually have been treated with the insertion of a shunt system, the treatment itself may lead to difficulties and complications. The tubes may need to be lengthened as the child grows or the shunt may become blocked and need to be replaced urgently. Occasionally, the tubes themselves may become disconnected, and need surgical correction. Low grade, persistent septicaemia, most commonly due to *Staphylococcus albus*, may occur and this is difficult to control until the valve is removed.

Social and psychological problems. Children with physical handicaps are not necessarily also emotionally disturbed, but research findings do suggest that these children tend to be less mature and more disturbed than those without any handicap. Mental handicap too may present a problem, although the intelligence level varies and is usually related to the type of defect.

HYDROCEPHALUS

Hydrocephalus is the name given to an excessive accumulation of cerebrospinal fluid within the skull. The resulting pressure causes the skull bones to separate, the skull circumference to increase, the ventricles to become distended and the substance of the brain to be compressed.

The excess accumulation is produced by obstruction of the flow or absorption of the fluid, due to congenital malformation, birth injury, inflammatory processes or pressure from a tumour.

In the *communicating type* there is a block within the subarachnoid space although there is free communication between the ventricular system and the spinal theca.

In the *non-communicating type*, the outflow from within the brain to the subarachnoid space is blocked.

In some cases the abnormality is slight and may arrest spontaneously.

Presentation

1. Increased intracranial pressure from obstruction of cerebrospinal fluid circulation leads to separation of the skull sutures and increasing skull circumference measurement.

2. The skull appears abnormal in shape and size, with a bulging brow which often seems to dwarf the face.

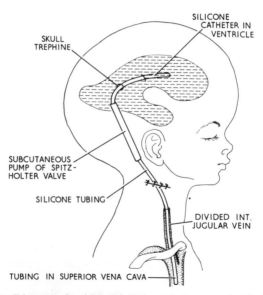

FIG. 33   Diagram of a child with hydrocephalus treated with the aid of a Spitz-Holter valve.

3. The fontanelles are tense and palpate.

4. The eyes show a downward deviation—the 'setting sun' sign, as the white of the sclera is visible above the iris.

5. Vomiting, failure to thrive and irritability, together with delayed development, are often noticed very early on in the condition.

Principles of care and treatment

After confirmation of hydrocephalus by radiography and other special investigations surgical treatment may be indicated. By means of a fine tube and a one-way valve, e.g. Spitz-Holter or Puderz valve, the cerebrospinal fluid is diverted from the ventricles into the blood steam or into the atria of the heart or peritoneal cavity.

Pre-operative care

If the child has been vomiting for some time, nutrition and hydration may be a problem. Offer small but frequent feeds with extra clear fluids.

In view of the raised intracranial pressure, minimum nursing care disturbance to avoid increasing irritability. Plan for care of pressure areas, eye care to be completed before feeding whenever possible.

Encourage parents to participate in care as much as possible. Provide facilities for parents to be resident if they wish to be. Answer all their questions about the care being provided, and explain the need for investigations and surgery. If the child is old enough explain all the treatments, etc. in a language he can understand.

Prepare for surgery as for any other operation that involves the use of general anaesthesia.

Shaving the child's head. In order to avoid undue distress for the child, the head is shaved in the anaesthetic room after the anaesthetic has been administered. The hair should be shampooed the day before operation and any scalp infection should be treated.

Post-operative care

Nursing action	Explanation
Frequent observations of pulse, respiration, temperature, blood pressure and neurological status.	Initially to detect signs of haemorrhage, shock and increased intracranial pressure. Later to indicate infection or blocked valve.
Change position of child every 2 hours.	To prevent pressure areas becoming sore.
Head of child should be raised.	To promote drainage of cerebrospinal fluid through shunt.
Avoid positioning of child on site of valve until wound is well healed.	To avoid damaging the overlying skin.
Nasogastric tube may be in situ on free drainage particularly if a rentriculoperitoneal shunt is performed.	To avoid abdominal distension.
Commence feeding gradually, 4–6 hours post-operatively. Administer intravenous fluids as prescribed. Measure and record fluid intake and output.	To maintain hydration and nutrition. Provide oral pleasure and comfort.
Frequent mouth and eye care.	To prevent dryness of mucous membranes and avoid infection.
Pump or 'milk' valve only as directed by surgeon.	To promote drainage where indicated.

Nursing action	Explanation
As child progresses plan play activities appropriate to interests and development.	To prevent mental stimulation.
Involve parents in care, giving explanation where necessary.	Preparation for discharge home.
Parents should be taught to detect complications and seek medical advice for fever, dehydration, redness/swelling of operation site and headache/irritability.	Infection. Shunt malfunction.

SOME BEHAVIOUR PROBLEMS

Enuresis

A child who repeatedly passes urine involuntarily at an age when the child is normally expected to be toilet-trained is said to be suffering from enuresis. The child may either never have been dry, or may have relapsed after a period of normal control of micturition. Wetting may occur several times a night, very occasionally, or perhaps once or twice per month.

Causes include renal infections, nephrosis, diabetes, psychological disturbances, congenital abnormalities of the urinary tract, spina bifida, neurological lesions, mental handicap, chronic constipation, and intestinal worms. A frequent cause is behaviour disturbance following the birth of a new baby, a change to a new school, a severe illness or other experience causing a loss of security.

A thorough physical examination, urinalysis and full investigations of the renal tract must be done to exclude organic disease, and if these are negative, psychological treatment may be advised. This will include full enquiry into home background, and the parents will be interviewed as well as the child. They may be advised to restrict fluid intake during the evening, to rouse the child and to offer a pot before they themselves go to bed and to leave a small light burning. Punishment and scolding are, as a rule, out of place, although an overworked exasperated mother may well be forgiven if she loses patience with the child. Constant wet sheets may be a great trial in a small town flat and criticism from neighbours is not easy to bear.

Every small improvement should be hailed as a hopeful sign and encouragement and praise given whenever possible. Sometimes drugs are used such as the tricyclic antidepressants. A 'conditioned reflex' can be created in older children by using a specially designed buzzer which goes off and rouses the child starting to void urine. Properly used these may score successes in 75% of cases treated.

Faecal Incontinence (Encopresis)

Faecal incontinence, i.e. soiling at an age when a child may reasonably be expected to be toilet-trained, may be due to a number of reasons. A common cause is constipation with overflow (Tripp and Candy, 1985), and reasons for this situation range from 'pot refusal' due to painful anal fissure in toddlers, to emotional disturbances, congenital abnormalities and bad housing conditions. Another example is the child who uses bowel function to attract mother's attention. Sometimes the lavatory itself is to blame: it may be situated on a dark landing in an old tenement building or in the garden, or it may be so high that the child dreads using it for fear of falling in.

The cause of faecal incontinence should therefore be investigated very carefully and patiently. Good teamwork between parents, paediatrician, child guidance clinic and health visitor will usually cure the condition.

MENTAL HANDICAP

Mental handicap or mental defect can be defined as inadequate mental development resulting in incapacity for independent social and intellectual adaptation in everyday life. There are many causes for this handicap which can be classified into the following groups:

1. Genetically determined, e.g. Down's syndrome.
2. Antenatal infection, e.g. rubella or syphilis.
3. Birth injury.
4. Postnatal, e.g. encephalitis, cerebral infection, trauma.

Mental handicap may also be associated with other handicaps, e.g. cerebral palsy or the child with hydrocephalus and myelomeningocele.

Only a few types of mental handicap are obvious at birth, such as Down's syndrome or microcephaly, whilst with others the condition may be unsuspected for several months. The first indication of this handicap in the young child is usually noticed in a delay by the child to reach the normal milestones in sitting, standing and walking; speech too is delayed. The child often appears placid and 'good' or conversely may appear hyperactive, restless and difficult to feed. Occasionally the handicap is only recognized when the child starts school and has difficulty in learning.

Whatever the cause and whenever it is diagnosed, the news will cause much anxiety and distress for the parents and the family. The parents may vacillate between extreme feelings of total rejection of their child to overwhelming possessiveness which may lead to neglect of their other children. The parents often try to find a cause for the handicap and may blame themselves. The nurse must recognize that these feelings are very real to the parents, who will need support and help in adopting a positive acceptance of their child's handicap. Many parents benefit from having contact with parents in a similar situation and help, both practical and emotional, is provided by voluntary agencies for the handicapped child.

The parents will have many questions to ask, wanting to know what their child's potential will be, how best to help him and what type of schooling will be needed? In order to answer these questions a complete assessment will be made by the multidisciplinary team concerned with the care for the child. Measurements of the intelligence quotient will be made by the clinical psychologist and compared with the chronological age; physical ability will be assessed by the physiotherapist, social behaviour by the nurse and the child's medical history thoroughly investigated by the paediatrician.

Even with this initial assessment it is difficult to forecast how the child will develop and progress. Assessment therefore should be carried out periodically in order that appropriate stimulation and training is given at the right stage of development.

Parents will need to know that their mentally handicapped child requires more and not less of the normal childhood pleasures and activities. It is through play, nursery rhymes, songs and stories that the young child learns. Children should be cuddled, praised and made a fuss of so that they feel secure and will want to do their best. As far as possible the parents should treat children normally whilst recognizing that because of this handicap they will be slower and less able than other children of the same age.

All children whatever their disability are able to go to school. Special schooling with small groups of children and specially qualified teachers that is geared to the individual child's needs and potential may be provided within the local school or in a special school (Warnock Report, 1978). It is now recognized that with training and care many mentally handicapped people can take their place in society where they may work in sheltered workshops and live in a hostel if there is no family home.

However, it is important to recognize that many children, because of their handicap or social background, may require admission into care where specialist expertise will provide an environment which will give the child the opportunity to learn social skills and to be cared for.

Respite care
Respite care has been defined by Sines (1988) as 'the means to give families some break or respite from the demanding routine of caring for their handicapped child'. Such care may also be needed as an emergency provision when, for example, a sudden death or illness of a parent occurs in a family. Respite care can be provided in a variety of settings and for a negiotated period of time, although this usually means for longer than a weekend or a few hours. For the child it means leaving family, friends and familiar environment to enter a residential care setting.

Phased respite care for a handicapped child provides a regular pattern of admission to a residential unit. The frequency of phased respite care may vary considerably and usually those parents using this service are making provision for their child or adolescent to be gradually introduced to a long-term care setting. Such care provision needs to be seen as part of a co-ordinated community approach to integrated services for children with handicaps through health, education and social services.

As with all children the mentally handicapped child may need admission into the paediatric unit with a superimposed medical or surgical condition. The nurse should especially remember how distressing this situation will be for the child. In order to avoid too much bewilderment and distress the child should, whenever possible, be looked after by 'their nurse'. Every effort should be made to follow the child's home routine whilst in hospital in order to maintain progress. Facilities for mother or father to be resident should be provided.

REFERENCES

Simpson, D. and Reilly, P. (1982). Paediatric coma scale. *Lancet* **ii**, 450.

Sines, D. (ed.) (1988). *Towards Integration: Comprehensive Services for People with Mental Handicaps*. London: Harper and Row.

Tripp, J.H. and Candy, D.C.A. (1985). *Manual of Paediatric Enterology*. London: Churchill Livingstone.

Warnock Report (1978). *Special Educational Needs. Committee of Enquiry into the Education of Handicapped Children and Young People* (H.M. Warnock, Chairman). London: HMSO.

FURTHER READING

Cunningham, C. (1988). *Down's Syndrome*, 2nd edn. London: Souvenir Press.

Drillien, C.M. and Drummand, M.B. (1977). *Neurodevelopmental Problems in Early Childhood*. Oxford: Blackwell Scientific.

Evans, O.R. (1987). *Manual of Child Neurology*. London: Churchill Livingstone.

Hopkins, A. (1981). *Epilepsy*. Oxford: Oxford University Press.

Hosking, G. (1982). *An Introduction to Paediatric Neurology*. London: Faber & Faber.

Purchese, G. and Allan, G. (1984). *Neuromedical and Neurosurgical Problems*, 2nd edn. London: Baillière Tindall.

Till, K. (1975). *Paediatric Neurosurgery*. London: Blackwell Scientific.

13 The child with dermatological problems

ECZEMA

Eczema is an allergic skin condition seen in varying degrees of severity. There is no cure for eczema. However, atopic eczema in the majority of children is self-limiting and often disappears within a few years. In mild cases only the flexor surfaces of the legs and arms are affected; in severe cases the rash may cover most of the body including the cheeks, forehead and scalp.

Eczema is common in childhood but estimates as to its incidence vary from 1 in 20 to as many as 1 in 8 (Breeze, 1990) having atopic tendencies. Commonly there is a familial history of asthma or hay fever. Boys are more frequently affected than girls and the babies are often blue-eyed, fair-haired and frequently delightful patients to look after. Allergy to certain foods such as eggs, fish, cow's milk and certain pollen or household dust can sometimes be found, either by taking a careful history or by performing intradermal tests.

Signs and symptoms
The rash is commonly first noticed over the forehead, cheeks and scalp but the areas around the mouth stay clear. As the eczema spreads the flexures of the elbows and knees and the folds behind the ears become affected and patchy areas may occur in any part of the body.

Initially the skin is red, hot and scaly but soon papules and vesicles appear and as they break down clear serum exudes from the lesion. This is known as weeping eczema and at this stage the skin easily becomes infected. Irritation is intense and it may be almost impossible to stop the infant from scratching. As the exudate dries up thick crusts are formed. In spite of the extensive lesions, eczema leaves no scars.

Treatment
Treatment often includes a full investigation of the possible exciting causes. Intradermal tests with specific proteins, pollen or dust may show a positive reaction to a certain agent which can then be eliminated from the diet or the child's environment.

Local treatment and principles of care
This includes the use of coal tar preparations, calamine lotion with or without an oily base and the addition of a mild antiseptic. Ointment containing hydrocortisone may be ordered for local application. This should be applied with care remembering that absorption of cortisone can lead to dangerous complications. Unguent emulsifications may be added to bath water or alternatively applied to lesions. This preparation whilst replacing soap allays irritation, is soothing and assists with the separation of crusts. The child usually enjoys the bath, giving mother an opportunity to make a special fuss of her child. A soft towel should be used for drying. The skin is gently dabbed and never rubbed as this is abrasive to healing skin.

The local applications vary according to the stage of the rash. When dry and scaly, emollients are usually ordered. They are either applied direct to the skin and left exposed, or spread thinly onto gauze and bandaged in place with an open-weave bandage. Tubular gauze is also useful for keeping a dressing comfortably in place. Infected areas may be treated with antiseptic lotion and an appropriate systemic antibiotic after a swab test has identified the organism.

General principles of care

Nursing action

Keep the child cool. Clothing should be light and made of cotton. Cotton mittens should be worn at night. Alternatively child may be left without any clothing on. Ambient temperature should be 70°F to avoid hypothermia.

Nails kept clean and short. Children should be encouraged to rub instead of scratch the skin (Breeze, 1990).

Occupation. Suitable play activities and education as appropriate should be provided according to the individual child's needs.

Parental participation. Every effort should be made to support and encourage the involvement of parents in care. Facilities for the mother or father to be resident should be provided.

Diet. A nursing/medical history will indicate any allergy to specific foods, e.g. eggs or cow's milk.

Explanation

Will help to relieve irritation and incidence of scratching. Scratching of the skin produces further damage to the epithelial cells and increases the risk of introducing infection.

To prevent secondary infection.

Will help to divert the child's attention from the skin irritation whilst helping to meet normal developmental needs.

Important to the child's normal emotional developmental needs. Will help to allay anxiety and frustration, thus reducing the likelihood or further scratching and will help to promote healing.

Eliminate those items from the diet to help reduce extent of the eczema.

Nursing action	Explanation
Sedatives. Antihistamines may be prescribed.	Will reduce irritation.
Information. Put parents in touch with the National Eczema Society.	This will help to allay parental anxiety and provide family support through its befriending service.

Immunization and vaccination

Children with eczema can be treated as any others with regard to immunization programmes in the United Kingdom (Department of Health, 1990).

ACNE VULGARIS

This very common and distressing condition occurs at puberty. It is due to an excessive output and overgrowth of sebaceous glands particularly on the face, chest and shoulders. Blockage of sebum occurs and a comedo or 'black head' is produced.

Treatment

It is of utmost importance to reduce the greasiness of the skin. The face should be washed in hot water as often as possible and the comedos removed with a comedo extrator. Calamine lotion with 3% sulphur is then applied and rubbed in well. Topical peroxide preparations or vitamin A acid have in some instances been helpful.

Long-term tetracycline therapy has been found to be of value in severe cases. The patient is always very self-conscious about these spots and will need constant reassurance that once puberty is over these lesions will disappear, but that squeezing of the spots produces scars and should be avoided.

General preventative guidance

Wash the face gently at least twice daily.

Shampoo hair daily or as frequently as possible.

Continue the above regimen even after the face clears.

Diet does not appear to make any difference, but occasionally a patient may feel that a certain food worsens the condition, e.g. chocolate, which is then best avoided.

IMPETIGO CONTAGIOSA

Impetigo is a skin infection caused by the streptococcus or staphylococcus. It is very common in children of school age and spreads easily, particularly in overcrowded homes with poor hygiene. The organism enters the skin through a crack or a scratch and for that reason is often associated with an infested head.

At first small vesicles appear and as they break the lesion becomes red and weeping and as the exudate dries up thick crusts form. Typical sites are on the scalp, the chin and around the lips. The crusts have the appearance of being 'stuck on'.

Local treatment

Local treatment consists in softening the crusts with warm saline bathings or a solution of potassium permanganate 1 : 4000. The skin may be painted with an antiseptic preparation such as boracic cream or an antibiotic cream. Occasionally antibiotics may be ordered by mouth if the infection is severe or fails to respond to local treatment.

The child suffering from impetigo is likely to infect others and if admitted to hospital should be nursed with barrier precautions. Crockery and cutlery should be sterilized until the last lesion has healed. Scratching is prevented in the same way, as in the case of infantile eczema (see p. 341).

The condition may clear within a few days and rarely leaves any scars. Recurrence should be prevented by giving the mother guidance with regard to personal hygiene and building up the child's general resistance, by good diet, exercise in the fresh air and an adequate vitamin intake.

N.B. If the child is being cared for at home he should be kept away from his school or playgroup until the lesions have healed. Inform the health visitor or school nurse when the diagnosis has been made.

BURNS AND SCALDS

Burns and scalds are among the most frequently occurring accidents in childhood and they are the more tragic, because so many of them are preventable.

Common causes of burns and scalds in children

1. Open fires left unprotected.
2. Mirrors, pictures and attractive ornaments placed above electric fires or open fires attract children to reach for them.
3. Saucepans containing hot fluids with their handles left jutting out on stoves within the reach of children.
4. Tablecloths which can be pulled by a young child so that the items on the table fall over, including teapots, cups, etc. containing very hot fluids.
5. Baths filled with hot water before cold so that the young child is scalded on buttocks or feet on immersion into the bath.
6. Playing with matches.
7. Playing with fireworks.

Prevention

1. A fire should always be guarded when young children are about.

2. Advise parents to remove items from above a fireplace.

3. Always invert saucepan handles on any stove.

4. With young children in a family tablecloths should not be used. The table may be protected either with place mats or with a short plastic non-slip cover.

5. Always fill a bath with at least 1 inch of cold water before running in the hot. Herd *et al.* (1986) recommended that domestic hot water thermostats should be reduced to 35°C to reduce incidence of bath time scalds.

6. Never allow children to handle matches until old enough to be instructed in their proper use.

7. Ensure that all young children using baby walkers are adequately supervised, as they may tip into a fire which is inadequately guarded.

8. Firework parties should always be supervised and managed by responsible adults. Children should never have free access to loose fireworks.

Classification of burns and scalds

Modern surgery refers to only two degrees of burns and scalds: superficial burns, and full thickness or deep burns. As a rule *superficial burns* may be expected to heal with little scarring, while *full thickness* burns are slow to heal and may cause scarring, crippling contractions and loss of function, and usually require skin grafting and prolonged and repeated treatment in hospital.

The extent of the burn is as important as the depth. For purposes of classification the 'Waller Method' is frequently used. The body surface is divided into sections of 9% of the total and thus, with reference to a chart, it is

FIG. 34 The Lund and Browder method of measuring burns (From Lund and Browder, 1944).

easy to estimate the extent of the burn as being a multiple of 9%. The seriousness of the burn or scald is often far more dependent on the extent of the affected area, than on the thickness. A child may die with an 18% superficial burn but an older patient may be expected to survive deep burns covering 50% of the body surface.

The Lund and Browder method of estimating the extent of burns is shown in Fig. 34. As in Waller's 'Rule of Nines' method, the body is divided into areas each of which is given a percentage value, but the values of certain areas alter with age as the proportions of the child's body are changed by normal growth.

Treatment for shock
No time should be lost in treating shock, even if the usual symptoms may at first not be evident because shock is delayed. Shock is always directly proportionate to the area involved, as the loss of salts, protein and fluids into

TABLE 12   Table showing how the extent of a burn in certain areas of a child's body changes with age.

Areas affected by growth	Age				
	1 month	1 year	5 years	10 years	15 years
A = half of head	9½	8½	6½	5½	4½
B = half of one thigh	2¾	3¼	4	4¼	4½
C = half of one lower leg	2½	2½	2¾	3	3¼

the tissue spaces and onto the body surface reduces the volume of circulating blood. The body reacts to this by a drop in blood pressure, subnormal temperature, pallor, thirst, restlessness and failure to secrete urine.

Intravenous therapy. This should be started immediately in all cases in which the area involved exceeds 9% of the body surface. It is usual to take blood for grouping and haemoglobin estimation before starting the infusion.

Plasma or dextran are the fluids of choice, although fresh blood may be given according to the level of the haemoglobin which should never be allowed to fall below 70%.

The rate of fluid loss is estimated by repeated haematocrit readings, the haemoconcentration and the amount of urinary output. On the first day approximately two-thirds of the fluid loss is replaced in the first 8 hours after admission. After that, chemical tests of both blood and urine are done at least daily and the findings are taken as a guide for further intravenous therapy.

Oxygen therapy. Shock and the loss of red blood cells from the burnt surface may cause sufficient reduction

FIG. 35 Extensive burns. Child being nursed using the exposed method on foam pads which are changed frequently.

in the oxygenating power of the blood to make oxygen therapy necessary. This is usually best given by mask as oxygen given by means of a tent interferes with local treatment and influences bacterial growth.

General principles of care

Admission. The child should be admitted to a warmed cubicle as heat loss can exceed heat production (Bruce, 1989), and barrier techniques used in order to protect the child from infection.

Swabs for laboratory culture should be taken from the burned areas. Sterile bed linen should be used. The child's weight should be recorded as the basis for calculating drug dosage and intravenous therapy.

At this stage the child should never be left alone. The parents will need considerable support and reassurance during this time, especially as it is likely they will be suffering some shock themselves as a result of the accident.

Nursing observations. Observations of the child's appearance, pulse rate and blood pressure should be made frequently, as they are of considerable importance in assessing the child's general progress. In addition any girl with extensive burns (more than 10% surface area) should have an in-dwelling catheter in the bladder, and any boy should have Paul's tubing attached to the penis, so that urine output can be measured and recorded hourly. A rising pulse rate, hypotension and oliguria are all indications that the infusion rate should be increased to meet the body's fluid requirements. The nurse should realize that shivering and vomiting in these children are more likely to be due to inadequate fluid replacement or infection than to their being cold.

Diet. Oral fluids should be commenced as soon as possible after admission to the ward and are best given at this stage as 5% glucose 40 ml/kg/24 hours. It may be necessary to pass a nasogastric tube in order to avoid disturbing the child too much. Once the shock associated with the injury has passed, usually in about 2–3 days, the child should be given a diet high in protein and kilojoules. It may be necessary for this to be continued for several weeks, for much protein is lost from the burns and healing is delayed by malnutrition. Initially the child may be given a fortified milk preparation if necessary through a nasogastric tube.

Iron is necessary to combat anaemia. As soon as the patient can tolerate it, a full diet is given which is augmented by eggs, milk, vitamins and foods which are rich in iron. Such foods are red meat, liver, kidney, sardines, black treacle, wholemeal and rye bread and

Bovril and Marmite. As most of these foods are both palatable and colourful, there should be little difficulty in arranging attractive meals. The food intake must be measured accurately and the amounts taken should be known and supplemented by tube feeding if necessary. Much patience and ingenuity may be needed to achieve the necessary fluid and kilojoule intake.

Drug therapy. A broad spectrum antibiotic or a combination of one of these with penicillin is given prophylactically for the first 24 hours. The drug may then be changed according to the sensitivity report.

Pain relief. Diamorphine (0.075 mg/kg body weight) and Trineprazine (3 mg per kg body weight) are suitable sedatives and analgesia to give to the child who will be frightened as well as in pain. This should always be relieved, as pain does exacerbate shock. These drugs should not be given subcutaneously for the first day or so, as in the presence of shock they may not be adequately absorbed until later, with dangerous results. Initially the intravenous route is used.

Usually by 48 hours pain subsides and drugs such as codeine or phenobarbitone are effective. Elixir Phenergan has a sedative effect and at the same time reduces tissue swelling and may need to be continued for some time.

Local treatment and principles of care
Treatment of the burnt area depends upon the extent of its surface and the part of the body involved. Prevention of infection, healing and early grafting, leading to early functioning of the part affected, are the desired goals.

Two methods may be used, the exposed or the closed method.

Wound care. After adequate sedation the affected area and surrounding skin is cleansed. Large, heavy blisters may be punctured and drained but small ones are left and dead skin is not removed unless it is very dirty.

A hard, dry crust of plasma exudate or eschar usually forms within 24–36 hours and provides a sterile covering for the underlying surface. Air is allowed to circulate freely to aid the drying process and for that purpose special beds, polyurethane pads, extensions and slings may be used and the patient's position changed according to need. Using an aerosol spray, topical antibiotics can be applied, e.g. polymyxin and bacitracin. Systemic antibiotic therapy is usually prescribed. Pressure on the affected part must be avoided as a good blood supply is essential to healing.

After about 7–10 days the crust begins to separate and then needs to be gently lifted away. The cleansed wound is covered with a single layer of paraffin gauze, e.g. Jelonet overlapping the area by 5 cm to allow for slippage (Bruce, 1989). The area is then covered with layers of gauze and a light conforming cotton bandage. A single layer of gamgee and a crêpe bandage may then be applied. For superficial wounds the dressing may be left intact for 10 days if the child remains well, apyrexial and there is no evidence of exudate through the dressing.

Full thickness burns are treated in the same way initially, but after 1–2 weeks the child is taken to the theatre for thorough examination and wound toilet. It is then possible to decide how much of the tissue is dead and consequently incapable of primary healing. As a rule partial thickness burns may be expected to heal in 3–4 weeks, but full thickness burns will require grafting and are usually associated with some degree of deformity. Any sloughs are removed and skin grafting is undertaken. Loss of blood may be considerable and blood transfusion may be necessary.

The nurse during the healing phase should watch any exposed and pendant parts (the extremities particularly) for oedema and bleeding. Either must be reported at once. The bandaging requires great skill as considerable pressure is required in order to prevent blood or exudate from lifting the graft off its bed. At the same time it is obviously dangerous to apply the crêpe bandages too tightly. Oedema may be severe and may cause the bandage to become tight and impede circulation with consequent death of the skin graft. Nursing methods, such as elevating the part supported by foam wedges, with padding of neck or axilla if these are affected, helps to promote comfort and reduce any swelling.

Complications

Damage of liver and kidneys, pneumonia, reactions to blood transfusion, sepsis, uraemia and psychological disturbances are common. Awareness of these at the earliest stage is essential to provide effective treatment. Local complications may arise from sloughs and crusts which by their position or extent may restrict chest movement or the blood supply to extremities, causing chest complications or thrombosis and gangrene of the parts. Burns and scalds of the eyelids are likely to cause contractions followed by exposure of the cornea, resulting in keratitis. Careful swabbing may prevent complications but in some cases it is deemed best temporarily to stitch the upper and lower lid margins together or to excise the contracted lids and graft them.

Burns of the hands and external genitalia present further problems which have to be dealt with as the individual case demands. Warm baths will help the child to 'kick out' any contractures although splinting may still be necessary. Pressure garments are also beneficial. The application of an oily cream will help to soften healed areas.

Lesions of groins, neck and armpits should be prevented from contracting by separating them or extending them fully with the aid of pillows or rolls of polyurethane foam. Scalds of face, neck and tongue may require tracheostomy.

Psychological care

These children are usually severely shocked and numbed in the first hours but after this initial stage they need a great deal of assurance, company and occupation. They are frightened by the accident and the sudden admission to hospital and often haunted by memories of the burst of flames and by feelings of guilt. Flame burns in particular, cause severe nightmares after 2 or 3 days, and the children easily develop feelings of resentment and a poor relationship with their parents.

The presence of the mother for as much time as possible is of great psychological value. Any relatives or neighbours involved in the accident should be allowed to visit and speak to the child in order to reassure. The parents can be encouraged to feed and play with their child, and sometimes may help their child to sleep when it is wakeful or frightened. *It is in these first, initial stages that comfort from the parents is so important.* It is useless to cure a child physically while allowing psychological damage to persist or to develop.

Although a physiotherapist will carry out daily treatment to prevent and correct contractions and bad posture, mothers can often be taught to assist, e.g. when games are played to encourage deep breathing and so help to prevent chest infections. As soon as possible full occupation is needed to keep these patients happy.

Boredom encourages scratching and picking at the crusts, both of which may lead to infection, delayed healing and unnecessary scarring. Adequate occupation and company are far better means of preventing this than sedation or restraint. Toys and occupational material may at first need to be of the sterilizable kind. In situations of stress such as this, the child should not be deprived of a loved toy and if this cannot be sterilized even a teddy bear can be covered by a clean polythene bag.

Children nursed by the exposure method often miss their usual coverings at first and if cold, can be covered by sterile towels and wear sterilized bootees and mittens. Little girls enjoy wearing pretty hair ribbons even if this is the only 'clothing' they are allowed. The young patients soon get used to their nakedness and although they may at first feel cold when transferred to the open ward they then often dislike being dressed.

Consideration for the mental welfare of the parents is as important as for the child. Parents often blame themselves in some way for the accident and some time may have to be spent with anxious parents outlining the treatment, the probable outcome of the illness and the degree of scarring and length of hospitalization to be expected. Siblings should be encouraged to visit. Parents of newly admitted children should be encouraged to speak to those of convalescent patients as they may be able to give them comfort from their own experiences.

REFERENCES

Breeze, E. (1990). Management of atopic eczema. *Primary Health Care*, Jan/Feb, pp. 12–13.

Bruce, E. (1989). Thermal injuries in paediatrics. *Paediatric Nursing*, **1**(9), 8–9.

Department of Health (1990). *Immunisation against Infectious Disease*. London: HMSO.

Herd, A.N., Widdowson, P. and Tanner, N.S. (1986). Scalds in the very young, prevention or care. *Burns*, **12**, 246.

Lund, C.C. and Browder, N.C. (1944) Estimation of areas of burns. *Surgery, Gynaecology and Obstetrics*, **79**, 352–358.

FURTHER READING

Dickson, D.S. (1983). *Nursing and the Management of Burns*, 5th edn. London: Faber and Faber.

Jackson, R.H. (1977). *Children, the Environment and Accidents*. London: Pitman Medical.

Murray, D. (1981). *The Anti-Acne Book*. London: Arlington Pocket Books.

Verbov, J. (1979). *Modern Topics in Paediatric Dermatology*. London: Heinemann Medical.

14 The child with orthopaedic problems

MUSCULAR DYSTROPHIES (MYOPATHIES)

A number of variants of the myopathies exist which all have the characteristics of progressive, degenerative changes in the muscle fibres, leading to wasting and weakness. The nerves are not affected in this group and there are neither sensory changes nor paralysis. The diseases are often hereditary and familial and usually lead to early death due to intercurrent infection such as pneumonia. A proportion of children with muscular dystrophy are mentally handicapped but the majority are of normal intelligence.

The various types of myopathies affect different muscle groups in particular, causing degenerative changes in the muscle fibres and their replacement by connective tissue and fat. Whole groups of muscles may thus be weakened and although the process may be a very slow one, it is always progressive and the patient eventually becomes completely incapacitated and crippled.

Diagnosis
Diagnosis is confirmed by electromyography, by which means the changes can be differentiated from those in other diseases of muscles. The destruction of muscle causes excretion of creatinine in the urine.

Pseudohypertrophic Muscular Dystrophy

The most common of the myopathies in childhood is pseudohypertrophic muscular dystrophy so called because of the enlargement of certain muscles in this condition.

Signs and symptoms

The child may be normal up to school age but gradually it is noticed that he or she tires easily, prefers to sit about rather than play with other children, and finds it difficult to walk up stairs without the help of the banister. The gait becomes unstable and the child is easily pushed over in play. The muscles of the shoulder girdle may become so weak that the child cannot raise his arms above his head and when the doctor places her hands underneath the arms to lift the patient, the child literally slips through.

Weakness of the muscles of the pelvic girdle and the spine lead to kyphosis and lordosis. The gait is waddling at first and later becomes impossible. When the child tries to rise from the lying position, it is necessary to roll on to the front and then rise onto hands and knees; by gradually moving one hand after the other up the legs and above the knees, the child eventually succeeds in rising to the upright position. This manoeuvre is very characteristic of the disease.

As the muscular weakness progresses the child becomes bedridden and deformities through contractions may develop.

Treatment

Treatment aims at preventing crippling and wasting by massage and exercises. Movement should be encouraged as disuse leads to more rapid wasting. Pneumonia usually causes death after a few years.

Other types of the myopathies
These affect specific muscle groups in particular. The rate of progress may vary greatly and in spite of crippling the patient may survive into middle age. The more common varieties are the facioscapulohumeral type and myotonia congenita. As the name implies, the muscles affected in the facioscapulohumeral type, are those of the face, arms and shoulder girdle. The first signs may be difficulty in sucking and in closing the eyes completely. The handicap is, as a rule, slight and a fairly normal existence is possible. Myotonia congenita causes voluntary muscles to go into protracted contractions followed by slow relaxation. Muscle biopsy shows enlargement and thickening of muscle fibres. Muscle biopsy and electromyography are usually carried out to confirm diagnosis as the changes in the electrical activity in the muscle and those in the structure of the muscle are characteristic of the various types of the disease.

Genetic counselling should be offered to all such parents considering enlarging their family.

PERTHES' DISEASE
(Syn: Legg–Perthes' disease, Legg–Calvé–Perthes'
disease, Coxa plana)

Osteochondritis is a fairly common abnormality of growth and development of the epiphyses in children. The most common of the diseases in this group is Perthes' disease. This disease affects boys more frequently than girls and develops between the ages of 4 and 8 years (Gartland, 1979). It is usually unilateral.

The cause is a disturbance in the blood supply to the epiphysis, which leads to deformity of the epiphysial plate and in the later stages, if untreated, to collapse of the head of the femur and arrest of the development of the epiphysis.

Examination reveals that the range of movement is limited in all directions. Occasionally a bone scan may be used to differentiate the disease process from toxic synovitis of the hip, septic hip joint or osteomyelititis. Changes may not show up on radiographs for some time; after a while there may be wasting of the leg and in some cases shortening. The latter is due to collapse of the head and later premature epiphysial arrest. The child may complain of pain in the groin.

Treatment

There are two distinct approaches to the treatment of Perthes' disease. Some surgeons consider that prolonged immobilization with traction is required to prevent osteoarthritis in later life. Others believe that once the early stage of muscle spasm is passed, ambulation with the aid of crutches is all that is required. If the disease process affects the entire femoral head osteotomy may be necessary. To avoid the effects of prolonged hospitalization these children, where possible, should be cared for at home with the support of the community nursing services.

Principles of care

Those children who are treated by bed-rest combined with traction and splinting, and those with calipers, have to be given special care of skin and pressure areas to prevent soreness. With the surgeon's permission groin and any other straps should be released twice daily and the skin washed and carefully dried.

General muscle tone should be maintained by giving daily massage and exercises. As the stay in hospital may extend over several weeks, schooling and play activities should be made available and whenever possible outings or a weekend visit home should be arranged.

Prognosis
The prognosis is excellent provided adequate early treatment is given but some children may develop degenerative disease of the hip joint in later life.

CONGENITAL DISLOCATION OF THE HIP JOINT

Children with congenital dislocation of the hip joint have an abnormally shallow acetabulum which causes the femoral head to be displaced upwards and backwards when the child begins to put weight upon the limb. The neck of the femur may be shortened and the capsule becomes stretched. Sometimes the femoral head lies outside the acetabulum at the time of birth. The child walks with dips on the affected side or has a waddling gait if the dislocation is a bilateral one. Because the pelvis is tipped forward, lordosis develops.

Congenital dislocation of the hip joint is a fairly common condition. Successful treatment depends on an early assessment and this should not be delayed beyond the first week of life.

The abnormality occurs most in girls; the condition runs in families and although usually present at birth it is often not noticed until the child begins to walk. The dislocation may be unilateral or bilateral and it may be partial or complete.

Signs and symptoms
The observant midwife, mother or nurse may notice that one leg is shorter than the other and that the perineum is wider than usual. A telescoping movement of the leg may be possible. When the baby lies prone, the gluteal crease

on the affected side is higher than that on the good side and the buttocks may be flattened.

When the baby is being medically examined he or she is placed on her back with the legs towards the examining doctor with hips and knees flexed at right angles. The middle finger of each hand is placed over the great trochanter while the flexed leg is contained in the palm of the hand and the thumb on the inner side of the thigh opposite the lesser trochanter. Keeping the legs flexed at 45° abduction the middle finger of each hand is pressed on the great trochanter to test whether or not the femoral head can be lifted into the acetabulum. If the test is positive, a click will be heard. This is known as the Ortolani sign.

Not in all cases in which the test is positive will treatment be necessary. An orthopaedic surgeon must however be asked to see the baby without delay.

Treatment

Treatment should be started as soon as the condition has been recognized, as its duration and success depend on the age of the child. In very young babies a double nappy may give sufficient abduction to provide effective treatment. In more severe cases a harness splint may be used to maintain continuously the abducted position of the hips.

Older children may be placed on a special abduction frame and skin traction is applied to bring the head of the femur into position opposite the acetabulum. The legs are gradually abducted at intervals of 2 or 3 days to allow for gradual stretching of the muscles. When both legs have been abducted to right angles to the trunk (Fig. 36), the child is taken to the theatre.

Tenotomies may be necessary to obtain a fully abducted position of the hip joints in children over 18 months of age.

FIG. 36 Nurse renewing bandages following daily inspection of skin for child on hoop traction.

Two different methods of treatment are then commonly used, depending on the age of the child, radiograph appearance and the surgeon's wishes:

1. The dislocation is reduced and the legs rotated to bring the femoral head into the acetabulum. The legs are

FIG. 37 Batchelor plaster showing wide abduction.

fixed externally rotated and in full abduction with the knees flexed at right angles to the femora. A so-called *'frog plaster'* is applied, which reaches from the nipple line to the ankles.

2. The dislocation is reduced, the femora internally rotated and the legs fully abducted from the knees downward. A plaster, reaching from the groins to the ankles enable the child to move freely in the hip joint while maintaining flexion and extension. A wooden crossbar is incorporated into the plaster from one knee across to the other: this is called a *Batchelor plaster* (see Fig. 37). After a time the child learns to move about and even to 'walk' using knees.

In either case treatment has to be continued for a year

to 18 months and during that time the child may be discharged home and brought back for changes of plaster at intervals of approximately 3 months. Occasionally neither of these methods is successful and open reduction and rotation osteotomy to correct the angle of the femur on the hip may be necessary. This would not be done until the baby is at least 1 year old. In very persistent cases shelf operation, acetabuloplasty, is performed to deepen the acetabulum, and a hip spica applied.

During the stage of abduction the child suffers considerable discomfort and frustration due to the immobility and her position on the frame. A great deal of individual attention and occupation help to comfort the child. The child is best served if the mother can be resident. In the initial stages sedatives should be given generously. Patience and imagination will be required to get the child to take fluids and food in this position and to teach her to pass urine and faeces without unduly soiling the padding of the frame. The bandages are taken off the legs daily and the skin inspected for reactions to strapping. They are washed and powdered before reapplying the bandages. The frame padding or plaster can be protected by thin plastic sheeting or waterproof adhesive tape.

Principles of care following manipulation and application of plaster

Nursing action	Explanation
Plaster is exposed to allow for drying naturally. Patient turned 2- to 4-hourly.	Drying plaster quickly causes cracking. Allow for drying of plaster back and front.
Turn, using palms of hands only whilst plaster is still damp.	Avoids indentation of plaster which weakens it.

Nursing action	Explanation
Observe toes for signs of plaster being too tight.	Tight plaster will obstruct blood supply (on digital pressure skin should flush quickly).
Apply bootees and mittens.	Extremities become cold quickly.
Support arms and feet with pillows.	Can cause discomfort.
Observe for pressure sores where child uses joints to move himself.	Elbows and heels become red and sore.
Adjust child's position with bean bags and/or foam wedges to allow participation with surroundings. When plaster is dry the child can be taken for walks in a twin pushchair.	Child will become frustrated and irritable if isolated by position.
Provide suitable play activities.	To encourage normal development and allay boredom.
Observe for the indications of plaster sores (restlessness, itching, fretfulness and slight rise in temperature).	The signs appear as the sore develops. Once the sores are established pain disappears. There may then be staining of the plaster.

The child is usually sent home and only readmitted for change of plaster and reassessment at intervals of 2–3 months. The mother is taught how to keep the plaster clean and to provide all care for her child. Before discharge home the family health visitor should be informed in order to provide on-going support and counselling to the mother and the family.

Treatment continues over a period of 1–2 years depending in part on the age of the child, as the longer the condition has been left untreated the more difficult is successful treatment. When the plaster is eventually re-moved the child is at first allowed the freedom of the bed. Daily physiotherapy is given and after about 3 weeks, if X-ray appearance is satisfactory, the child is allowed to start weight-bearing. In early, successful cases walking should be normal and a complete, permanent cure can be expected.

TALIPES

Talipes may occur on one or both sides and is often associated with other congenital abnormalities such as spina bifida. There are variants in severity and in the type of deformity. Usually several joints of the foot are in-volved, often causing inversion of the forefoot, internal rotation of the tibia and plantar flexion of the ankle joint. There are four types, and any may be seen in varying degrees of severity.

1. *Talipes equinovarus* (*clubfoot*). The deformity con-sists of inversion (turning in) of the forefoot, internal rotation of the tibia and plantar flexion of the ankle joint.

2. *Congenital talipes calcaneovalgus*. The deformity consists of eversion (turning out) of the foot and dorsiflex-ion at the ankle joint. The tendon Achillis is lengthened. This deformity is less severe and yields more easily to treatment than the equinovarus deformity. In mild cases it may be sufficient for the mother to stretch the foot into equinus and varus position several times before each feed. She will also have to do this in cases which require surgery.

3. *Talipes equinovalgus*. In this deformity there is eversion and plantar flexion.

4. *Taliper calcaneovarus*. In this deformity there is inversion and dorsiflexion.

The two last-mentioned deformities are usually seen in children with paralysis and/or cerebral palsy.

Treatment of talipes equinovarus
This should be commenced within 36 hours of birth and its success depends greatly on the promptness with which it is started. The foot is manipulated manually until the little toe touches the peroneal surface of the leg. The over-corrected position is maintained by adhesive strapping, splints or Plaster of Paris. Manipulation is repeated weekly at first. Kicking and standing on the splints when the child is old enough are encouraged as this helps to develop the leg muscles.

Manipulation often causes reactionary swelling and as treatment is often given in the out-patient department, full instructions to bring her baby back if there is reason for concern, should be given to the mother.

If treated from birth, correction may be complete by the age of 6 months or a year but a special night boot is usually worn for another year or two. Occasionally the outside of the shoe heel is raised or an inside iron with a 'T' strap fixed to the shoes when the baby starts to walk.

Long-term care
Cases treated less promptly may need many years of treatment, and cure may not be permanent. Parents are usually very pleased with the initial improvement and it may be difficult to impress on them the importance of continuing treatment for a number of years. Sometimes manipulation, stretching and splinting fail and operation becomes necessary. This may be either open or closed tenotomy, or, as a last resort, Steindler's operation or triple arthrodesis.

FIG. 38   Mobile with the aid of a wheelchair.

OSTEOMYELITIS

Osteomyelitis is an infection causing acute inflammation beneath the periosteum, resulting in an abscess and sequestrum formation (death of the bone).

The disease attacks children between the ages of 2 and 12 years, although babies in the neonatal period may be affected. The femur, humerus, clavicle and maxilla are common sites of infection and there may be evidence of a recent knock or injury. There is frequently a history of infected tonsils, boils or septic spots and the causative organism is often the staphylococcus.

Signs and symptoms

The onset may be acute with hyperpyrexia, tachycardia, headaches, rigor, toxaemia or septicaemia, but at times it can be quite insidious. Infants appear to have little pain, but the general disturbances include vomiting and diarrhoea, causing dehydration, In older children pain can be very severe until tension subsides following treatment with antibiotics which reduce the infection.

The limb is held immobilized in a relaxed position and occasionally the condition may be mistaken for some form of paralysis. Any handling is deeply resented. The skin over the affected area may be found to be red, shiny and hot, although it may take a day or two for the inflammation to become obvious. The white cell count is high (mainly polymorphonuclear cells) and blood culture is sometimes positive. X-ray appearance is rarely abnormal before the second or third week.

Treatment

Large doses of antibiotics together with immobilization, may bring about a cure, but sometimes the child does not respond well. Analgesia should be given whenever needed.

The usual antibiotics in this case are penicillin, kanamycin and cloxacillin, given by injection. Surgery may become necessary to either drain an abscess that has formed, or to remove damaged bone.

Principles of care
As there may be exquisite pain, jarring of the bed must be avoided and for that reason the bed should be situated in a corner of the ward in the acute stage. Analgesia should be given as required. Temperature, pulse and respirations are taken every 4 hours and fluid intake and output charts kept up to date. Abundant fluids are given and as the child is often negative and reluctant to drink, it is important to vary the drinks by using different flavours and by alternating hot and cold drinks.

Once the fever has subsided, a nourishing, high protein diet is given to build up the child's general health. Small pillows, sand-bags and air rings should be used to ensure a comfortable position and rest for the affected part.

Every effort should be made to maintain as many of the child's normal activities as possible, e.g. schooling and play activities.

N.B. In the presence of any draining wound the child should be isolated and nursed with full barrier precautions.

SYNDACTYLY

Syndactyly or webbing of the digits of the hands and feet may be partial or complete. The underlying bones and joints may be normal, or sections may be missing or fused. The plastic surgeon may be able to separate the digits and to give the hand an aesthetically good appearance, without much difficulty. Or it may be necessary to utilize one of the fingers as a thumb by transplanting muscles in such a way as to bring a digit into apposition to the others to make gripping possible. Occasionally skin grafting is undertaken to supply skin for the surfaces between the divided digits.

In looking after these patients post-operatively it is important to watch for signs of impaired circulation, sometimes a difficult task as the entire hand or foot may be covered in a tight crêpe bandage.

OSTEOGENESIS IMPERFECTA
(FRAGILITAS OSSIUM)

As the name suggests, the bones in fragilitas ossium are fragile and fractures occur on the least provocation. There are two main types of the disease. In the antenatal variety most of the bones of the fetal skull and skeleton have sustained fractures before birth. Callus formation causes the bones to be thickened and deformed. Babies with this complaint have markedly blue sclerotics. The condition is familial and severe cases become seriously handicapped, while others die at birth due to fractures occuring during labour.

In the second variety the fractures occur mostly after the first year of life. The bones are porous and the teeth translucent. Although the fractures heal rapidly, deformities inevitably result and these children lead sheltered lives with schooling frequently interrupted by treatment or admissions to hospital. Occasionally the condition improves at puberty. Neither the cause nor any effective treatment are known.

CORRECTION OF DEFORMITIES CAUSED
BY PARALYSIS

The abnormal and imbalanced pulls of certain muscle groups against others weakened by paralysis can cause severe and progressive deformities in the growing child. Surgical treatment is often necessary to prevent deformity and to stabilize joints and so to improve function. The results of congenital abnormalities of the spine (e.g. myelomeningocele) and cerebral palsy are examples.

Corrective operations include transplantation of tendons in the leg or foot. This transplantation aims at counteracting an abnormal pull from a group of healthy muscles which would lead to deformity. Transplantation of the tendons of the hamstring muscles, for instance to the back of the femur, may enable a child with spastic paralysis to straighten his knees and to walk almost normally.

Tenotomy may be performed to lengthen certain tendons, e.g. a contracted Achilles tendon in the child with cerebral palsy in order to promote mobility.

REFERENCE

Gartland, J.J. (1979). *Fundamentals of Orthopaedics*. Philadephia: Saunders.

FURTHER READING

Brunner, L.S. and Suddarth, D.S. (1986). *The Lippincott Manual of Paediatric Nursing*. London: Harper & Row.
Lloyd-Roberts, G.C. and Ratliff, A.H.C. (1978). *Hip Disorders in Children*. London: Butterworth.
Powell, M. (1986). *Orthopaedic Nursing and Rehabilitation*, 9th edn. London: Churchill Livingstone.
Roaf, R. and Hodkinson, L.J. (1980). *Textbook of Orthopaedic Nursing*, 3rd edn. Oxford: Blackwell Scientific.

15 The child with genitourinary problems

The kidney excretes waste products of metabolism, and acts as a filter and reabsorbs certain substances necessary to the body. The nurse caring for children needs to understand the importance of any abnormalities in the urine and to use her powers of observation in recording any change in colour, odour and quantity. Her careful reporting may help the paediatrician who relies on the accuracy of her reports and tests.

Observations should be recorded clearly and accurately on the patient's chart and abbreviations should be avoided as they may easily lead to misinterpretations or misunderstandings.

Methods of Collecting Clean and Ordinary Specimens of Urine

Even newborn babies may show signs of renal damage due to abnormalities present *in utero*, e.g. back pressure caused by inadequate relaxation of the bladder neck or sphincter or inadequate muscle action in the bladder wall or ureters. Interuterine surgery is being developed to prevent the resulting damage which is frequently irreversible.

Infection in infancy, caused by ascending bacterial invasion or by deformities such as double ureters, neurogenic bladder, horseshoe kidney, etc., may lead to permanent renal damage in later life unless treated at the

FIG. 39 Urine collecting bag (*left*), in position (*right*). The bag may be used for either boys or girls for obtaining single specimens, or for 24-hour collections.

earliest possible moment. Careful collection of urine for examination is therfore of very great importance.

Accurate measurement of the urinary output and drainage is of paramount importance as it may be an aid to diagnosis and lead to the prevention of serious complications. Where appropriate the nurse should state whether the urine came from a nephrostomy, perineal or suprapubic or urethral catheter or if it was passed normally per urethram.

It may be difficult to collect urine from babies and toddlers. The container should be of appropriate size for the amount of urine collected (e.g. 10-ml bottles are quite adequate for babies). Special plastic urine collecting bags may be used both for boys and girls (Fig. 39). Where these are not available the following techniques can be used:

Baby boys. Urine may be collected by strapping Paul's tubing to the penis. If the specimen is for bacteriological investigation, an aseptic technique should be used. A tray with receivers and sterile cotton wool swabs, saline or a mild antiseptic solution, a sterile Paul's tubing, and four lengths of 6 mm strapping is required. The penis is well cleaned, where possible the foreskin retracted and the glans gently swabbed before fixing the tube in position. Paul's tubing, previously sterilized, is easy to use and very effective.

Baby girls. Baby girls present a much more difficult problem. It may be advisable to wash and swab the buttocks and genitalia carefully before commencing a feed and then to sit the baby on a sterile receiver while she is feeding. Babies often pass urine during a feed.

Alternatively, a sterile receiver may be placed inside a well fitting air-ring and the baby nursed sitting upright over the opening.

Catheterization
Catheterization in young children should be avoided whenever possible. Sometimes catheterization may have to be carried out for diagnostic purposes, to relieve retention of urine, and in certain post-operative cases. Children with paralysis of bladder muscles may be taught to self-catheterize as a routine method of emptying the bladder.

Basically the requirements are the same for children as for adults. It is, however, essential to have at least one assistant or whenever possible the mother present, to ensure that the child maintains the correct position without struggling and who can reassure and talk to the child.

Little girls should have their buttocks raised on a sand bag or rolled towel. When the buttocks are thus elevated the catheter should be directed downwards rather than at right angles to the perineum, as it would be with an adult. As the urethra is short urine should be obtained after passing only 2.5–5 cm of the catheter. It is important to wash the groins, thighs and genitalia with soap and water before starting the actual catheterization. When the procedure is completed the surrounding skin should be carefully dried. A pot or bedpan should be offered as catheterization leaves the patient with a feeling of irritation and an apparent desire to pass urine.

Suprapubic aspiration in order to obtain sterile urine specimens is often carried out instead of catheterization. This procedure is performed by a doctor with a fine needle and syringe. By this means the specimen obtained is not contaminated with other organisms, and there is less likelihood of introducing infection into the bladder.

Mid-stream specimens

With older children, capable of co-operation and control in passing urine, this method can replace catheterization in many cases. After cleaning the genital area in the method described above, the child is asked to pass some urine in order to flush the urethra. After approximately 30 ml has been passed the stream is interrupted and the remaining urine collected in a sterile container with clear indication that the specimen was a mid-stream one.

Twenty-four-hour specimens

To estimate accurately the volume of urine passed or the amount of a particular constituent in 24 hours, the following procedure is adopted. In young children 12 hour specimens may be considered acceptable.

The patient is asked to empty the bladder at 08.00 hours and this urine is discarded. All urine passed in the following 24 hours is then collected. The patient is asked to pass urine at 07.55 hours the following day and this specimen is added to the total collected.

Retention of Urine

This, irrespective of the cause, may produce restlessness in unconscious patients and may disturb sleep. Simple nursing measures may relieve retention. The mother or nurse can sit the patient in a warm bath, allow small boys to stand up while using a bottle, and run a nearby tap. Such nursing attention is infinitely worthwhile and may make painful, complicated measures such as catheterization unnecessary.

Investigations of the Urinary Tract

Intravenous pyelography

Intravenous pyelograms are done to outline the urinary tract and demonstrate the efficiency of renal function. Fluids are withheld for the 6 hours preceding the test but dry foods may be given.

A straight radiograph is taken first, in order to ascertain that no gases will obscure the picture. If this is satisfactory a radio-opaque dye is then injected into a vein. In most cases the median basilic vein is chosen for the injection but with babies it may be necessary to use another vein if possible, but occasionally it is necessary for the medium to be subcutaneously combined with hyaluronidase in order to speed up and facilitate absorption. The dye is rapidly excreted by the urinary tract.

N.B. *Iodine sensitivity*. A test dose of 1 ml is injected intravenously. If no reaction occurs in 1 minute the full dose of the opaque medium can be given. *Sensitivity reaction*: nausea, vomiting, urticaria, flushing and restlessness.

Immediately after the injection the child is given a 'fizzy drink' or an infant is given a feed. This allows for the demonstration of the left kidney on X-ray behind the gas bubble formed in the stomach.

Serial pictures are taken, usually at 3, 8, 15 and 30 minutes after the injection and the progress of the dye is watched. Any abnormalities in the filling of the renal tract or in excretion are demonstrated on the radiograph.

Micturating cystogram
Co-operation will be needed from the older child during this procedure, so the mother or nurse should carefully explain what is involved prior to catheterization. If possible the mother should accompany the child. A small child may have the examination carried out under a general anaesthetic. The child is usually catheterized in the ward, before transfer to the X-ray department. Following introduction of the contrast medium through the catheter, this is then removed and the child encouraged to pass urine. As the bladder contracts X-rays are taken. If the cystogram is being carried out under a general anaesthetic, suprapubic pressure is needed to empty the bladder.

Cystoscopy
Cystoscopy is exactly the same as with adults except that children are given a light anaesthetic. Cystoscopy is usually done to examine the bladder, urethra, and ureteric openings into the bladder for congenital abnormalities.

Retrograde pyelography
Retrograde pyelography is sometimes needed to ascertain further evidence, particularly if, due to poor renal function, the intravenous pyelogram has failed to yield adequate information.

For this procedure a lighter anaesthetic has to be given

but otherwise preparation is the same as for intravenous pyelogram, and the procedure is similar to that used in adults.

Cystography
Cystography may be done in order to determine the capacity and outline of the bladder or to demonstrate the presence of urethral valves and vesico-ureteric reflux.

Renal biopsy
Renal biopsy is carried out under a general anaesthetic as an aid to the assessment and progress of renal tissue, particularly for those children suffering from nephritis or nephrosis. It may also be performed following a kidney transplant.

Following return to the ward after the procedure, nursing care should monitor the following:

Nursing action	Explanation
Pulse and blood pressure.	Any increase may indicate haemorrhage into the renal tissue.
All urine passed is measured and examined for blood.	Some haematuria is usually present for 24 hours. If persistent or excessive, report to doctor.
Pain related to site of puncture, backache and dysuria.	Some discomfort expected initially, prescribed analgesia should be given. If persistent or excessive, report to doctor. May indicate renal damage.
Puncture site should be left exposed to observe for swelling, discoloration and haemorrhage.	Report any change. May indicate damage to other tissues or renal haemorrhage.

Renal Function Tests

Urea clearance test
A comparison is made between the amount of urea present in the circulation and urine respectively. The test demonstrates the extent of healthily functioning substance in the kidney, following disease.

Urea concentration test
This is a test of the kidneys' ability to excrete urea, one of the end products of protein metabolism. The child has nothing to eat or drink for 12 hours (usually overnight) before the test.

Urine is then collected, following which a dose of urea is given. A further 3 specimens of urine are collected at hourly intervals.

Ureatine clearance test
A 24-hour collection of urine is commenced. During this period a specimen of blood is obtained. The laboratory staff will need to know the child's age, sex, height and weight in order to assess glomerular function in the excretion of ureatine, a breakdown product of protein metabolism.

ACUTE PYELONEPHRITIS (PYELITIS)

This is essentially an infection of the renal parenchyma and the pelvis of the kidney. The disease is a very common one in childhood, affecting girls rather more often than boys and it occurs frequently in young infants.

Mode of infection
The infection may reach the kidneys via the blood stream, from the bowel via the lymphatic system or as an ascending infection from the bladder and urethra. In many cases

the infection is caused by a malformation in the urinary tract, such as a kink in one of the ureters which causes the urine to be dammed back, to stagnate and to become infected.

In about 70% of cases the causative organism is the *Escherichia coli* (bacterium), but streptococcal and staphylococcal infections also occur.

Signs and symptoms
As a rule, the onset of the disease is a very sudden one. One of the earliest symptoms is vomiting, soon followed by a rise in temperature to between 39.4° and 40.6°C (103°–105°F); rigors and meningism are common. The child is pale and ashen in colour, with flushed cheeks and dark rings round the eyes. The child is irritable and suffering from spasmodic, colicky pain, which is a constant feature. With young babies diarrhoea occurs and this together with the vomiting soon causes dehydration. The urine is scanty, strongly acid and may have a curious fishy smell. The tongue is dry and thirst is marked. If old enough to do so the patient complains of dysuria.

Investigations
Examination of a clean specimen of fresh urine under the microscope will reveal the presence of pus cells, albumin and organisms. The prognosis is as a rule a good one, recovery taking place in 3 days to a week. Recurrent cases are often due to malformations in the urinary tract and therefore X-ray investigations are carried out. The prognosis depends on the underlying cause.

Nursing care
The nursing care during an attack of pyelitis is mostly symptomatic. In order to reduce the temperature, the

bedclothes are cradled and a fan may be used to cool and circulate the air. Tepid sponging is soothing but must not be done without medical permission. If the patient is incontinent the buttocks should be washed frequently as the acid urine is liable to excoriate the skin. It may be helpful to apply a soothing emollient cream. The mouth easily gets dry and dirty, and careful mouth toilet is essential.

Temperature, pulse and respirations are taken and recorded 4-hourly and a strict intake and output record is important. If vomiting persists and dehydration becomes marked, fluids may have to be given intravenously.

Drugs
According to the sensitivity of the causative organism, various drugs such as sulphonamides and nitrofurantoin are administered.

Diet
In the majority of cases the patient should be given liberal amounts of fluids. For babies, milk is withheld as long as vomiting persists. Once the acute stage of the illness is passed, children quickly regain their appetite and no special diets need be given.

NEPHRITIS

A variety of classifications of nephritis have been used in the past, but the term nephritis is now used for those conditions in which inflammatory changes predominate in the renal substance. Nephrosis or nephrotic syndrome is characterized by degenerative changes in the renal tubules. Sometimes it is difficult to draw a distinction between the two conditions and in the sub-acute phase the term 'nephrotic-nephritis' may be used.

TABLE 13 Comparison between nephritis and nephrotic syndrome

	Nephritis	Nephrotic syndrome
Onset	Very sudden	Insidious
Cause	Streptococcal infection 10–14 days previously in 75% of cases	Unknown in many cases, in others associated with renal disease
Age	Commonly 3–8 years rarely in infancy	All ages
Haematuria	Present	Rarely present
Proteinuria	Moderate degree	Considerable
Urinary output	Diminished	Variable
Oedema	Of short duration if it occurs	Persistent
Blood pressure	Raised at onset	Usually normal
Diet	Restricted protein, low salt if oedema present	High protein, low salt

Nephritis

Acute post-streptococcal glomerulonephritis; acute hae-morrhagic nephritis.

Definition

A disease of sudden onset, usually following a strep-tococcal infection (most commonly tonsillitis) 10–14 days prior to onset of haematuria, hypertension and acute renal inflammation.

Pathology
Both kidneys are affected, but are of normal size. Microscopical appearance shows minute haemorrhages blocking the glomeruli which means that the filtering capacity of the kidneys is interfered with; small areas of necrosis may also be seen.

Age
Affects most commonly the age group 3–8 years; rarely in infancy.

Clinical presentation
Haematuria is often the presenting symptom, it may be very obvious or only minimal giving a 'smoky' appearance to the urine. This may last for a few days or for many weeks. Urinary output at onset of the disease is usually diminished. The child appears 'off colour', uninterested in his normal play activities and very lethargic. Headache and vomiting frequently occur at onset of the disease. Oedema is common, and is especially noted in the eyelids and the pendant parts, but is of short duration. It is associated with an increase in weight. In cases of streptococcal infection the antistreptolysin titre is raised. The temperature is elevated and the blood pressure may remain normal but more commonly it will also be raised Thompson and Woodhouse (1987).

Investigations
These will include daily tests of urine; quantitative daily albumin estimations may also be recorded. Laboratory examinations of the urine to detect the presence of cells and casts will be required at frequent intervals, but less often once the haematuria has disappeared. As the kidney cannot clear the waste products in the normal way, the blood urea level may rise about 7.47 mmol/litre (45 mg/

100 ml) or more, and creatinine and phosphorus levels are also higher than usual. Culture of throat swabs and a full blood count will also be made. X-ray of the sinuses and examination of the tonsils and teeth are carried out in order to discover any foci of infection.

Treatment
Diet, rest and nursing care are the main forms of treatment. Penicillin may be prescribed for any latent streptococcal infection. Anaemia is treated with iron therapy. Sulphonamides may be ordered.

Nursing care
Children suffering from nephritis should have reduced activity until urinary output and blood pressure are normal, and the haematuria has subsided. The child should be kept warm, comfortable, resting, and yet able to watch the life of the ward around him (Whaley and Wong, 1987). A daily bath is given. If constipation is troublesome a mild aperient may be given.

The mother or nurse should make time to play and read stories in order to relieve the monotony of bed rest and to promote development. Visiting should be enouraged to enable the child to maintain family contacts, and to adjust to hospitalization. The child will be able to take part in the activities of the hospital school.

Observations

1. Temperature, pulse and respiration are recorded 4-hourly initially as any change may be the first indication of complications developing, e.g. further infection.

2. Fluid intake and output should be recorded with accuracy.

3. Frequent recordings of the child's weight are made; it is most useful to chart this as a graph to show progress, as it is a good guide to the amount of oedema present.

4. Blood pressure readings are taken twice daily initially, then less frequently if good progress is made. Any rise in the blood pressure readings must be reported immediately.

5. The appearance of an early morning specimen of urine should be noted daily.

6. Note of the child's general appearance must also be made, e.g. looks and interest in surroundings. Any observation of twitching of the limbs should be reported immediately as this may be an indication that hypertensive encephalopathy, a serious complication, is developing.

Diet

In order to rest the kidneys the fluid intake is usually restricted during the initial phase; the amount allowed varies according to the child's weight.

Examples of the amount of fluid allowed in 24 hours

5 years	18 kg (40 lb)	Basic allowance	360 ml (12 oz)
10 years	30 kg (66 lb)	Basic allowance	480 ml (16 oz)

Added to the basic allowance would be an amount equal to the volume of urine passed during the previous 24 hours.

For the first 3 or 4 days the child's diet consists of drinks with added glucose. Orange juice should be avoided in view of its relatively high potassium content. The nurse should remember that the child will enjoy variety, and hot drinks as well as cold should be offered to relieve the monotony of the fluid diet. When diuresis occurs a light diet is gradually introduced, the protein of which is restricted until the urine tests show an improvement in the cell count. While any oedema is present, salt intake too will be restricted.

Prognosis

1. The majority of cases are uncomplicated and usually resolve in about 6 weeks.

2. Rarely, hypertension may lead to cardiac failure and encephalopathy. A few patients progress into the nephrotic syndrome. If anuria develops the outlook is grave.

NEPHROSIS, NEPHROTIC SYNDROME (LIPOID NEPHROSIS, SUBACUTE NEPHRITIS)

Definition
This condition is manifested clinically by insidious onset of gross generalized oedema, and by proteinuria, associated with low plasma proteins.

Pathology
Both kidneys are affected and appear very pale and swollen.

Age
Pure nephrosis or lipoid nephrosis, starts in children below the age of 5 years. Nephrotic syndrome, associated with a variety of other kidney conditions is seen in older children.

Clinical presentation
The child appears irritable, listless and pale with no interest in food. Oedema affects the face, legs and abdomen leading to weight gain. Urine output is reduced and pro-

teinurea is present. Haematuria may occur and usually indicates a poor prognosis. Blood pressure initially is normal.

Investigations
Daily testing of urine and estimation of the amount of protein lost in the urine. Frequent laboratory examination of the urine for cells and casts, also culture for evidence of infection in the urine is required. Blood investigations needed will include a total blood picture, urea levels which are normal until the terminal stages, total plasma proteins which are low, serum cholesterol which is usually raised, and the ESR which may be elevated. Serum electrolytes should be estimated frequently. Renal biopsy may be performed to confirm the diagnosis if there is any doubt about this.

Drugs
Steroid therapy in the form of prednisone or prednisolone is of great value to the child with nephrosis; initially doses are high, the amount given being reduced after 10 days until a maintenance dose is reached to prevent the return of proteinuria. This maintenance dose may need to continue for as long as 6 months, but unfortunately relapses are common so that a return to higher dosages may be necessary. The long-term effect of steroids is to produce dwarfism, obesity and adrenal failure. The child receiving long-term steroids may need to receive antibiotics as a prophylactic measure as these children are especially prone to infection.

In steroid resistant cases, the diuretic chlorothiazide may be combined with spironolactone (Aldactone A) in a dosage of 25 mg four times daily. Potassium chloride should be given during therapy with chlorothiazide to prevent a potassium deficiency occurring. Cyclophosphamide

(3 mg/kg) is sometimes combined with steroids for those children liable to relapse (Whaley and Wong, 1987). The child and the parents should be warned that this drug may produce baldness, but that the hair will quickly grow again once the course of treatment has been completed. Meanwhile a wig can be worn if necessary.

A blood transfusion is given occasionally to correct anaemia and to improve the child's general condition.

Nursing care
The basic nursing care is the same as that for the child with nephritis, but as the oedema may be causing respiratory embarrassment the nurse will have to use her skills in making the patient comfortable with extra pillows. Support for the scrotum may be necessary if the patient is a boy. As the child with gross oedema will be unable to move much, conscientious care of the skin and pressure areas is important. Small pillows and bed cradles should be used to prevent foot drop and to take the weight of the bed clothes off the patient's limbs. The peripheral circulation is often poor and oedematous limbs may be cold and discoloured; warm blankets and woollen socks may help to keep the feet warm. Care must be taken when using hot-water bottles as the oedematous limbs are relatively insensitive, and burns could occur easily.

Because of the loss of gamma globulin together with oedema, there is a great tendency to infection and evidence of sepsis such as septic spots on the skin should be reported immediately.

Observations
Observations are the same as for the child with nephritis except that it is not usually necessary to record the blood pressure as frequently unless it is found to be raised.

Diet

As a great deal of protein is lost in the urine, a high protein diet is given as soon as the child is well enough to eat it. Estimations of the blood urea will act as a guide to tolerance of this regimen; if the blood urea rises excessively it may be necessary to restrict protein intake. Restriction of salt to less than 2 g daily is also necessary while there is evidence of oedema. Paediatricians vary as to the need to restrict fluids, some allow 600 ml a day, others relate the fluid intake to the urinary output, while others do not restrict fluids at all.

Anorexia is frequently a problem, and the nurse needs to use skill and ingenuity to tempt the child's appetite by serving meals as attractively as possible. When a precise amount of protein is sent up from the diet kitchen the amount of food rejected should be recorded after every meal, so that the amount of protein refused can be accurately measured.

Prognosis

The long-term outlook is not good despite the use of steroids. Approximately 30% of patients die from complications, e.g. intercurrent infections or peritonitis. Some children after a variable period become symptom free, in others the oedema persists.

RENAL FAILURE

Renal failure occurs when the kidneys are unable to maintain regulation of the composition or the volume of the body fluids. With acute renal failure the child's condition deteriorates rapidly in a few days. The chronic form of renal failure may take several months. The main causes of renal failure are:

1. Shock associated with major injury or haemorrhage.
2. Burns involving more than 15% of the body surface.
3. Gastroenteritis resulting in severe dehydration.
4. Septicaemia.
5. Renal disease.
6. Obstructed urinary flow.
7. Mismatched transfusion, ingested poisons, anaphylactic shock.
8. Hypoxia in the neonatal period.

Signs and symptoms
The usual presenting symptom in acute renal failure is oliguria, but occasionally the child will be observed to pass dilute urine in large quantities. Drowsiness, headache, loss of appetite, pallor, vomiting, sore dry mouth, pyrexia, diarrhoea and convulsions are all common and may occur simultaneously or at different times. Blood pressure and intracranial pressure are high and there may be visual disturbances and retinal haemorrhages. The pulse rate is rapid and the volume poor.

Treatment
Uraemic children are particularly prone to infection, and the appropriate antibiotics will be ordered. These may need to be given in reduced dosage, as some reach dangerous blood level concentrations if given in the normal amounts when the kidneys are not properly functioning, e.g. gentamycin, streptomycin, kanamycin and the sulphonamides. Intravenous fluids will be required for some children depending on the primary cause of the renal failure. For the severely anaemic child blood will be required and will usually be given as packed cells in order to avoid overloading the circulation. Peritoneal dialysis or haemodialysis is sometimes indicated if the child's condition continues to deteriorate and the blood urea level rises

above 65 mmol/litre (400 mg/100 ml). Haemodialysis is the most effective method but requires special facilities that are not available in all units. For most children peritoneal dialysis is effective and can be used even in young children. Kidney transplant operations in children are now carried out most successfully in a few specialized units. This offers a new life to these children but unfortunately there are not yet enough suitable donors and there are still many technical problems to overcome.

Nursing care
The aim of nursing care throughout this illness is to make the child comfortable by anticipating needs, alleviating symptoms and providing the nurse's prescription of t.l.c. (Tender Loving Care).

Accurate records of the intake and output must be carefully maintained. The basic fluid intake should be totalled together with the output of the previous 24 hours and calculated to allow for insensible loss through the skin and lungs which the nurse should remember will be greater during a heatwave or if the child is pyrexial. Because of the poor kidney function only small amounts are allowed. An average daily fluid intake allowance would be:

Infants   12 – 15 ml/kg/24 hours.
Older children   10 ml/kg/24 hours.

The mouth will be dry and careful mouth toilet is essential. Frequent mouth washes can be given providing the older child knows now to swallow any of the glycothymoline or whatever fluid is being used. Sucking fruit pastilles slowly, will also help to keep the mouth moist as well as providing extra calories. Adequate calories must be given in the diet to minimize further protein breakdown. A pleasantly flavoured glucose concentrate such as

'Hycal' (25 ml = 60 calories approx.) can be given. Some first-class protein will also need to be provided in the diet to prevent further breakdown of body protein and so increase the blood urea. Occasionally if the child is comatosed 'Aminosol' or 'Intralipid' will be given intravenously to meet essential nutrition requirements. Daily weight should be recorded ideally using a weighing bed, taking care that the bedclothes remain the same weight. Temperature, pulse and blood pressure readings should be recorded frequently and any changes reported.

Peritoneal dialysis
In peritoneal dialysis, fluid is run into the peritoneum via a catheter. Waste products of metabolism such as urea, potassium and solutes move across the peritoneal membrane from their high concentration in the blood to a low concentration in the dialysis fluid by diffusion and osmosis. The fluid with the waste products is then drained away and the cycle repeated.

There are basically two types of peritoneal dialysis used for children: Intermittent Peritoneal Dialysis (IPD) and Continous Ambulatory Peritoneal Dialysis (CAPD). Preparation of the child and family for both these techniques are similar. The procedure should be carefully explained to the child and parents before the treatment commences. Wherever possible families should be introduced to other children having the same form of treatment (Jepson, 1989). The child should also empty his bladder and be weighed. A sedative may be required. Strict asepsis is observed throughout the procedure. The abdominal skin is cleaned and the doctor will infiltrate a local anaesthetic of 1% lignocaine into the skin midway between the umbilicus and symphysis pubis. A stab incision is made through which a 'Trocath' at permanent Tenchkoff catheter is introduced under general anaesthesia and a catheter is pushed gently into the pelvis and connected to the previously prepared dialysing set.

Continuous ambulatory peritoneal dialysis

The amount of dialysing fluid run in depends on the age and weight of each child. Small infants will accommodate 150–200 ml each run, but a child of 12 years may take as much as a litre. The first run is drained immediately but in subsequent cycles the fluid is allowed to remain in the peritoneal cavity for 30 minutes. Dialysis is used continuously until the plasma electrolytes are more or less normal. Throughout this procedure the nurse must observe the child most carefully, noting any difficulty in respiration, nausea or vomiting. Care should be taken to prevent kinking of the tubing. If the flow diminishes it can often be rectified by changing the child's position or repositioning the catheter. If the catheter becomes blocked, the doctor will need to syringe it through with heparinized saline, or replace it with a new one.

Intermittent peritoneal dialysis

Following insertion of the Tenchkoff or permanent catheter the child is connected to the dialysis machine and the dialysing fluid at a rate of 30 ml per kilogram of body weight is flushed into the peritoneum. Flushing is continued until the used fluid is no longer blood-stained and therefore unlikely to clot. Heparin 500 units per litre of dialysate is also added to prevent clotting inside the catheter (Jepson, 1989).

Regular cycles of dialysing are continued, during which time observations of the child's condition are regularly recorded to include pulse, blood pressure, weight and body temperatures using both central and peripheral temperature probes. The frequency of these recordings can be reduced once the child's condition is stable. Monitoring of urea, creatinine and electrolytes will also be carried out so that any adjustments necessary to the fluid dialysing cycle can be made.

Complications include infection and strict asepsis always needs to be observed whenever diaylsis lines, bags or dressings are changed.

Long-term follow-up care
All children receiving dialysis and their families require considerable support. Parents need to be encouraged to become involved in the treatment regimen for its satisfactory performance at home, enabling the child to lead a fairly normal life at school and at play. Although Jepson (1989) states that renal transplantation is the most economical treatment for end stage renal failure and remains the ultimate aim, CAPD is cheaper than any other form of hospital dialysis and gives the child relative freedom, enabling him to stay at home.

SURGICAL CONDITIONS OF THE GENITOURINARY TRACT

In childhood the majority of operations performed on the genitourinary system are to correct congenital abnormalities. These are often the cause of recurrent urinary tract infections, colicky pain, and failure to thrive. In extreme, untreated cases, uraemia and death may result.

In investigations and treatments of the urinary tract the danger of ascending infection must constantly be borne in mind. Catheterization, the use of in-dwelling catheters, is only ordered if there is no other alternative. When drainage tubes are in use it is the task of the nurse to watch the tube carefully. Kinking or compression of the tube may lead to damming-back of urine and as a child is unlikely to voice a complaint it is the nurse's responsibility to appreciate that there is something wrong by noticing the patient's restlessness or by noticing an abnormal output of urine. Accurate measurement of the urinary drainage and output is more important if serious complications are to be prevented. Operations on bladder or kidney may result in bleeding and clot formation. Morphine may be given to lower blood pressure and relieve pain, and lavage may have to be employed to dissolve clots and prevent the child from straining in an attempt to pass the clot per urethram. At operations which may be expected to cause post-operative bleeding, the surgeon usually stitches a drainage tube into the wound, the substance of the kidney or the bladder to allow blood to escape. These tubes or drains call for careful nursing attention and vigilance.

Movement of the patient need not be restricted and change of position from side to side is helpful in promoting drainage and preventing chest complications.

Congenital Abnormalities and their Treatment

Agenesis of the kidney
Failure of development of the kidney is as a rule unilateral. In that case the other kidney may hypertrophy and take over the total renal function and no treatment is necessary. Bilateral agenesis is incompatible with survival beyond the neonatal period.

Horseshoe and double kidney
A horseshoe kidney is formed by the union of the lower poles of the two kidneys, and may remain symptomless. The abnormality may be found accidentally in the course of a routine abdominal X-ray examination, or in other instances the child has recurrent urinary tract infections or attacks of pain and vomiting. A double kidney shows up

plainly when pyelography is performed and it is often associated with double ureters. in long-standing cases hydronephrosis may develop. One of the ureters may have a kink or stenosis and if this is the cause of the recurrent infection or pain, it is removed.

Hydronephrosis and megaureter or hydroureter

Recurrent infections, obstructions and congenital abnormalities of urethra, ureters or renal pelvis may cause dilatation of one or both ureters or renal pelves. The patient suffers severe, recurrent pain and vomiting. The obstruction may be due to abnormally situated blood vessels which press on the ureters, stenosis of the ureter, ureteric or urethral valves, obstruction in the bladder neck and neurological causes. The obstruction may be unilateral or bilateral. If the cause of the obstruction can be removed, the ureters may regain their tone and return to a normal size. Nephrostomy and pyeloplasty are performed to relieve the condition.

Vesico-ureteric reflux

Some infants suffer from a maldevelopment of the ureteric orifices leading into the bladder. Every time the bladder contracts as the patient passes urine, urine flows back into the ureters and kidney causing disease and infection. The condition may rectify itself as the structures grow larger; alternatively re-implantation of ureters has to be carried out.

Urethral valves

Urethral valves occur only in boys. They may obstruct the urinary outflow and eventually cause renal failure. The bladder becomes distended and in babies this may cause a grossly enlarged abdomen. There is a constant trickle of urine so that the napkins are wet all the time. This may lead to the condition being missed for some time. The baby may, however, be observed to strain on passing urine and later there is enuresis both day and night. A catheter can be passed quite easily as the valves merely act as an obstruction to the outflow. Urinary tract infections are common as the bladder cannot empty adequately.

The presence of valves can be demonstrated by carrying out a voiding urethrogram. A catheter is passed into the bladder and a radio-opaque substance run in. After removing the catheter radiographs are taken while the patient voids urine and dye and empties the bladder. Ultrasound scanning and a DTPA (99^{m}Te-Diethylenetri-aminepentacetic acid) isotope scan may also be carried out on an outpatient basis (de Sousa, 1989).

In some cases the urethra can be sufficiently dilated to relieve the obstruction, but often the valves have to be excised via a perineal urethrostomy using diathermy. The prognosis depends on the amount of renal damage caused through infection and back pressure.

Neuromuscular incoordination of bladder and bladder neck

Neuromuscular incoordination causes incontinence, back pressure of urine and eventually hydronephrosis. Children and parents are taught routine catheterization to prevent these complications occurring. If the hydronephrosis is bilateral, it may be necessary to transplant the ureters into a resected loop of ileum opening on to the abdominal wall. A well-fitting appliance is made to fit over the stoma and urine is collected into a bag. The mother and child must be taught to keep the stoma clean and dry. The surrounding skin needs protection by painting it with tincture of benzoin. The bag should be emptied every 4 hours and the appliance renewed as necessary and at least once a week. If disposable bags are not worn, the bag should be washed in soapy water in order to eliminate odour. The mother is given several bags to use and told to report to the hospital if the urine becomes scanty or offensive, of it the child seems off colour or is vomiting.

Ureterocele
It sometimes happens that part of the mucous lining of the bladder prolapses into it and causes obstruction of ureteric or urethral openings. This leads to stagnation of urine, back pressure, hydroureters and hydronephrosis. Treatment consists of diathermy to the prolapsed mucosa through a cystoscope or cutting and re-implanting the ureters.

Circumcision
Surgical removal of the foreskin is done either if it is abnormally tight (phimosis), for recurrent balanitis or for religious reasons. In the neonatal period the prepuce normally adheres to the glans penis and only begins to separate after some months. Attempts to retract the foreskin routinely at bath time should therefore not be made during the first 2 or 3 years of life as forceful retraction may cause tears, infection and scarring.

Circumcision should always be carefully considered. Some authorities believe that any operation in this area should be avoided if at all possible on account of the psychological implications. Post-operatively, severe haemorrhage occurs easily and irritation of the glans, ulceration of the urethral opening from friction, ammoniacal dermatitis and meatal ulcers causing scarring and stricture are complications which result fairly frequently.

The child is admitted to hospital as a day patient and discharged towards evening. The mother is instructed to call her own doctor or bring the child back to hospital in the event of bleeding or if the child fails to pass urine. She should also be given clear instructions regarding hygiene of the area.

Post-operatively the wound edges are often covered with ribbon gauze soaked in compound tincture of benzoin and left in place for approximately 1 week. After that time it is soaked off in a bath and routine washing is all that is required. Very occasionally the ribbon gauze has been put on too tightly and congestion and oedema of the glans result. This requires urgent relief by sitting the patient in a warm bath of potassium permanganate (two crystals to each half litre of water) and peeling the dressing off gently. Failure to do this may result in gangrene. Some surgeons leave the penis uncovered but spray the wound with Nobecutane, allowing the child to have a bath as usual from the second day. Others apply antibiotic ointment or powder instead.

During the immediate post-operative period these children are often very restless and miserable and a sedative should be given. The mother or a nurse should be available to pick the baby up and comfort him as much as possible. In uncomplicated cases there is no difficulty of micturition but the first time the child passes urine should always be noted.

Paraphimosis
Occasionally children are brought to hospital with a grossly swollen or discoloured penis caused by a tight foreskin which has been retracted but could not be returned to its normal position. Relief is a matter of urgency as the blood supply is partly cut off. Cold packs or a bath may make it possible to reduce the condition and circumcision may be undertaken at a later date. Alternatively immediate operation may be necessary if other methods fail. The skin is divided and the constriction relieved. A watch should be kept for retention of urine.

Hypospadias
Malformation of the penis and urethra may cause the
urethral opening to be somewhere on the undersurface of
the penis and in extreme cases it may be at the juncture of
penis and scrotum. Plastic surgery aims at straightening
the penis and making a new urethra from flaps of skin.
The operation is usually done in two or three stages and
not started until the child is about 18 months old, although
meatotomy may have to be performed sooner to enlarge
the urethral opening. Oedema following operation may be
severe and for that reason an incision is sometimes made
on the dorsum of the penis to prevent constrictive swelling
and the formation of a haematoma, by allowing for adequate drainage.

The stitches are as a rule left exposed and are kept dry
by dusting with an antiseptic powder. Some surgeons
secure the sutures with glass beads. During the second
stage, when the urethra is newly constructed, the site of
operation is kept dry by the use of an in-dwelling catheter
which is passed into the bladder through the perineum
immediately behind the scrotum. The catheter and tubing,
leading to the underwater drain containing a mild antiseptic solution, should be watched for any kinking and drainage has to be carefully measured morning and evening.

After 8–10 days the patient is allowed to pass urine
through the urethra while the catheter is still in position,
but spigoted and as soon as he can do so satisfactorily the
in-dwelling catheter is removed. The perineal wound
heals without suturing.

Following any operation on the penis or urethra, the
urinal used by the patient should be sterile until the
wound is healed.

All operations on the penis are extremely painful and
distressing and every effort should be made to alleviate
apprehension and discomfort. Sedatives should be given

generously, penis and scrotum carefully supported by small pillows, the weight of the bedclothes taken by a cradle and great care taken not to pull at the catheter during bedmaking. Pressure areas need careful attention and the bowels should be watched as constipation is common and causes additional discomfort.

Undescended testicle

The testes undergo migration in fetal life from a position high up in the abdomen through the inguinal canal and into the scrotal sac. They usually reach this final position by the time of birth. In some cases, however, migration is incomplete on one or both sides. On examination it is usually possible to determine the exact position of the testicle and the length of the spermatic cord. In many cases the testicle is retractile, that is to say it lies subcutaneously near the opening of the inguinal canal and can be brought down without difficulty. Although it may retract again it can be expected to descend by the time puberty has been reached. In other cases it is ectopic and has to be brought down surgically and stitched into the scrotal sac. This is usually done at the age of 6–8 years and always before the onset of puberty. Unfortunately the testicle may be malformed and atrophic. In these cases it is removed as there is a danger of malignancy if this is not done. There may be an associated hernia, which can be repaired at the same time.

Post-operatively nursing care usually presents no problems. Sometimes hormone therapy with human chorionic gonadotropin (HCG) replaces operation. Rezvani (1987) reports a successful outcome in 20% of patients treated with HCG.

Long-term follow-up. Discussion on the importance of long-term follow-up of these boys should always be dis-

cussed with the parents. Even after successful orchidopexy fertility is reduced in later life and the risk of
developing malignant testicular tumour is increased in
the third or fourth decade of life. Those who remain untreated or those who had corrective surgery during or
after puberty are at greatest risk.

Exomphalos with or without ectopia vesicae
If the anterior abdominal wall is absent or if fusion of
the abdominal muscles is incomplete, the abdominal and
pelvic organs may be only thinly covered by amnion or
peritoneum or even lie on the surface at the time of birth.
The pubic bones are separated and the hip joints are
abnormal. Malformation of this kind may be asociated
with malformations of the penis or the vagina and with
absence of the urethra or bladder wall or eversion of the
bladder. If this is the case, the ureteric openings can be
plainly seen and there is a constant trickle of urine.
Ammonia dermatitis and excoriation of the surrounding
skin develop and may lead to an ascending infection of the
renal tract. Where possible surgery will be undertaken in
the neonatal period but if operation is not possible until
the child is older (6–12 months of age) the skin should be
protected by sterile ointments and barrier creams. Moist,
sterile pads with protective covering are applied to absorb
the urine. These should be changed at frequent intervals.

After performing an osteotomy to approximate the
pubic bones it may be possible to suture the skin and
bladder wall, but it is often necessary to leave the repair of
muscle to a later date. If there is a normally functioning
urethra, repair is comparatively successful, but often
urethra and sphincter control are defective or absent and
transplantation of the ureters into the sigmoid colon,
ileum or rectum is necessary. The abnormal bladder is
then removed at the same time. Alternatively the surgeon

may divert the urine through a loop of bowel isolated from the ileum and brought on to the abdominal surface. A stick-on ileostomy bag catches the urine. It can be emptied or changed as required.

Hydrocele
A hydrocele is a swelling of the scrotum caused by fluid which accumulates in the scrotal sac. It may be unilateral or bilateral. The hydrocele may close spontaneously in the first year of life. Because of this, operation is usually delayed unless the swelling causes discomfort or embarrassment. Aspiration of the fluid is obviously useless. If operation becomes necessary, the sac is incised and the opening closed by tying off the remnant of the processus vaginalis which is present and emptying the sac.

The operation is a simple one which causes little discomfort and few problems in the after care. The child may be treated as an outpatient or as a day case.

Transplanation of ureters
The operation of transplanation of ureters may have to be considered in cases in which there is either an abnormal or diseased bladder or an absence of sphincter control. This is frequently associated with malformation of the vagina, such as rectovaginal fistula.

The operation is a difficult one and as a result is often disappointing. For this reason it is more usual to create an ileal loop bladder.

The ureters are brought out on to the abdominal wall and each allowed to drain into a collecting bag.

Alternatively a loop of ileum is cut off from the alimentary canal and utilized as a reservoir, an opening made on to the surface and urine drained into a colostomy bag. This method lessens the risk of infection.

Nephrostomy
Drainage of the pelvis of the kidney is called nephrostomy. It is performed when some obstruction in the urinary tract has caused long-standing back pressure and dilatation of the ureters and renal pelvis (hydro-ureter and hydronephrosis) or when oedema following operation on the ureters obstructs the normal urinary flow.

A nephrostomy tube drains the renal pelvis of urine and is attached to a collecting bag. This tube may remain in place for up to 4 weeks but before it is removed the child will have an intravenous pyelogram or ultrasound scan to ensure there is free drainage of urine from the renal pelvis. When the tube is removed initially there may be drainage of urine from the site, but this usually dries up quickly. Children often find this tube uncomfortable, as they are unable to lie on their backs to sleep and dressing may be difficult (de Sousa, 1989).

The skin around the wound should be carefully cleansed and protected against excoriation by the application of a barrier cream. Extra lengths of drainage tube are often used to allow for free movement without pulling on the tube, when this kind of drainage is used in children.

Nephrectomy
The removal of a kidney is never considered unless full investigations have shown that the other kidney is healthy and capable of taking over the total renal function. The tests carried out include intravenous pyelography, retrograde pyelography and excretion tests. It is also usual to ensure that the remaining kidney will not be at risk from the presence of infection elsewhere in the body.

Reasons for undertaking nephrectomy include congenital abnormalities of the ureters or kidney, hydronephrosis and Wilms' tumour. Tuberculosis of the kidney is rare in childhood. The child is usually admitted several days prior to operation to allow him to get used to the ward. Fluid intake and output are carefully measured for comparison with the post-operative fluid balance. In the case of Wilms' tumour, operation may be considered urgent and no time may be allowed for any special preparation unless a course of radiotherapy is given initially.

Wilms' tumour (nephroblastoma)
Wilms' tumour, which arises from the kidney, is the most commonly occurring malignant growth of childhood.

Signs and symptoms
Frequently the first signs noticed are an enlargement of the abdomen. Pain, haematuria and suppression of urine together with general malaise, anaemia and failure to thrive occur rather later and these children do in fact remain surprisingly well for a long time despite the great malignancy of the condition and its tendency to form metastases in other parts of the body, particularly the lungs. The tumour is as a rule unilateral.

Treatment
This should be started without delay. A minimum of palpation for diagnostic purposes is allowed as there is a danger of dispersing the tumour cells into the renal vein and so encouraging spread. An intravenous pyelogram or body scan will reveal distortion of the renal pelvis and displacement of the kidney. A radiograph of the chest should be taken to ensure that there is no secondary spread of the tumour to the lungs. Operation to remove the affected kidney should be performed as soon as possible, blood transfusion is usually required during operation. Radiotherapy combined with cytotoxic drugs is ordered post-operatively, reducing the risk of metastases. With prompt treatment the prognosis is usually good.

REFERENCES

Blandy, J.P. and Moore, J. (1989). *Urology for Nurses*. Oxford: Blackwell.

de Sousa, M. (1989). Renal tract problems. *Paediatric Nursing* **1**(7), 11–12.

Jepson, S. (1989). Peritoneal dialysis. *Paediatric Nursing* **1**(5), 22–23.

Rezvani, I. (1987). Cryptorchidism: a paediatrician's view. *Paediatric Clinics of North America*. **34**, 735–746.

Thompson, F.D. and Woodhouse, C.R.J. (1987). *Disorders the Kidney and Urinary Tract*, pp. 57–70. London: Edward Arnold.

Whaley, L.F. and Wong, D.L. (1987). *Nursery Care of Infants and Children*, 3rd edn, pp. 1260–1270. Washington, DC: C.V. Mosby.

FURTHER READING

Blandy, J. (1982). *Lecture Notes on Urology*, 3rd edn. Oxford: Blackwell Scientific.

Cameron, S. (1981). *Kidney Disease*. Oxford: Oxford University Press.

Innes-Williams, D. and Johnson, J.H. (1982). *Paediatric Urology*, 2nd edn. London: Butterworth.

Kelalis, P.P. and King, L.R. (1976). *Clinical Paediatric Urology*, Vols 1 and 2. London: W.B. Saunders.

Morgan, R. (1981). *Childhood Incontinence*. London: Heinemann Medical.

16 The child with infection problems

SCABIES (SARCOPTES SCABIEI)

Scabies is a skin infection caused by a minute parasite. The female mite burrows into the skin, most commonly between the fingers, and lays her eggs; it is usually possible to see the burrows with the help of a magnifying glass. As the eggs hatch, the larvae move to the hair follicles. Intense irritation results and this is particularly marked when the skin becomes warm at night. In young babies the soft skin allows for access in any part of the body and lesions can be found anywhere. In those babies who have not started walking, lesions may even occur on the soft skin of the soles of the feet. Secondary infections are common as a result of scratching. The infection occurs as a result of direct contact with an infected person or through indirect contact with soiled bed linen, clothing, etc.

Treatment
The child is given a warm bath which softens the skin and opens the burrows to allow penetration of the prescribed lotion; the skin is then dried and allowed to cool before treatment. The lotion is applied—0.5% malathion or 1% gamma benzene hexachloride (e.g. lindane)—taking care to work in between the toes, fingers and other flexures. Gamma benzene hexachloride is contraindicated for infants, breast-feeding mothers and pregnant women (Robinson, 1986).

A single application is usually sufficient to achieve a cure but those areas of the skin that are washed within 24 hours of the scabicide being applied should have the lotion reapplied. This is particularly important to remember when the hands are washed.

All clothing, underwear and bed linen should be changed. All members of the family should be treated at the same time.

It is not necessary to send blankets or other garments for disinfection but all clothing, underwear and bed linen should be laundered.

It is important to tell the parents that the lesions may persist for several months despite successful treatment— irritation too may continue. Calamine may be applied to ease this irritation.

HEAD LICE (PEDICULOSIS CAPITIS)

Infestation of the hair by head lice should be suspected if the child is noticed to be scratching the scalp frequently, particularly at the back, as the head lice tend to inhabit the occipital region rather than the front part of the scalp. Secondary infection of the scratches on the scalp may produce a coincident impetigo. In some children, where infestation is severe, cervical adenitis associated with malaise and pyrexia may occur as a result of secondary infection.

The louse reproduces by means of hatching shiny, oval eggs which are attached to hair follicles close to the scalp by means of a 'cement-like' substance. This makes the removal of the eggs or 'nits' (the empty egg shell) difficult. The nit can only be removed from the end of hair.

Treatment
The basis of successful treatment is both educational and

practical. It is essential that the whole family be treated and this should include all the adults as well as any pre-school children.

Pediculosis capitis may be treated with Malathion or Carbaryl according to the manufacturers' instructions. A hairdryer should not be used to dry the lotion on the head (Caddow, 1989). Twelve hours after the use of either preparation, the hair is shampooed and combed with a fine comb whilst still wet.

Swimming should not be allowed for 24 hours after treatment as chlorine effectively destroys the potency of the pediculocide. Equally if the patient has been swimming within 72 hours before treatment the hair should be washed throughly and dried before treatment.

It is not necessary after treatment to comb out the 'nits' or eggs, which can be uncomfortable for the child. These eggs die and any eggs found more than half an inch away from the scalp are harmless.

Prevention

Parents should be advised to inspect their child's hair as part of a regular routine for early detection and treatment of head lice. Grooming of the hair at least twice a day with an ordinary comb is also fatal to head lice, as they are unable to regenerate injured tissue (Caddow, 1989).

CATSCRATCH FEVER

Probably a bacterial (Margileth, 1984) infection following a scratch or bite of an animal, especially a cat—the cat apparently healthy. A few days after the scratch an ulcer or sore develops. A week or two later the regional lymph nodes become very enlarged and there is some fever. Nodes may suppurate or adenitis persist for some months.

Pus is sterile and white cell count normal. May be treated with broad-spectrum antibiotic to prevent suppuration.

TOXOCARIASIS (VISCERAL LARVA MIGRANS)

Toxocariasis is an infection caused by the transmission of the visceral larvae migrans. These are deposited in the soil from dog and cat faeces. Children 1–4 years of age are the most likely to be infected. The infection is transmitted by direct contact of hands from contact with dog, cat, objects from the soil, or soil itself. It may also be transmitted by ingestion of the soil. When the ova are swallowed, the larvae hatch in the intestine, pass through the intestinal wall and wander through the viscera. They pass first to the liver and then to other intestinal organs, where they may produce granulomas. These are most commonly found in the liver but can also occur in the kidney, heart, striated muscle, brain and eyeball. Common presenting symptoms are fever, skin rash with general malaise and anorexia. As the larvae migrate, haemorrhage, granuloma formation and chest infections with enlarged tender liver and spleen occur. Ophthalmitis may occur in severe infections. There is an associated eosinophilia. Diagnosis is difficult although a standardized skin test is available. Treatment is symptomatic.

Prevention

All dog and cat owners should periodically 'deworm' their pets. Dogs should be kept away from public parks, etc. where children play, especially unescorted pets who are likely to defaecate indiscriminately. Enforcement and public education are needed to prevent canine soiling of footpaths and public places.

INTESTINAL PARASITES

Threadworms (Pinworms—*Enterobius vermicularis*)

Threadworm infestation is exceedingly common in children, and entire families may be affected.

The threadworm normally inhabits the large intestine but the female migrates to the anal region where she deposits her eggs. Irritation, particularly during the night, causes the child to scratch and reinfect himself through his finger nails. Sharing beds and towels is an obvious way in which infection is spread to others.

Signs and symptoms

The most general symptom is itching and this in turn may cause restless sleep and irritability. Scratching and irritation may cause inflammation of the perineum, vulvovaginitis, bed-wetting and occasionally diarrhoea or rectal prolapse.

The tiny worms may first be noticed in the course of a toilet round, although the worms remain on the surface of the stool only momentarily and then disappear into its substance. Alternatively the mother may describe symptoms which suggest the diagnosis.

Diagnostic test

In order to prove the presence of threadworms a simple test can be done. A piece of Sellotape 2.5 cm wide and 7.6 cm long is placed, sticky side down, on the perineum immediately on waking. It is then transferred to a microscope slide, again sticky side down and labelled and sent to the laboratory. The threadworm ova are obvious under the microscope. As the procedure is such a simple one it can easily be carried out by an outpatient's mother.

Treatment
Careful hygiene is the first essential. Finger nails should be kept short and hand washing before meals should be enforced. Pyjamas should be worn in preference to night gowns and both pyjamas and day knickers should be washed in a hot cycle of a washing machine daily. At night cotton mittens can be worn to prevent infecting the finger nails. A bath taken immediately after rising will remove ova laid during the night and limit their dissemination. The local application of an analgesic ointment is useful to relieve rectal irritation.

Drug therapy
Piperazine hydrate (0.25–2 g twice daily for 7 days) may be given. It is effective when given in one single dose. However, in order to exclude possible reinfestation, a second dose is often given after a week or 10 days. Alternative preparations include Mebendazole (for all ages over 2 years). All members of the family should be treated together.

Prevention
Reinfection is common. Threadworm ova are able to survive on many surfaces in the home. Bedrooms and bathrooms should be vacuumed and all surfaces cleaned regularly. Care should be taken to avoid scattering ova from bed linen and clothing onto the floor. All family members should be encouraged to wash their hands with the aid of nail brush after using the toilet and before meals.

RINGWORM (DERMATOPHYTES)

Ringworm fungi (or dermatophytes) are able to invade the skin, nails or hair. Table 14 gives details of ringworm

TABLE 14 Ringworm infections

Type/Organism	Presentation/Diagnosis	Treatment/Nursing interventions
Tinea capitis (ringworm of the scalp) *Microsporum audouinii*	Lesions on scalp—pruritic—may extend to neck. Characteristic scaly, circumscribed patches of alopecia. Examination under a Wood's glass filter shows a characteristic green colour.	Oral griseofulvin. The child should know that he should not share combs, brushes or headwear with others. Treatment may be required for several weeks and the nurse will need to stress the importance of compliance with treatment. Drug side-effects include: gastrointestinal upset, headache and photosensitivity, but are uncommon.
Tinea corporis (ringworm of the body) *Microsporum trichophyton*	Lesions spreading peripherally—generally round, red, scaly and may involve the nails. (tinea unguium) Direct microscopy of scales necessary to cofirm diagnosis. N.B. Usually of animal origin.	Oral griseofulvin. Topical antifungal preparations may be applied. Keep separate towels. Emphasize good health and personal hygiene.
Tinea pedis (athlete's foot) *Epidermophyton floccosum/ interdigitale*	Most commonly seen in adolescents. Areas of sodden, macerated cracks and fissures appear between toes and on soles of foot. May be very sore and pruritic. Diagnosis confirmed by direct microscopy of skin scrapings.	Oral griseofulvin and the application of topical antifungal preparations. Keep separate towels. Advise patient to wear cotton socks and well ventilated shoes. (Reduce perspiration and temperature of feet.) Not as contagious as once thought.

N.B. It is important to remember that fungal infections are frequently associated with poor lost resistance, which should if possible be corrected otherwise drug therapy may fail. Similarly, treatment may fail unless the animal source has also been treated or removed.

infections involving the head, body and feet, and outlines the treatment and nursing care necessary.

COMMUNICABLE DISEASES

Table 15 gives details of the incubation periods, sources, causative organisms, modes of spread, and the sign and symptoms of common communicable diseases. Nursing intervention, treatment and other relevant information is also given.

PAEDIATRIC HUMAN IMMUNODEFICIENCY VIRUS INFECTION (AIDS)

Acquired Immunodeficiency Syndrome (AIDS) is a new disease in mankind. It was first reported in adults in 1981 and in children in 1982 (Centers for Disease Control, 1982). This virus has now been identified as a retrovirus. Retroviruses are able to make a DNA copy of their RNA (with the assistance of a special enzyme, known as reverse transcriptase) which is then inserted into the nucleus of the cells they infect. HIV infection in children remains at present a rare condition but throughout the world increasing numbers of children with HIV infection are being reported (Mok, 1988; WHO and ICN, 1988).

Transmission
HIV is a blood-borne infection. The virus can be found in the blood and most body fluids of people infected with the virus. This means that the virus can be transmitted to the child in the following ways:

1. through being born to an HIV-positive mother;
2. being breast-fed by an HIV-positive mother;
3. through exposure to contaminated blood or blood products or unsterile needles/syringes;

TABLE 15 Communicable diseases

Disease	Incubation period	Organism, source and mode of spread	Signs and symptoms	Nursing interventions, treatment and complications	Other remarks
Mumps	14–21 days	Virus. Saliva of infected person. Droplet or direct contact with infected person.	Fever, malaise, stiff jaw, swelling of salivary gland—parotid and submandibular. Unilateral or bilateral. Trismus. Pain on eating—especially sugars. Furred tongue, mouth dry—diminution of saliva. Moderate lymphocytosis.	Symptomatic. Mouth care—drink with straw. Avoid foods which are sweet and stimulate salivary glands. Analgesia for pain. Mastitis, oophoritis, prostatitis, pancreatitis (all rare), meningitis, encephalitis (may lead to permanent deafness), facial paralysis. Orchitis at or after puberty.	Complement fixation test reaction to confirm diagnosis—rarely necessary.
Glandular fever (infectious mononucleosis)	2–6 weeks	Epstein-Barr virus (EBV). Droplet. Direct intimate contact with infected person.	Lassitude, anorexia, general malaise, pyrexia, headache, sore throat with tonsillar exudate which separates easily without bleeding. May be petechiae on palate.	Symptomatic. Treat general debility and depression—prolonged convalescence. Treat secondary infections—hepatitis, meningitis, encephalitis.	Relapses common, but complete recovery eventually.

Disease	Incubation period	Causative organism	Mode of spread	Clinical features	Complications / Treatment	Prevention / Notes
			Low infectivity.	Enlarged lymph nodes and spleen. Transient macular rash—chest trunk, limbs and particularly dorsum of hands and feet. Leucocytosis with raised monocytes (atypical). Paul Bunnell test may be positive.	Nephritis.	
Diphtheria	2–7 days	*Corynebacterium diphtheriae*	Droplet. Nasal and mucous discharges from infected person.	Malaise, headache, rapid, feeble pulse, some rise in temperature, toxic. Albuminuria, exhaustion. *Faucial:* Slight sore throat, continuous greyish membrane spreading to soft palate and pharynx, which bleeds when attempt made to remove. Glands of neck very enlarged, 'Bull neck', myocarditis. *Nasal:* Thin bloodstained nasal discharge with offensive smell. Crusting of external nares.	Diphtheria antitoxin if any question of infection possible. Absolute bed rest, mouth care, tube feed if necessary. Tracheotomy may become necessary. Antibiotics to treat secondary infection. Mechanical ventilation will be necessary if diaphragm paralysed. Physiotherapy after acute stage. Myocarditis, paralysis of limbs, palate, diaphragm, ciliary muscles and external rectus muscles, nephritis, peripheral neuritis.	Notifiable. Follow up contacts and possible carriers. Treat carriers with antibiotic. Immunization advisable to prevent infection and epidemics. Schick test to assess immunity—negative if immune.

TABLE 15 *continued*

Disease	Incubation period	Organism, source and mode of spread	Signs and symptoms	Nursing interventions, treatment and complications	Other remarks
			Laryngeal: Croupy cough, laryngeal stridor, loss of voice, asphyxia.		
Acute infectious gastroenteritis	Incubation period variable depend upon the organism. Organism spread most commonly by the faecal–oral route. Affects all ages but most common (and usually more severe) in young bottle-fed infants.	*Escherichia (Bacterium) Coli, Salmonella, Campylobacter.* Dysentery bacillus, *Shigella* Adenoviruses Rotavirus	Acute diarrhoea—green stools. May be associated with vomiting/nausea Abdominal pain and discomfort. Dehydration. Fever or hypothermia in the young infant.	Fluid therapy to correct fluid and electrolyte loss. Appropriate antibiotics. Symptomatic. Care of mouth and skin (sore arms). Oral feeds/fluids reintroduced gradually. Oral thrush. Secondary infection.	Often has a seasonal incidence.

Disease	Incubation period	Cause/Source	Symptoms and signs	Treatment	Notes
Brucellosis (undulant fever)	1–3 weeks	*Brucella abortus* (cattle). *Brucella melitensis* (goats). *Brucella suis* (pigs). Infected, unpasteurized milk, meat, dairy products. Infected hides and carcases.	Headache, malaise, anorexia, constipation, fever—settles by lysis in 10 days, but recurs. Cough, backache, profuse sweating, palpable spleen. Transient arthritis. *Abortus fever* (chronic brucellosis). Insidious, milder and more prolonged. Recurrent night sweats without serious general ill health. (*In both*) Blood culture may be positive. Rising agglutination titre. Leucopenia, mild anaemia.	Tetracycline streptomycin, vitamin B. Symptomatic—treat debility with long convalescence. Disinfect excreta—especially urine.	Notifiable. Recurring at short intervals for many months. Pasteurization of milk, clean water and destroying infected animals prevents disease.
Roseola infantum (exanthema subitum, sixth disease, pseudorubella)	8–15 days	Virus. Source unknown. Droplet.	Fever, macular rash—appears immediately temperature fallen, fades on pressure. On trunk, neck, proximal part of limbs; *not* face. Lasts 1–3 days. Little malaise. Catarrhal pharyngitis, cervical lymphadenopathy. Neutrophil leucopenia with relative lymphocytosis.	Symptomatic. Convulsions due to high fever.	Practically confined to children between 6 months and 3 years of age.

TABLE 15 *continued*

Disease	Incubation period	Organism, source and mode of spread	Signs and symptoms	Nursing interventions, treatment and complications	Other remarks
Measles (morbilli)	10–14 days	Virus. Source from respiratory tract secretions, blood and urine of infected person. Droplet.	Running eyes and nose. Dry, irritating cough. Conjunctivitis. Photophobia. Pyrexia. Transient prodromal rash. Koplik spots—white on red base on buccal mucous membrane. 3rd day: temperature subsides. 4th day: rash appears—dusky red macular rash behind ears → face, trunk, limbs. Temperature again elevated. Rash becomes large irregular blotchy areas of darker red.	Bed. Symptomatic. Antibiotic for secondary infections. Otitis media. Blepharitis. Corneal ulcerations. Bronchopneumonia. Collapsed lobe of lung. Bronchiectasis and lung abscess (if collapse insufficiently treated). Tuberculosis. Encephalitis and encephalomyelitis (gastroenteritis in infancy).	Notifiable. Segregate until rash fades. Passive immunity for 3 months after birth (if mother has had measles)
German measles (rubella)	14–21 days	Virus. Nasopharyngeal secretions of infected person, also virus present in faeces, blood and urine. Droplet.	Mild malaise and pyrexia day before rash. Generalized tender lymphadenitis especially posterior cervical and occipital. Rash: pink macules and papules at first discrete then confluent.	Very little necessary— symptomatic. Occasionally: Encephalitis. Arthritis.	Danger to fetus during first 14 weeks in utero if mother affected. Baby may be born deaf, with cataract, glaucoma, or heart disease (also risk of abortion). Mother should be given gamma globulin.

	Incubation	Organism / Source	Signs and symptoms	Treatment / complications	Notes
Scarlet fever (scarlatina)	1–7 days	Haemolytic streptococci (Lancefield Group A). Usual source is from the nasopharyngeal secretions of infected persons. Droplet, fomites, milk.	Headache, vomiting, pyrexia. Sore throat—soft yellow exudate. 'Strawberry tongue'. Polymorphonuclear leucocytosis. Raised antistreptolysin titre. Cervical lymphadenitis. Rashpunctuate erythema, bright scarlet, behind ears and sides of neck → whole body except circumoral pallor. Desquamation after 1 week.	(Septic and toxic forms very rare.) Bed. Penicillin and sulphonamides. Fluids. Mouth care. Pneumonia. Septicaemia. Otitis media. Acute nephritis and rheumatism. Anaphylactoid purpura. Sinusitis. Encephalitis. Quinsy. Retropharyngeal abscess. Cervical adenitis and abscess.	Notifiable. Dick test for diagnosis—rarely used. Possibility of cardiac lesions from acute rheumatism.
Whooping cough (pertussis)	7–14 days	Bordetella (Haemophilus) pertussis. Discharge from respiratory tract of infected person. Droplet or direct contact.	Cold → chest infection → cough which becomes paroxysmal with vomiting and may end with a whoop. Ulcer on fraenum. Lymphocytosis. Low erythrocyte sedimentation rate. Baby vomits, cyanosed, limp, no paroxysms.	Feed after vomiting. Sedation. Broad-spectrum antibiotics for secondary infections. Deal with debility—long convalescence, high-calorie diet. Otitis media. Bronchopneumonia. Pulmonary collapse. Bronchiectasis. Tuberculosis. Subconjunctival haemorrhage. Cerebral anoxia or haemorrhage. Convulsions. Rectal prolapse. Hernia. Spontaneous pneumothorax.	Notifiable. No passive immunity in babies. Mild abortive case in immunized child, but equally infectious. Child often 'whoops' for months after attack—not infectious. Routine immunization. Resuscitation equipment and oxygen available in case a severe apnoeic attack should occur.

N.B. For the infant under 3 months the best protection against whooping cough is the vaccination of all siblings.

TABLE 15 *continued*

Disease	Incubation period	Organism, source and mode of spread	Signs and symptoms	Nursing interventions, treatment and complications	Other remarks
Chickenpox (varicella)	14–21 days	Virus. Respiratory tract secretions from infected person; also early skin lesions (not scabs). Contact and droplet.	Minimal malaise and headache. Fever. Transient prodromal rash. Main rash appears in crops—mainly on face, head and trunk (centripetal) oval, unilocular papules → vesicles → pustules → crusts. Irritating rash. Lymphocytosis.	Prevent from scratching to avoid scarring. Baths. Calamine. Keep cool. Short nails. Elbow splints if necessary. Antihistamines. Antibiotics for secondary infections—impetigo, boils, cellulitis, conjunctivitis, polyneuritis, encephalitis, transverse myelitis.	Herpes zoster closely allied. Severe or fatal if child has leukaemia or is on steroid therapy. Segregate until scabs dry.
Poliomyelitis	5–35 days	Virus, through gastrointestinal tract.	Sore throat, headache, stiff neck. Muscle weakness.	Bed rest. Symptomatic treatment. Paralysis.	Vaccination available.

Disease	Incubation period	Causative organism / Transmission	Signs and symptoms	Treatment / Nursing care	Prevention
Tuberculosis	3–12 weeks	*Mycobacterium tuberculosis*. Close contact with infected person. Droplet.	The majority of children show little clinical upset. Vague and non-specific. Fever, loss of appetite and weight, lassitude and headache. However, specific symptoms will vary according to system attacked.	Nursing care aimed at symptomatic relief. Long-term chemotherapy with antituberculous drugs.	Prophylaxis with BCG.
Tetanus	3 days to 3 weeks	*Clostridium tetani* found in soil. Through break in skin.	Fever, feels unwell. Stiffening of jaw. 1–2 days later spastic rigidity of the body.	Bed rest in quiet dark room. Reduce muscle spasms, maintain hydration. Clean wound. Convulsions leading to death.	Tetanus immunoglobulin or antitoxin. Very rare in United Kingdom due to effective immunization programmes and prophylactic treatment at time of injury.

4. through penetrative sexual contact, e.g. child sexual abuse by an HIV-positive individual;

5. through skin piercing procedures, tattooing (blood brother/sister games) etc. with contaminated implements.

The major risk factors for children have been identified as:

1. Having a mother with a known infection or at increased risk of infection.

2. Receiving a transfusion of infected blood or blood products.

Diagnosing HIV infection in children

It is important for nurses to understand the basis for which the diagnosis of HIV infection in children is made in order to be of the best help, support and counsel to the child's parents.

For infants and children under the age of 15 months with perinatal infection, HIV culture in blood as well as clinical symptoms suggestive of HIV disease are better criteria for HIV infection than the HIV antibody test alone. In these children, a positive antibody test is an accepted criterion for infection only in the presence of both cellular and humoral immune deficiency, or the presence of clinical symptoms.

Infants less than 15 months old who have been exposed perinatally are classified as of 'indeterminate infection' if no other tests apart from an antibody test have been performed.

This group of children will need to be medically followed up at regular intervals to determine both HIV and general health status.

For older children with perinatal infection and those with HIV infection acquired through other modes of transmission, the diagnosis is based on one or more of the following:

- the identification of HIV in blood or tissues;
- the presence of HIV antibody (positive screening test plus confirmatory test) regardless of whether immunological abnormalities or clinical signs or symptoms are present; or
- the confirmation that the child's symptoms meet the CDC classification for paediatric AIDS.

Classification for paediatric HIV infection
In 1987, the Centers for Disease Control, Atlanta, Georgia, USA developed a classification system for HIV infection in children under the age of 13 years. This new classification (see Table 16) recognizes the differences of HIV infection in children from that of adults (Centers for Disease Control, 1987).

Clinical presentation
The onset of HIV infection in children produces a widespread clinical picture and the child will often be a

---

TABLE 16   Classification for paediatric HIV infection (from Centers for Disease Control, 1987)

P–0	Indeterminate infection
P–1	Asymptomatic infection
	A Normal immune function
	B Abnormal immune function
	C Immune function not tested
P–2	Symptomatic infection
	A Non-specific findings
	B Progressive neurological disease
	C Lymphocytic interstitial pneumonitis
	D Secondary infectious diseases
	E Secondary cancers
	F Other diseases attributable to HIV

member of a 'sick family' as one or maybe both parents will also have the disease. Mok (1988) estimates that in the United Kingdom 80% of children acquire the infection from their mothers. Nurses seeing children with non-specific symptoms or clinical signs should bear in mind the possibility of HIV infection, especially if either parent is known to have 'at risk' behaviour or if the child has received blood or blood products in the past which may have been contaminated.

Whilst 75% of children infected with HIV will present with non-specific symptoms, common presentation patterns included repeated episodes of infection especially diarrhoea or candidiasis in associated with repeated upper respiratory tract or ear infections and lymphadenopathy. Failure to thrive and neurological abnormalities with developmental delay may also be seen.

Treatment and nursing interventions

Caring for HIV-infected children requires close observation of the health authority's control of infection policies for blood and body fluids. These principles apply whether the child is cared for at home or in the hospital ward. No cases of transmission caused by casual contact are known (Fisch *et al.*, 1987), therefore continue to hug, cuddle and comfort the child in the normal way and encourage others to do so. Individualized care plans will identify particular needs for each child and his family, and nursing interventions should be implemented to meet them.

Long-term follow-up

Whilst the diagnosis of Acquired Immunodefieciency Syndrome (AIDS) in children carries a high mortality with a median survival of nine months following diagnosis, less is known about the prognosis for those children who have minimal symptoms of the disease and very little about those children who remain asymptomatic. It is conceivable that many HIV-positive children will live for many years, perhaps with episodes of acute life-threatening illness and chronic disability (Weller, 1989).

Normal immunizations should not be withheld from a child with HIV or from siblings—recommended guidance is issued by the Department of Health (1990).

PROTECTIVE ISOLATION NURSING MANAGEMENT

The aim of care is to prevent the spread of infection from the infected child to another using isolation nursing techniques. For other children who are susceptible to infection, e.g. those with immunosuppressive problems, the aim is to protect the child using reverse barrier nursing techniques. Nursing policies will vary from unit to unit but the following principles will apply.

Ideally nursing care should take place in a cubicle with its own hand basin, soap and hand towel dispenser, where the child can be observed easily through glass panes and also see out easily for himself. All equipment and furniture in the cubicle should be easy to clean and maintain. The doors to the cubicle should preferably be of the swing type so that entering and leaving can be made easily without contamination of the hands.

Physical isolation can be a bewildering and frightening experience for a child and an explanation should always be given. Protective isolation need not exclude resident parents and opportunities for mother or father to live in should be offered. Visitors, too, should be welcomed, although initially it may be necessary to restrict these to family members. A joint care plan should be drawn up where possible with the parents who will need to be kept fully informed regarding the procedures to be observed.

Other members of staff, play workers, teachers, etc. will also need to be made aware of 'protective isolation' protocol.

Equipment in cubicle

1. Bins and plastic bin-liners with good seals, for soiled hand towels, linen and disposables.
2. Basic items for physical examination, e.g. spatula, tape-measure, stethoscope, etc.
3. Small amount of clean linen.
4. Cleaning equipment.

Nursing records and charts are best left outside the cubicle except for those charts needed for immediate recording of frequent observations.

Gowns
Gowns or plastic aprons should be worn if the child, bed, bedding or clothing is handled. When worn, these should be put on and taken off correctly.

Masks
Incorrectly used, masks do more harm than good and they should only be worn when the health authority policies indicate that they are necessary either to protect the wearer or the patient. They cease to protect once they are wet. Following use, masks should be held only by the tapes and discarded.

Hand washing technique
Hands are the most important vehicle of infection, and a careful hand washing technique by all members of the staff is essential. This has been shown to be the single most important factor in reducing the spread of infection (Taylor, 1987). The method of hand washing which in-

cludes the palmar surfaces, fingers thumbs and the inter-digital webs is crucial if hand washing is to be effective. Careful drying of the hands and the use of a hand lotion will reduce soreness, chappedness, and cracks in the skin surface.

Parents and other visitors will need careful instruction and supervision in hand washing techniques. Staff must be repeatly reminded of the importance of good hand washing techniques (Christensen *et al.* 1982).

Cleaning
Particular attention should be paid to the cleaning of all hand basins and water outlets and all other services. These should be cleaned by a member of the domestic staff who has been carefully instructed in the technique to be followed.

Disposal of excreta
1. Infants should wear disposable nappies which can be sealed in the appropriate bag and disposed of according to the health authority policy.
2. Usually excreta in bed pans/potties can be disposed of using the bed pan sterilizer in the normal way. However, if the infection is due to typhoid or polio the faeces should be soaked, e.g. with an appropriate disinfectant, for one hour. The bed pan is then disinfected and cleaned in the usual way.

Disposal of foods and feeds
Wherever possible disposable utensils should be used. Left over scraps of food can be disposed of in the appropriate bin. Left over milk feeds or fluids can be disposed of down the sink.

Following discharge of the patient from protective isolation, all equipment within the cubicle should be dealt with according to health authority policy. It is usually considered sufficient following cubicle clearance that all walls, surfaces and furniture are washed, dried and the room left to air for several hours.

REFERENCES

Caddow, P. (1989). *Applied Microbiology*. London: Scutari.

Centers for Disease Control (1982). Unexplained immunodeficiency and opportunistic infection in infants. *Morbidity and Mortality Weekly Report* **31** (49), 665–667.

Centers for Disease Control (1987). Classification system for human immunodeficiency virus (HIV) infection in children under the 13 years of age. *Morbidity and Mortality Weekly Report* **36** (15), 225–236.

Christensen, G.D., Korones, S.B., Reed, L. *et al.* (1982). Epidemic *Serratia marcescens* in a neonatal intensive care unit. *Infection Control* **3**(2), 127–133.

Department of Health (1990). *Immunisation against Infectious Disease*. London: HMSO.

Fisch, M.A., Dickinson, G.M. *et al.* (1987). Evaluation of heterosexual partner's children and household contacts of adults with AIDs. *Journal of the American Medical Association* **257**, 640–644.

Margileth, A.M. (1984). Cat-scratch disease update. *American Journal of Disease in Childhood* **138**, 711–713.

Mok, J.Y.Q. (1988). HIV infection in infants and children. *Medicine International*, September, pp. 2360–2363.

Robinson, R. (1986). Scratching the surface. *Journal of Infection Control. Nursing Times* **82**, suppl. 71–72.

Taylor, L.J. (1987). An evaluation of hand washing techniques. 1 and 2. *Nursing Times* **74**(2), 54; **74**(3), 108–110.

Weller, B.F. (1989). Children and HIV Infection. *Nursing Standard* **4**(3), 50–52.

WHO and ICN (1988). *Guidelines for Nursing Management of People Infected with Human Immunodeficiency Virus*. London: HMSO.

FURTHER READING

Christie, A.B. (1980). *Infectious Diseases*. London: Churchill Livingstone.

Department of Health and Social Security (1981). *Whooping Cough*. Report from the Committee on Safety of Medicine and the Joint Committee on Vaccination and Immunisation. London: HMSO.

Department of Health (1990). *Immunisation Against Infectious Disease*. London: HMSO.

Illingworth, R.S. (1981). *Infectious Immunisation of Your Child*. London: Churchill Livingstone.

Appendix 1
Safety

Prevention of accidents

Dangers	How to guard against them in home and hospital
	Fires
Electric fires, gas fires, coal fires	Efficient guards fixed to fire surround. Fix on wall whenever possible. Wire netting fixed to fire.
	Electricity
Sockets	Locked sockets prevent children from poking fingers or pointed articles into the holes. 'Baby Guards' can be obtained to fit over all 5, 13 and 15 amp British plugs.
Flexes	Short flexes prevent accidents, i.e. tripping over them. Long flexes tempt children to pull on them, e.g. flex from electric iron.
	Hot water
Water taps	Fix out of reach if possible. Never leave child alone in bathroom.
Baths	Run cold water in before the hot to prevent floor of bath from getting too hot.
Bath water	Mix well, test with elbow.
Hot-water bottles	Use tap (not boiling) water. Cover completely with two protective layers. Never give hot water bottles to unconscious or paralysed patients.

Scalds

| Teapots, kettles | Point spout away from table or stove edge. Drinking from the spouts of teapots and kettles seems attractive to the very young child. Oedema of the mouth, larynx and oesophagus may necessitate tracheostomy. Keep well out of the way. |

Tablecloths — Tablecloths should not be used or should at least not exceed the size of the table surface. If allowed to hang over table edge the toddler may tug on them when wanting to reach something on the table. Serious scalds may result if there is a teapot on the table.

Saucepans — Saucepan handles should always be directed backwards or inwards. Safety rails for stoves are available. The child may reach for the handle in an attempt at 'peeping inside' to see what is cooking.

Buckets — Buckets filled with scalding water should never be left standing on the floor unguarded. The young child may fall or plunge his hands into it.

Swallowing and inhaling

Toys — Toys should be large enough to make it impossible for younger children to swallow or inhale them.

Beads, nails and small marbles should not be given to very young toddlers.

Toys should not have sharp edges—danger of cuts and abrasions.

They should be coloured with vegetable (not lead) paint.

Suffocation

Pillows — Should not be used in cots before the age of 1 year or until the child can safely move himself. They are particularly dangerous if they are soft.

Plastic bibs — Avoid. They may fall over the baby's face and interfere with breathing.

Plastic bags — Children should never be allowed to play with these.

Prevention of accidents—contd.

Dangers	How to guard against them in home and hospital
Mittens	*Gangrene* These are best avoided. A thread of cotton or strand of wool hanging off the inside edge of the mitten has been known to wrap itself round the tip of a finger causing constriction and gangrene.
Small objects	*Foreign bodies* All body orifices offer opportunities for young children to push beads, peas, ball of paper, etc., into them. Sepsis and foul-smelling discharge will result. The observant and watchful mother or nurse should spot the toddler doing this sort of thing before the harm is done.
Knives, saws, axes, scissors	*Sharp things* All these should be kept out of harm's way. If left lying around they are likely to be misused and dangerous. Playing with them should be forbidden, while very young. When a little older their use should be supervised. The 'first' scissors should have rounded ends and they should not be too sharp. A child who has 'his own' will not want adult ones.
Safety pins	Should always be fastened when not in use. If in use they should be inaccessible to the child. On napkins they should be pinned horizontally.
Pin boxes, needle books	Should be kept well out of reach.
Matches	*Fire and burning* Children should be taught to respect matches as dangerous.
Matchboxes	Should not be left lying around the house.
Lighters	The same applies to them as to matches.

Fireworks and bonfires	Children should know that both may be enjoyed only while supervised by adults.
Clothing	Pyjamas are preferable for girls as well as boys as their closer fit diminishes the danger of catching fire.
	Flame-proofed materials are obtainable, their advantages greatly outweigh the extra cost.
Mirrors, pictures	Should not be fixed over fireplaces. Clothes easily catch fire as one leans over the fireplace to look in the mirror.

Windows

Guards	Safety guards should be fixed on windows of any rooms in which young children may have to be left alone.
Chairs, step ladders	May invite the child to climb on to them and lean out of the window. If unguarded this may have serious results.

Stairs

Safety gates	When there is a toddler in the house stairs should be made safe by placing safety gates at the top and bottom of flights of stairs.

Poisoning

Solvents	Young people should be aware of the health problems of 'glue sniffing'. Counselling and support groups should be provided for adolescents to discuss the hazard of solvent abuse.
Disinfectants	Should be kept locked away or out of reach even if the toddler climbs to get at them.
	They should always be clearly labelled, but it must also be remembered that the child may not be able to read. Disinfectants should not be stored in old fruit-juice bottles which still have the original label on.
Pills tablets, medicines	As the young child loves putting things in his mouth, pills, etc., should be inaccessible to him. These should be kept in a locked cupboard.

Prevention of accidents—contd.

Dangers	How to guard against them in home and hospital
Berries	A firm warning against picking and eating berries must be given in early days.
Cosmetics	Cosmetics should be kept out of reach of toddlers as some are harmful when taken internally.

Water safety

Paddling, swimming	Young children should be taught to swim early in life. The child should be shown danger spots such as sudden drops in depth, dangerous currents and outlets from drains. When on holiday by lake, sea or river, children should wear safety belts or jackets. Parents should insist on children paddling or swimming where other people are about.

Road safety

Road deaths and injuries	The Safety Code should be taught untiringly by parents and in schools.

Appendix 2
'Play Matters'

PLAY MATTERS—THE NATIONAL TOY LIBRARIES ASSOCIATION AND ACTIVE

The first toy libraries were set up in 1967 by groups of parents of children with physical, mental or multiple handicaps. To-day toy libraries cater for all children in the community, including those with special needs, so that they may benefit from playing with a selection of carefully chosen toys.

Why Toy Libraries?

Children learn through play. The right play material at the right time is not only enjoyable but also encourages a child's development in the vital early years of life; play can help children who have disabilities to reach their full potential.

Good toys, however, are often expensive. Even if they can afford to buy, many parents and carers find it difficult to choose appropriate toys; they may hesitate in case the toys they have chosen are not suitable for their child's needs. A toy library, from which toys can be borrowed, gives a child a chance to experiment with a wide selection of carefully chosen toys. Favourites may then be bought with confidence and appropriate toys are available for each successive stage of play. At some toy libraries large toys which may be too big or too expensive for home use are available for play sessions.

A toy library provides good quality (and sometimes specially adapted) toys which may be borrowed and taken home. A lonely child may be an unhappy child and a toy library provides an opportunity to play with other children in an exciting but caring environment. It is also a meeting place where parents and other carers, volunteer helpers and professionals can meet informally. A growing number of toy libraries have a link with a professional—physiotherapist, social worker or health visitor—thus providing the parents or carers with an opportunity to talk over and share any worries they may have about a child's development.

Toy Libraries in Hospitals

Many health authorities now provide a toy library service for children who are either inpatients or outpatients. 'Play Matters' is always pleased to provide advice and support for any health authority that wishes to establish a toy library and can also provide details of the nearest toy library in health authority premises (which may be in a hospital or clinic) for information regarding day-to-day administration.

For young people and adults with a mental handicap who are being cared for in the community 'Play Matters' is developing the concept of the leisure library. Leisure libraries loan equipment for recreation and leisure activities which are age appropriate; like toy libraries they also provide a meeting place.

How to Find Your Nearest Toy Library

Write to: 'Play Matters'/The National Toy Libraries Association, 68 Churchway, London NW1 1LT. (An SAE is always appreciated.) Should there not be a toy library in your neighbourhood the organization will be pleased to give advice and support in helping you to start one.

Courses are held regularly both in London and in the regions on starting and running a toy library and on various aspects of play. The organization also publishes a range of books, many concerned with play for children with special needs. (Publications list available from the address above.) The magazine *What Toy*, published annually in October, features about 500 'new-on-the-market' toys which have been appraised in toy libraries for their play value.

Membership of 'Play Matters' is open to individuals as well as to toy libraries. Local toy libraries may make a nominal charge for borrowing a toy and/or for annual membership per child or per family.

Appendix 3
Useful addresses

Association of All Speech Impaired Children (AFASIC), 347 Central Markets, Smithfield, London, EC1A 9N11. (071 236 3632).

Association of Brain-Damaged Children, Mrs Betty Lale (Secretary), 24 Robert Road, Exhall, Coventry, CV7 9GU (serving Coventry area only). (0203 313817).

Association of British Paediatric Nurses, The Hon. Secretary, c/o Ms Linda Bushell, 101 Salisbury Road, West Ealing, London, W13 9TT. (071 405 9200 Ext. 5845).

Association for Spina Bifida and Hydrocephalus, 42 Park Road, Peterborough, PE1 2UG. (0733 555988).

BLISS (Baby Life Support Systems), 17–21 Emerald Street, London, WC1N 3QL. (071 831 9393).

British Diabetic Association, 10 Queen Ann Street, London, W1M 0BD. (071 323 1531).

British Epilepsy Association, Ansley House, 40 Hanover Square, Leeds, LS3 1BE. (0532 439393).

British Heart Foundation, 14 Fitzharding Street, London, W1H 4DH. (071 935 0185).

British Kidney Patient Association (BKPA), Borden, Hants. (042047 2021).

Brittle Bone Society, 112 City Road, Dundee, DD2 2PW. (0382 67603).

Chest, Heart and Stroke Association, CHSA House, 123–127 Whitecross Street, London, EC1Y 8JJ. (071 490 7999).

Child Growth Foundation, 2 Mayfield Avenue, Chiswick, London, W4 1PW. (081 995 0257/994 7625/995 9075).

Cleft Lip and Palate Association (CLAPA), 1 Eastwood Gardens, Kenton, Newcastle-upon-Tyne, NE3 3DQ. (091 285 9396).

Colostomy Welfare Group, 15 Station Road, Reading, Berkshire, RG1 1LG. (0734 391537).

Cystic Fibrosis Research Trust, 5 Blyth Road, Bromley, Kent, BR1 3RS. (081 464 7211/2).

Down's Syndrome Association, 155 Mitcham Road, Tooting, London, SW17 9PG. (081 682 4001).

Foundation for the Study of Infant Deaths, 35 Belgrave Square, London, SW1X 8QB. (071 235 1721).

Genetic Counselling: every General Practitioner should hold a list issued by the Department of Health.

Haemophilia Society, 123 Westminster Bridge Road, London, SE1 7HR. (071 928 2020).

Handicapped children, supplies and equipment:
   E.J. Arnold & Son Ltd, Buttersley Street, Leeds.
   James Galt & Co. Ltd, Brookfield Road, Cheadle, Cheshire.
   Task Master Ltd, Morris Road, Clarendon Park, Leicester.

Lady Hoare Trust for Physically Disabled Children, Mitre House, 44–46 Fleet Street, London, EC4Y 1BN. (071 583 1951).

Leukaemia Research Fund, 43 Great Ormond Street, London, WC1N 3JJ. (071 405 0101).

Muscular Dystrophy Group of Great Britain, Nattrass House, 35 Macaulay Road, London, SW4 0QP. (071 720 8055).

National Association for the Education of the Partially Sighted, Joseph Clark School, Vincent Road, Highams Park, London, E4 9PP. (081 527 8818).

National Association for Gifted Children, Park Campus, Boughton Green Road, Northampton, NN2 7AL. (0604 792 300).

National Association for Maternity and Child Welfare, Strode House, 46–48 Osnaburg Street, London, NW1 3ND. (071 383 4541).

National Association for the Welfare of Children in Hospital (**NAWCH**), Argyle House, 29/31 Euston Road, London, NW1 2SD. (071 833 2041)

National Children's Bureau, 8 Wakeley Street, London, EC1V 7QE. (071 278 9441).

National Deaf Children's Society, 45 Hereford Road, London, W2 5AH. (071 229 9272/4).

National Eczema Society, Tavistock House East, Tavistock Square, London, WC1N 9SR. (071 388 4097).

NSPCC, 67 Saffron Hill, London, EC1N 8RS. (071 242 1626).

Royal National Institute for the Blind, 224 Great Portland Street, London, W1N 6AA. (071 387 1266).

Royal National Institute for the Deaf, 105 Gower Street, London, WC1E 6AH. (071 387 8033).

Scottish Council for Spastics, 22 Corstorphine Road, Edinburgh, EH12 6HP. (031 337 9876).

Scottish Society for the Mentally Handicapped, Head Office: 13 Elmbank Street, Glasgow, G2 4QA. (041 226 4541).

Spastics Society, 12 Park Crescent, London, W1N 4EQ. (071 636 5020).

Terence Higgins Trust, BM AIDS, London, WC1N 3XX. (071 242 1010, between 3pm–10pm).

Appendix 4
Normal values and conversion tables

(Normal values)

Haemoglobin
New born   16.6 g/dl

Age 12 years $\begin{cases} 13.8 \text{ g/dl girls} \\ 14.0 \text{ g/dl boys} \end{cases}$

Red blood cells
Newborn $4.5–5.0 \times 10^{12}$/litre
Age 12 years $4.2–5.4 \times 10^{12}$/litre

White blood cells
Newborn $16–20 \times 10^{9}$/litre
Age 12 years $4–12 \times 10^{9}$/litre

Platelets
$200–500 \times 10^{9}$/litre

Sedimentation rate (Westergren)
$2–10$ mm/h

Total protein   5.2–7.8 g/litre
Albumin   3.5–5.0 g/litre
Globulin   1.7–2.8 g/litre
Fibrinogen   0.2–0.4 g/litre
Bilirubin   0.1–0.5 mmol/litre

Serum electrolyte

Sodium	136–143 mmol/litre
Potassium	4.1–5.6 mmol/litre
Chloride	98–106 mmol/litre
Bicarbonate	21–25 mmol/litre
Urea	2.5–6.7 mmol/litre

Blood sugar

Serum glucose (fasting)	3.4 to 5.6 mmol/litre

Cerebrospinal fluid

Pressure	50–150 mmH$_2$O (7.5–20 kPa)
Sugar	3.9–4.8 mmol/litre
Total protein	10–30 mg/litre
Cells	<5 lymphocytes/mm^3

Urine (24-hour content)

Protein (total)	30–50 mg
Urea	200–500 mg/kg body weight/day

Average blood pressures

	Systolic		Diastolic	
Age	(mm Hg)	kPa	(mm Hg)	(kPa)
Birth	65–95	8.5–13	30–60	4–8
5 years	80–110	11–15	45–65	6–8.5
10 years	90–120	12–16	50–70	7–9

Normal distribution of body fluids—as percentage of body weight

	Premature infants	F.T. infants	Children	Adults
Body water (%)	75–80	70–75	60–70	55–60
Extracellular (blood and between cells)	40–50	35–40	30–50	20
Intracellular	30–50	35	30–50	40

Index

Accident prevention 432–6
Acholuric jaundice 213
Acne 296
Acne vulgaris 342–3
Acquired Immunodeficiency
    Syndrome (AIDS), *see*
    also HIV infection 217,
    415–27
ACTH (Adrenocorticotrophic
    hormone) 294, 297, 317
Acute appendicitis 253–7
Acute bronchitis 153–7
    complications 155
    principles of care 155–6
    signs and symptoms 154
    specific treatment 154–5
Acute encephalitis 322–3
Acute haemolytic anaemia
    212–13
Acute leukaemia 218–24
Acute lymphocytic leukaemia
    (ALL) 219
Acute myeloblastic leukaemia
    (AML) 219
Acute pyelonephritis 380–2
Acute rheumatic fever
    197–200
Acute virus hepatitis 261
Addison's disease 297
Adelaide scale 311
Adenoidectomy 138–40
Adolescence 17–18

illness in 81–2
Adrenal cortex 294, 297
Adrenal glands 295–6
Adrenaline 295
Adrenocorticotrophic
    hormone (ACTH) 294,
    297, 317
Adrenogenital syndrome
    296–9
Agenesis of the kidney 396
AIDS Related Complex
    (ARC) 217
Aldactone 179
Allergic bronchitis 154
Allergies 165
Alopecia 221
Ammonia dermatitis 32
Anaemia 208–18, 227, 297
    classification 208
    clinical picture of 208–9
Anaesthesia 299
Anal fissure 244
Anal stenosis 270–1
Anaphylactoid purpura
    204–5
Angiography 192, 313–14
Anorectal manometry 265
Antenatal care 3–4
Antigen-antibody reaction
    297
Anus 262–72
Aortic stenosis 183

Aphthous stomatitis 227–8
Aplastic anaemia 209
Apnoea 99
Appendicitis 253–7
Artificial feeding. *See* Infant
    formula feeding
Artificial ventilation 99
Assisted Ventilation 189–91
Asthma 165, 295, 297
    common causes of 165–7
    drug therapy 169
    home care 167–9
    principles of care 166–7
Asymmetrical tonic neck
    reflex 6
Atopic eczema 339
Atrial septal defects 183
Attachment 51
Azathioprine 207

Babinski's sign 6
Bacterial endocarditis 194
Barium enema 265
Batchelor plaster 363
Bathing 28–9, 48
BCG vaccination 24
Behaviour problems 333–5
Behavioural development 6
Benzene 209
Benzocaine 228
Benzoin 398
Bilateral agenesis 396
Bile duct, atresia of 261–2
Bilirubin 212
Birth 4–9
Birth marks 66–7
Bladder and bladder neck
    398–9
Blalock–Hanlon operation
    185

Blended family 20
Blood pressure 175, 299, 443
Blood sugar 443
Blood transfusion 71, 213, 389
Body fluids 443
Body scan 406
Boehringer meconium strip
    285
Bonding 6
Bone marrow puncture 210
Bone marrow transplantation
    210, 223–4
Bone scan 359
Bonjela 228
Bottles (feeding) 43
Bowel control 328
Bowel resection 251
Bradycardia 175
Brain scan 315–16
Breast-feeding 34–8, 58
    correct position for 36
    good reasons for 34–5
    management of 35–7
    problems associated with
        37
Bringing up wind 42
Bronchiectasis 157–60
Bronchiolitis 170–2
Bronchitis, acute. *See* Acute
    bronchitis
Bronchography 153
Bronchopneumonia 162–3
Bronchoscopy 152
Buffalo hump 296
Burns and scalds 344–54
    classification of 345–6
    common causes of 344
    complications 352–3
    estimating the extent of
        346
    full thickness 345

Burns and scalds *con't*
  general principles of care
    348–50
  local treatment 350–2
  prevention 345
  principles of care 350–2
  psychological care 353–4
  superficial 345
  treatment for shock 346–8

Candida (Monilia) albicans
    229
Carbamazepine 317
Carbaryl 410
Cardiac arrest 99
Cardiac catheterization 192–3
Cardiac massage 100
Cardiac surgery 186–9
Cardiopulmonary
    resuscitation
    (CPR) 101
Cardiovascular problems
    174–96
Care by parent schemes
    106–7
Care participation 51–2,
    85–7
Catarrhal stomatitis 227–8
Catheterization 375–6, 395,
    398
Catscratch fever 410–11
Cerebral palsy 324–5
Cerebrospinal fluid 329, 443
Chest physiotherapy 57
Chicken-pox 222
Child abuse 67–70
  prevention of 70
Child development. *See*
    Developmental
    considerations
Children Act 1989 22–3

Chloramphenicol 209
Chlorothiazide 388
Choanal atresia 130
Chorea 200–1
Christmas disease 218
Cigarette smoking 82
Circumcision 399–400
Cleanliness 59
Cleft lip 144–7
Cleft palate 144, 148–9
Clotting mechanism
    disturbances 217–18
Cloxacillin 370
Coarctation of the aorta 181
Coeliac disease 281–4
  complications 284
  diet 283–4
  investigations 282
  principles of care 283
  prognosis 284
  signs and symptoms 281–2
Collagen problems 197–207
Colon 262–72
Colostomy 266–7
Comatosed state, definition
    309
Common cold 129–30
Communicable diseases 415
Community paediatric nursing
    107–13
Complementary feeds 37
Congenital abnormalities 395
Congenital abnormalities and
    their treatment
    396–406
Congenital atresia of the bile
    duct 261–2
Congenital dislocation of the
    hip joint 360–6
  principles of care 364–6
  signs and symptoms 360–1
  treatment 361–6

Congenital heart disease
    180–5
Congenital hypertrophic
    pyloric stenosis 234–6
Congenital laryngeal stridor
    130–1
Congenital talipes
    calcaneovalgus 366
Consciousness, assessment of
    309–11
Constipation 242–51
    causes of 243
    collection of specimens 245
    observation of faeces 245
    principles of care 243–4
    with overflow 244–5, 334
Continuous ambulatory
    peritoneal dialysis
    (CAPD) 393–5
Convulsions 316–19
Cooley's haemolytic anaemia
    214
Copper 212
Corticosteroids 297, 299, 317
Cortisone 295–7
Cot 56
Cot sides 102
Craniotabes 275
Crohn's disease 251–3
Croup 131
Cushing's syndrome 295
Cyanosis 176
Cyclophosphamide 388
Cystic fibrosis 284–9
    principles of care and
        treatment 286–9
    signs and symptoms 285
    specific investigations
        285–6
Cystography 379
Cystoscopy 378
Cytotoxic drugs 221–3, 406

Deafness 140–1
Deficiency anaemias 209–12
Deformities caused by
    paralysis 371–2
Dental care 226
Dermatological problems
    339–55
Dermatomyositis 206
Dermatophytes 413–15
Developmental consid-
    erations 3
    at birth 4–9
    at 12 months 11–12
    at 2 years 12–14
    at 3 months 7–9
    at 3 years 14–15
    at 5–7 years 15–16
    at 6 months 9–11
    at 8–11 years 16–17
    at adolescence 17
    newborn infant 6–7
Diabetes insipidus 294
Diabetes mellitus 299–307
    checklist 306–7
    diet 301, 302
    education 305
    general points 303
    injections 302–3
    international classification
        system 299
    investigations 300
    nursing goals 301
    points of importance 306
    signs and symptoms 300
    signs of oncoming coma 305
    treatment 300–3
    see also Insulin
Diabetic coma 305
Diamorphine 350
Diarrhoea 252
Digoxin 178, 200
Discharge home 47–8

Double kidney 396–7
Down's syndrome 335
Drainage tubes 395
Drugs in heart failure 178–9
DTPA (99mTe-Diethylenetri-
    aminepentacetic acid)
    isotope scan 398
Duodenal atresia 249
Duodenal intubation 286
Dwarfism 294
Dying child 118–22
    meeting the needs of other
        children 121–2

Ear mopping 143
Echocardiogram 193
Eczema 339–42
    local treatment 340
    principles of care 340–2
    signs and symptoms 339–40
    treatment 340
Education 21–2
    in hospital 21–2
Electroencephalogram
    314–15
Electromyography 356, 358
Elixir Phenergan 350
EMLA cream 222
'En face' position 7
Encephalitis 294, 322–3
Encopresis 334–5
Endocarditis 194, 199
Endocrine problems 291–307
Enterobius vermicularis 412
Enuresis 333–4
Environmental temperature 7
Epanutin 317
Epilepsy 308, 316–19
    general principles of care
        318
    major 317

minor 317
Erythrocyte sedimentation
    rate 199
Escherichia coli 255, 381
Excretion tests 405
Exomphalos with or without
    ectopia vesicae 403–4
Extended family 19
Eye care 60

Factor VIII (blood) 217
Factor IX (blood) 217
Faecal fat estimation 281
Faecal incontinence 334–5
Fallot's tetralogy 184
Familial thrombocytopenic
    purpura 216
Family relationships 18
Family structures 19–20
Family unit 79
Febrile convulsions 316
Feeding methods 34–47, 59
    see also Breast-feeding;
        Infant formula feeding
Fetal development 4
Fever blisters 226
First-aid box 110
Folic acid 211–12
Fragilitas ossium 371
Freeze-dried factors 217
Frog plaster 363
Frusemide 178, 200

G6PD (glucose-6-phosphate
    dehydrogenase) 213
Galactomin 278
Galactosaemia 278–9
    diagnosis 279
    treatment 278
Gastric lavage 236–7
Gastritis 233–4

Gastrointestinal problems
222, 226–72
Gaucher's disease 279
Generation gap 18
Genetic counselling 358
Genitalia 296
Genitourinary problems
373–407
Genitourinary tract, surgical
conditions of 395–406
Gentamycin 391
Gigantism 294
Gingivitis 228–9
Glasgow coma scale 309
Glycogen storage disorders
279
Glycosuria 296
Graft versus host disease 223
Grasp reflex 5
Grommet tubes 142
Growth hormone deficiency
295
Guthrie test 51, 277

Haematocrit 193
Haematological
problems 208–25
Haematuria 384
Haemodialysis 391, 392
Haemoglobin 212, 442
Haemolytic anaemia 212–15,
297
Haemolytic disease of the
newborn 61–2
Haemolytic streptococci 131
Haemophilia 217
Haemophilus influenzae 131,
322
Haemorrhagic anaemias
215–18
Haemorrhagic disease of the

newborn 61, 217
Harrison's sulcus 276
Head lice 409–10
Health visitor 48, 50, 52,
107–13
Heart disease 176–95
Heart failure 176–80
drugs in 178–9
play activity in 179
Henoch-Schönlein's purpura
204–5, 216
Hereditary spherocytosis 213
Hernia 258–60
Herpes 226
Herpes simplex 227
Hiatus hernia 239
Hip joint, congenital
dislocation. *See*
Congenital dislocation
of the hip joint
Hirschsprung's disease 263–9
diagnosis 265
post-operative management
268–9
principles of care 263–5
surgical correction 267
surgical management 266
HIV infection 217–18,
415–27
classification 425
clinical presentation 425
diagnosis 424–5
long-term follow-up 426
major risk factors 424
treatment and nursing
interventions 426
Hodgkin's disease 224
Home nursing 107–13
Horseshoe kidney 396–7
Hospitalization 16–18,
89–107
accident prevention 103–6

Hospitalization *con't*
  administration of
      medications 95-9
  contact with home 92
  education 21-2
  nurses' uniform 90-1
  play 92-5
  preparation for 89
  routine 91
  safety measures 102
  visiting 91-2
Hot cross bun effect 275
Human chorionic gonado-
      tropin (HCG) 402
Human immunodeficiency
      virus (HIV). *See* HIV
      infection
Humidified air 155-6
Hydramnios 240, 249
Hydrocele 404
Hydrocephalus 329, 329-33
  communicating type
      329-30
  non-communicating type
      330
  post-operative care 332-3
  pre-operative care 331-2
  presentation 330-1
  principles of care and
      treatment 331
Hydrocortisone 297
Hydronephrosis 397, 398
Hydroureter 397
Hydroxystilbamidine 230
Hyperglycaemic coma 305
Hypertension 296
Hypogammaglobulinaemia
      279
Hypoglycaemia coma 305
Hypoplastic anaemia 209
Hypospadias 401-2
Hypothermia 47, 54, 191

Hypothyroidism 291-4
  investigations 292
  nursing care and
      observations 293-4
  signs and symptoms 291-2
  treatment 293

Idiopathic thrombocytopenic
      purpura 216
Immunization 23-4, 342
Immunodeficiency disease
      279
Imperforate anus 271-2
Impetigo contagiosa 343-4
Incubator 55-6
Infant at risk 50-78
  child abuse/non-accidental
      injury 67-70
  general care 58-60
  neonatal problems 61-7
  nursing environment 54-7
  nutrition 57-8
  paediatric procedures 70-7
  principles of nursing care 60
Infant feeding. *See* Breast-
      feeding; Feeding
      methods; Infant
      formula feeding
Infant formula feeding 38-45,
      58
  bringing up wind 42
  choice of formula 40
  correct procedure for 41
  difficulties associated with
      45
  discharge home 44, 47-8
  equipment 43
  preparation of feed 44
  ready-to-feed concept 40
  sterilization 43
Infantile spasms 316-17

Infection
  prevention 33–4
  risk of 222
Infective hepatitis 261
Inflammatory heart diseases 194
Inguinal hernia 258–60
Insulin 299, 302–3
  administering 306–7
  recommended regimens 304
  see also Diabetes mellitus
Insulin coma 305
Intal Co 169
Intelligence quotient 336
Intensive care 7, 50
Intercostal drainage 191–2
Intermittent peritoneal dialysis (IPD) 393–5
Intertrigo 31–2
Intestinal obstruction 245–51
Intestinal parasites 412–13
Intestine 242–62
Intracranial tumour 323
Intravenous infusions 70–1, 100
Intravenous pyelography 377–8, 405, 406
Intravenous therapy 347
  splinting for 72–5
Intussusception 250–1
Iodine sensitivity 377–8
Iridocyclitis 204
Iron deficiency anaemia 210–11
Iron supplements 211, 212
Isolation procedures 34

Jaundice 64, 260–2, 278
  due to sepsis 261
  haemolytic types 260

obstructive 261
Jejunal biopsy 282
Juvenile arthritis 201–4

Kanamycin 370, 391
Kernicterus 64–5
Kidney transplant operations 392

Laryngitis stridulosa 131
Laryngoscopy 152
Laryngotracheitis 131–2
Last offices 120
Learning difficulties 335
Leukaemia 218–24
  drug therapy 221
Lipoid nephrosis 387–90
Lipoid storage disorders 279
Lipoidosis 279
Lobar pneumonia 160
Low birthweight infants 53
Lumbar puncture 311–13
Lupus erythematosus 206–7

Malathion 410
Mantoux test 163
Measles 222
Mebendazole 413
Mechanical ventilation 56–7, 189–91
Meconium 32–3
Medical advice, when to seek (sick child at home) 109
Medications 95–9
  pain prevention 117
Medicine cabinets 109–10
Medullary tumours 295
Megacolon 262–3
Megaureter 397

Meningitis 319–22
  complications 322
  diagnosis 320
  presentation 319–20
  principles of care 321
  prognosis 322
  sub-acute form 322
  treatment 320
Meningocele 325
Meningomyelocele 325
Mental handicap 308, 316, 319, 335–8
  respite care 337–8
Mesenteric adenitis 257–8
Metabolic disorders 273–90
  symptoms 273
Metronidazole 228
Miconazole 230
Microcephaly 335
Micturating cystogram 378
Middle ear
  inflammation 141
  prevention of infection 142
Midstream specimens 376
Moon-faced appearance 296
Moro reflex 5
Morphine 179, 396
Mother/infant bonding 51
Mouth conditions 226–30
Mouth to mouth breathing 99–100
Mucoviscidosis 284–9
Muscle biopsy 358
Muscular dystrophies 356–8
Mustard Procedure 185
Myocarditis 194
Myopathies 356–8
  common varieties 358
  diagnosis 356
Myotonia congenita 358
Myringoplasty 144
Mysolin 317

Naevi (birth marks) 66–7
Napkin rash 30–1
Napkins 30–2
Nasogastric tube feed 237–9
National Society for the Prevention of Cruelty to Children (NSPCC) 69–70
Necrotizing enterocolitis 65
Needle phobia 222
Neocortef 227
Neonatal problems 61–7
Nephrectomy 405–6
Nephritis 297, 382–7
  age group 384
  classification of 382
  clinical presentation 384
  definition 383
  diet 386
  fluid allowed in 24 hours 386
  investigations 384
  nursing care 385
  observations 385–6
  pathology 384
  prognosis 387
  treatment 385
Nephroblastoma 406
Nephrosis 382, 387–90
  age 387
  clinical presentation 387–8
  definition 387
  diet 390
  investigations 388
  nursing care 389
  observations 389
  pathology 387
  prognosis 390
  treatment 388
Nephrostomy 397, 405
Nephrotic syndrome 382, 387–90

Nervous system, examination of 308–11
Neurological problems 308–38
Neurological procedures 311–16
Neuromuscular inco-ordination of bladder and bladder neck 398
Newborn infant 4, 26–49
  general points 26
  pulse 28
  respirations 28
  sore buttocks 30–2
  temperature control 27
  temperature recording 28
Niemann-Pick disease 279
Nitrofurantoin 382
Non-accidental injury 67–70
Noradrenaline 295
Nostril care 60
Nuclear family 19
Nurse, role model of 52
Nursery ambient temperature 54
Nurses' uniform 90–1
Nursing models 84–7
Nursing process 83–4
Nutramigen 278
Nutrition, infant at risk 57–8
Nutritional deficiency anaemia 210–12
Nystatin 230

Obesity 296
Observation of infant at risk 58
Obstruction, signs of 133–4
Obstructive jaundice 261
Oesophageal atresia 240
Oesophagus 230–42

abnormalities 240–2
One-parent family 19–20
Ophthalmia neonatorum 66
Orchidopexy 403
Orem model 85
Orthopaedic problems 328, 356–72
Ortolani sign 361
Osteochondritis 358
Osteogenesis imperfecta 371
Osteomyelitis 369–70
  principles of care 370
  signs and symptoms 369
  treatment 369–70
Osteoporosis 202
Osteotomy 403
Otitis media 41
Otorrhoea 143
Oxygen therapy 56, 154, 156–7, 179, 347–8

Paediatric procedures 70–7
Pain 113–18
Pain assessment 116
Pain management 116–18
Pain relief 142
Paralysis, correction of deformities caused by 371–2
Paralytic ileus 256–7
Paraphimosis 400
Parent/child attachment 6
Parental visiting 52
Partnership in care model 85–7
Patent ductus arteriosus 180
Paul's tubing 375
Pediculosis capitis 409–10
Pel-Ebstein fever 224
Pelvic abscess 256
Penicillin 228, 370, 385

Perforated appendix 254
Periarteritis nodosa 205–6
Pericarditis 194
Peritoneal dialysis 391, 393–4
Peritonitis 254, 255
Perthes's disease 358–60
  principles of care 359
  prognosis 360
  treatment 359
Petit mal 317
Phenobarbitone 317
Phenylketonuria 51, 277–8
  diet 277–8
  signs and symptoms 277
  treatment 277
Phthalysulphathiazole 267
Physical contact 51
Physical growth 81
Physiological jaundice 64
Pierre Robin syndrome
  149–50
Pinworms 412
Piperazine hydrate 413
Pituitary gland 294–5, 295
Placing and walking reflexes 6
Plantar reflex 309
Plastic surgery 296
Platelets 442
Play activity 110–13, 437–8
  in heart failure 179
  in hospital 92–5
  see also Toys
'Play Matters' 437–8
Pleurisy 163–4
Police 69
Polyarteritis nodosa 205–6
Posseting 45
Post-mature infants 54
Postural drainage of the lungs
  159–60
Potassium chloride 388
Pre-packed feeds 40

Pre-term infants, definition 53
Prednisolone 297, 388
Prednisone 207, 297, 388
Premature, definition 52
Primary nursing 87–9
Protective isolation nursing
  427–30
Pseudohermaphroditism 295
Pseudohypertrophic muscular
  dystrophy 357
Psychological problems 329
Puberty 17, 302, 342, 402
Puderz valve 331
Pulse rate 174–5
  newborn infant 28
Pupil reflexes 5
Purpura 215–17
  due to lack of essential
    constituents in the
    blood plasma 217
  due to platelet deficiency
    216
  due to vascular defects 216
Pyelitis 380–2
Pyelonephritis, acute 380–2
Pyeloplasty 397
Pyloric stenosis 234

Radiant warmer 55
Radio-opaque methods
  313–14
Radiotherapy 223, 406
Rashkind balloon atrial
  septostomy 184
Rectal biopsy 265
Rectal prolapse 269–70
Rectal temperature 106
Rectum 262–72
Red blood cells 212, 442
Reflexes 5, 309
Regurgitation 45

Rejection 52
Renal biopsy 379
Renal failure 390–5
  long-term follow-up care
    395
  main causes of 390–1
  nursing care 392–3
  signs and symptoms 391
  treatment 391
Renal function tests 380
Renal tract, infection of 403
Replacement transfusion
    76–7
Resection of bowel 251
Respiration 150
Respirations, newborn infant
    28
Respiratory assistance 56
Respiratory distress syndrome
    63–4
Respiratory problems 129–73
Respiratory Syncytial Virus
    (RSV) 171
Respiratory tract 150–3
  examination 151–2
  special investigations 152–3
Restrainers 102–3
Resuscitation 99–102
Retrograde pyelography 378,
    405
Reye's syndrome 203
Rhesus incompatibility 61–2
Rheumatic carditis 197–200
Rheumatic fever 197–200,
    297
Rheumatic problems 197–207
Rheumatoid arthritis 297
Rickets 273–6
  active 274–6
  prevention 274
  signs and symptoms 274–6
  treatment 276

Rickety rosary 276
Ringworm 413–15
Role model 7
Rooting reflex 6
Roper model 84
Rose Waaler test 201

Safety measures,
    hospitalization 102
Safety pins 106
Safety precautions 432–6
'St. Vitus' dance 200–1
Salicylates 199, 203
Sarcoptes scabiei 408–9
Scabies 408–9
Scalds. *See* Burns and scalds
Scalp vein infusion 72
Schuller-Christian syndrome
    279
Sclerema 62
Sedimentation rate 442
Sensitivity reaction 377
Serum electrolyte 443
Serum hepatitis 261
Servo Control 56
Sex determination 296
Sexual development 81
Sexual precocity 295
Shock 295, 297
  treatment for 346–8
Sick child 79–125
  home nursing 107–13
  nursing models 84–7
  nursing process 83–4
  stress effects 79–80
  see also Hospitalization
Sickle cell anaemia 214–15
Small-for-gestational-age
    infants 53
Social problems 329
Social services 69

Sodium cromoglycate 169
Solid foods 46
Spina bifida 325–9
  conservative care 327
  degree of handicap 328
  degrees of 325
  indications for surgery 325
  long-term care 328
  post-operative management
    and care 326–7
Spironolactone 179, 388
Spitz-Holter valve 331
Splinting for intravenous
    therapy 72–5
Splints 103
Staphylococcus 131, 343
Staphylococcus albus 329
Status asthmaticus 169–70
Steatorrhoea 280–1
  investigations 280–1
  signs and symptoms 280
Steindler's operation 367
Sterilization of equipment 43
Steroid therapy 388
Steroids 200, 203, 213, 296,
    297
Still's disease 201–4
Stomach 230–42
Stools 32–3
  collection for fat estimation
    281
  in infancy and childhood
    246–8
Streptococcal infections 138
Streptococcus 343
Streptococcus pyogenes 197
Streptococcus viridans 194
Streptomycin 391
Subacute nephritis 387–90
Subphrenic abscess 256
Sulphanamides 382
Sulphonamides 213, 385, 391

Supplementary feeds 37
Suprapubic aspiration 376
Suprarenal glands 295
Sweat test 286
Symptomatic thrombo-
    cytopenic purpura 216
Syndactyly 370–1
Syndenham's chorea 200–1

Tachycardia 175
Talipes 366–7
Talipes calcaneovarus 366
  treatment of 367
Talipes equinovalgus 366
Talipes equinovarus (clubfoot)
    366
Teats 43
Teething 229
Television viewing 16
Temperature control,
    newborn infant 27
Temperature recording,
    newborn infant 28
Tenotomy 372
Term, definition 52
Terminal illness 118–22
  meeting the needs of other
    children 121–2
Tetracycline 342
Thalassaemia 214
Threadworms 412
Thrush 229
Thrush septicaemia 230
Thyroid gland 291–4
Thyrotoxicosis 291
Tine test 163
Tongue tie 230
Tonsillectomy 138–40
Tonsillitis 136–7
Total protein 442
Toxocariasis 411

Toy libraries 437–8
Toys 110–13
  safety measures 105–6
  see also Play activity
Tracheo-oesophageal fistula
  240
Tracheostomy 133–6, 157
Transcultural aspects 20–1
Transplantation of tendons
  372
Transplantation of ureters 404
Transposition of the great
  vessels 184–5
Triamcinolone 297
Trineprazine 350
Triple arthrodesis 367
Tryptic activity 286
Tuberculosis 24, 163
Twenty-four-hour specimens
  376

Ulcerative stomatitis 227–8
Ultrasound scanning 398
Umbilical cord 30
Umbilical hernia 258
Undescended testicle 402
Unit policies 52
Urea clearance test 380
Urea concentration test 380
Ureatine clearance test 380
Ureterocele 399
Urethral valves 397–8
Urinary output and drainage
  374
Urinary problems 328
Urinary tract infections 398
Urinary tract investigations
  377–8

Urine 443
Urine collection 373–5
Urine retention 377

Vaccination 23–4, 342
Vaseline 228
Ventilator 56–7, 189–91
Ventricular septal defect
  181–3
Ventriculography 313
Vesico-ureteric reflux 397
Vincent's angina 228
Virilism 295
Visceral larva migrans 411
Vitamins 46–7
  B 212
  B_{12} deficiency 211–12
  C 212
  D 273, 274, 276
Voluntary organizations
  69–70
Volvulus 249–50
Vomiting 45, 230–4, 239, 249,
  256

Waller Method 345
Weaning 45–7
Welfare Food Scheme 47
White blood cells 442
Wilms' tumour 406
  signs and symptoms 406
  treatment 406
Withdrawal reflex 6

Xanthomatosis 279
X-ray examination 151